SOMATIC GROWTH OF THE CHILD

SOMATIC GROWTH OF THE CHILD

PROCEEDINGS
OF A BOERHAAVE COURSE FOR
POSTGRADUATE MEDICAL TEACHING

EDITED BY:

J. J. VAN DER WERFF TEN BOSCH, M.D.
AND A. HAAK, M.D. (UNIVERSITY HOSPITAL LEIDEN)

CHARLES C THOMAS · PUBLISHER
Springfield · Illinois U.S.A.

Published simultaneously

in the U.S.A. by
CHARLES C. THOMAS — PUBLISHER
Bannerstone House
301—327 East Lawrence Ave., Springfield, Illinois, U.S.A.

Printed in the Netherlands

PREFACE

This volume contains the proceedings of a postgraduate medical course which was held in the Department for Clinical Endocrinology and Diseases of Metabolism, Leiden University Hospital, in September 1964. The course covered a wide area and was intended to show: how a child grows and why it grows as it does; when growth may be considered abnormal and what may cause the abnormality; which types of treatment are available and how the effects of treatment can be evaluated. It was not intended to cover the entire field, but rather to deal through appropriate examples with fundamental problems of normal and abnormal growth and of the methods available for their study.

The course was generated and fostered within the Dutch Growth Club; many of its members also appeared as speakers. This course is the first in a series of annual public manifestations that the Dutch Growth Club has undertaken to arrange.

We are grateful to Professor A. QUERIDO, and to the members of the Board of the Boerhaave Courses for Postgraduate Medical Teaching, who enthusiastically endorsed the idea of organizing the course and provided the means to carry out the plans.

This book owes its completion to the willingness of the speakers to prepare manuscripts, to Miss Y. HUIZER who typed the discussions from tape, to Miss M. G. VAN DIJK and Miss J. E. VAN EGMOND who dealt with the manuscripts, and to Mr. W. ZUIDERVAART who prepared many of the illustrations.

On behalf of the contributors we wish to thank authors and publishers who have given permission to reproduce original figures.

THE EDITORS

SPEAKERS*

H. H. van Gelderen, Dept. of Paediatrics, Academisch Ziekenhuis, Leiden

A. Haak, Dept. for Clinical Endocrinology and Diseases of Metabolism, Academisch Ziekenhuis, Leiden

Z. Laron, Dept. of Pediatrics, Tel-Aviv University Medical School, and Pediatric Metabolic and Endocrine Service, Beilinson Medical Center, Petah Tiqva, Israel

W. A. Marshall, Institute of Child Health, 30 Guilford Street, London, England

F. Schwarz, Dept. of Clinical Endocrinology, Academisch Ziekenhuis, Utrecht

J. van der Sluys Veer, Dept. for Clinical Endocrinology and Diseases of Metabolism, Academisch Ziekenhuis, Leiden

E. H. Sobel, Dept. of Pediatrics, Albert Einstein College of Medicine, New York, U.S.A.

R. Steendijk, Dept. of Paediatrics, Binnengasthuis, Amsterdam

A. M. Thomson, Reproduction and Growth Research Unit, Princess Mary Maternity Hospital, Newcastle-on-Tyne, England

H. A. W. M. Tiddens, Wilhelmina Kinderziekenhuis, Utrecht

H. K. A. Visser, Dept. of Paediatrics, Academisch Ziekenhuis, Groningen

J. J. van der Werff ten Bosch, Dept. for Clinical Endocrinology and Diseases of Metabolism, Academisch Ziekenhuis, Leiden

J. F. de Wijn, Central Institute for Nutrition and Food Research TNO, Zeist

DISCUSSERS*

B. J. van de Berg, Leiden
P. O. Clignett, Den Haag
W. Croughs, Groningen
J. J. van Gemund, Leiden
K. F. Kerrebijn, Den Haag
F. P. G. M. van der Linden, Nijmegen
R. Luyken, Utrecht
A. J. B. Olthof, Steenbergen
H. A. Polman, Groningen
A. Prader, Zürich, Switzerland
A. Querido, Leiden
J. M. Smit, Rotterdam
G. B. A. Stoelinga, Nijmegen
M. J. van de Vooren, Middelburg
F. Wafelbakker, Amsterdam
H. J. van Wersch, Heerlen

* When country is not indicated, address in the Netherlands.

CONTENTS

CHAPTER IV

GROWTH IN CHILDHOOD

CHAPTER V

GROWTH AROUND BIRTH

CHAPTER VI

HORMONES, FOOD AND ACUTE NON-ENDOCRINE DISEASES

CHAPTER VII

ABNORMAL BODY SIZE

CHAPTER VIII

SOME TYPES OF ABNORMAL GROWTH

CHAPTER IX

GROWTH PROMOTING AGENTS

CHAPTER X

GROWTH INHIBITING AGENTS

CHAPTER I

COLLECTION OF INFORMATION CONCERNING GROWTH

BASIC ANTHROPOMETRIC MEASUREMENTS

W. A. MARSHALL

It is obvious that measurements of body size must be accurate if they are to be of any real value for either scientific or clinical purposes. Yet there are many physicians who will happily accept measurements of stature in which there is an error of 2 to 3 centimetres due to poor technique and to the use of inadequate apparatus. These same physicians would be horrified at the suggestion that, for example, blood sugar should be measured by unskilled observers using inferior equipment, but the accurate measurement of stature is just as important in the study of growth as the measurement of blood sugar is in the study of diabetes mellitus. The simplest and most useful indication of overall growth is obtained by the accurate measurement of standing height or stature.

The weights of children are often compared with their heights on the assumption that the relationship between these two measurements gives an indication of whether or not the growth of the body tissues in general is in proportion to the increase in height. Sometimes conclusions about growth are even reached on the basis of weight measurements alone. In fact, however, if we are told that a child's weight has increased we know nothing more than that he has become heavier. This may mean that he has grown satisfactorily with a normal increase in bone and muscle, or it may only mean that he has become excessively fat. Indeed he might not have gained any tissue at all, but simply have retained excessive amounts of fluid owing to some pathological condition. We must have some indication of the actual amount of fat on the body and this can easily be obtained by measuring the thickness of skinfolds, with their subcutaneous fat, on both the limbs and the trunk. If limb circumference is measured as well as skinfold thickness it is possible to estimate also the amount of muscle plus bone in the limb. The most useful anthropometric measurements therefore are those of height, skinfold thickness and limb circumference, provided the correct apparatus and techniques are used in taking them. Other measurements such as sitting height, shoulder width and hip width are also valuable, but are beyond the scope of the present discussion.

In order to measure height the subject's socks must be removed. Although socks do not significantly add to the height, they may conceal the fact that the subject has raised his heels slightly from the ground. The subject must stand so that his heels and back are in contact with the vertical surface. The heels must also be in contact with the ground and it may be necessary for an assistant to hold them there. The head should be held so that he looks straight ahead with the lower borders of his eye sockets in the same horizontal plane as his external auditory meati. A horizontal surface is then slid down the vertical one, in contact with it, until it touches the subject's head and the distance from the ground to the horizontal surface is measured along the vertical one. During the measurement the subject should be told to take a breath and stretch so as to be as tall as possible. The stretching should be assisted by gentle upward pressure, applied by the observer, to the mastoid processes of the subject. This stretching minimizes the variation in height which occurs during the day and may vary as much as 2 cm. Apart from correct positioning and stretching of the subject, accuracy depends on three factors. 1. The vertical surface must be truly vertical. 2. The horizontal surface must be truly horizontal and both long enough and wide enough to make sure that it makes contact with the highest point on the head. In the type of instrument commonly used in schools, the horizontal surface is represented by a rod, which can be moved through several degrees from the horizontal position and is so narrow that it is easy to place it on either side of the highest point of the head. This is quite useless. Far better results would be obtained by using the wall and a book. 3. It must be possible to read the final measurement accurately. Industrial psychologists have shown that many fewer errors are made in reading numerals which appear in a fixed window than in reading other systems, such as pointers moving on scales or dials (2). The ideal instrument for measuring stature should therefore incorporate a device for reading the final result of numerals seen in this way as, for example, the Harpenden Stadiometer. With a suitable instrument and a skilled observer the range of error in the measurement of stature can be reduced to 3 mm.

The usefulness of skinfold measurements depends on the fact that in many parts of the body the skin and subcutaneous tissues are only loosely attached to underlying structures and can be pulled up between the thumb and fore-finger into a fold. The thickness of this fold of skin can be measured by applying some form of caliper on either side of it and gives a good indication of the amount of subcutaneous fat. The caliper must be designed to give constant pressure between the jaws at all openings. The Harpenden Skinfold Caliper (1, 3) is the most accurate at present available. Older calipers of the Franzen type produce a large increase of pressure as the spring is stretched by increasing the opening of the jaws and it is therefore difficult to interperate the readings obtained. The correlation between measurements taken with the Harpenden Caliper and direct measurements taken of fat width by x-ray is 0.85—0.9, which shows a very good agreement between the two methods. The pressure exerted on the skinfold at the caliper face is 10 grammes per square millimetre at all openings from 2 mm to at least 40 mm, in accordance with international agreement. There is no agreement yet as to the most desirable area and shape of the jaw face. The Harpenden Caliper has a rectangular face with an area of 90 sq. mm. The jaws of some American calipers are circular and of smaller area. The skinfold should be picked up between the thumb and fore-finger of the measurer's left hand, which should first be placed on the subject's skin just far enough apart to allow the full fold to be pinched up from the underlying tissues. The fold must be held firmly by the finger and thumb while the measurement is being taken. The calipers are applied to the fold at a short distance from the fingers, so that only the calipers' faces and not the fingers are exerting a pressure at the point where the measurement is taken. The fingers of the right hand are then released from the handle of the caliper, so that it can exert its full pressure on the fold. The dial is then read to the nearest 0.1 mm. For readings of less than about 20 mm the needle usual becomes completely stationary as soon as the full force of the caliper has been applied. With thicker folds and occasionally with thin ones, the reading may continue to decline slowly and it is less easy to obtain a precise reading. With experience, however, one learns to distinguish a period of rapid movement of the needle before the full force of the caliper has been applied from the period of slow decrease in the reading which may follow this. The reading should be taken at the end of the period of rapid movement, that is as soon as the full force of the caliper has been applied. Usually, the slow decline in the reading can be abolished by taking a firmer grip in the skinfold with the fingers and applying the calipers again.

The usual sites for taking skinfold measurements are as follows: 1. *Triceps* — this measurement is taken half way down the left arm between the tip of the acromium and the head of the radius, felt in the anticubital fossa. The subjects arm should hang relaxed at the side and the fold is picked up in a line passing directly up the arm from the tip of the olecranon process. It is convenient to mark the level with a pen before picking up the fold. 2. *Biceps* — this fold should be picked up at the same level as and exactly opposite the triceps fold on the left arm. 3. *Subscapular* — picked up just below the angle of the left scapula with the shoulder and arm relaxed. The fold should be picked up parallel to the natural cleavage line of the skin. 4. *Supra-iliac* — just above and parallel to the anterior end of the iliac crest on the left side. If a large number of skinfold measurements are taken it is found that they do not follow a normal distribution and that the error of measurement is proportional to the absolute measurement recorded in each case. So that simple statistical techniques can be employed it is necessary that a normal distribution should be obtained and for this purpose the measurements should be transformed according to the formula, skinfold transform = 100 log (reading in $^1/_{10}$ mm — 18). A table of this transform is given by EDWARDS, HAMMOND, HEALEY, TANNER and WHITEHOUSE (1955). In comparing a reading with the standards published by TANNER and WHITEHOUSE (1962) for triceps and subscapular folds, it is unnecessary to apply this transform as this is done automatically by the scale against which the standards are plotted. The accuracy of skinfold measurements taken with the Harpenden Caliper is such that a trained individual should duplicate his readings to within + or — 0.3 mm two thirds of the time at an opening of 8 mm. At greater openings the absolute error is greater but the percentage error between duplicate readings stays constant at about + or — 5 % for two thirds of the repeat readings. Differences between observers may be much greater than this, however, unless great care is taken in training the observers together and in keeping them trained. This variation between individuals is due to differences in the manner of locating and picking up of the skinfold.

Upper arm circumference should be measured in the horizontal plane at the same level as the triceps skinfold. A metal tape measure must be used (other materials are liable to stretch) and should be in contact with the skin all the way round the arm. The pressure applied by the tape should not be sufficient to indent the skin.

For the measurement of calf circumference the subject should sit with his leg hanging freely and relaxed from the knee down while the thigh is supported by the surface on which he is sitting. The measurement is taken in the same way as the upper arm circumference is measured.

More valuable information will be obtained from the few measurements discussed above if they are properly made than will be derived from many more measurements made less accurately.

REFERENCES

1. Edwards, D. A. W., W. H. Hammond, M. J. R. Healy, J. M. Tanner and R. H. Whitehouse, Design and accuracy of calipers for measuring subcutaneous tissue thickness, *Brit. J. Nutr.* 9: 133—143, 1955.
2. Gidds, C. B., Psychological aspects of machine design, *Machinery*, 8 pp., May 6, 1955.
3. Tanner, J. M. and R. H. Whitehouse, The Harpenden Skinfold Caliper, *Amer. J. Phys. Anthrop. N. S.* 13: 743—746, 1955.
4. Tanner, J. M. and R. H. Whitehouse, *Brit. Med. J.* i: 446—450, 1962.

TECHNICAL ASPECTS OF THE MEASUREMENT OF LENGTH IN INFANTS

R. STEENDIJK

Considering the number of data in the literature on the growth of the young child and adolescent, there is a conspicuous scarcity of similar data obtained during the first year of life. In view of the rapid rate of growth in this period (25 cm per year), it would appear that deviations from the normal rate could be established in less time than at a later age when growth rate is much slower, and therefore, that the first year of life would be a good period for the study of the effect of short-term illnesses or nutritional disturbances on growth. Our knowledge on this subject is still very poor. At first glance, this may seem surprising; however, it should be remembered that it is more difficult to obtain accurate measurements of the length of infants than of older children. This is not so much due to the fact that one has to take the measurements with the subject in the recumbent position as to the complete absence of co-operation on the part of the infant, which often has to be restrained with some force during the procedure. In addition, the growth rate declines so rapidly during the first year of life, that short-lasting deviations from the normal are difficult to ascertain.

The purpose of this paper is to illustrate some of the difficulties adherent to the technique of measurement and to give a rough sketch of the quantitative aspects involved.

The type of instrument needed for the measurement of infants has been described by HINDLEY in 1953 (2). The board used in the present study is shown in plate 1. It consists of a fixed head-board and a movable foot-board, which slides on the horizontal board. Head- and foot-board are exactly parallel and both are at right angles to the horizontal board. A ruler or tape-measure is fitted along the edge of the latter. The technique has been well described by FALKNER (1) and the following paragraph is quoted almost verbatim from his directions.

Two people are required to measure the recumbent length of babies and young children. The baby is placed on his back along the long axis of the board. One person firmly holds the crown of the head against the head-board in such a way that the upper margin of the external auditory meatus and the lower margin of the orbit of the eye are perpendicular. The second person now grips both ankles and places the soles firmly against the foot-board which is being manipulated with the other hand. The knees will often be bent in protest, but they may be firmly pressed down with the left hand. Once the feet are in position, it is usual for the head-holder to remark that the head is no longer against the board. This is good, for the head is now gently but firmly brought back to the head-board, the foot-holder not giving way too much. This means that the baby is stretched very gently, which is exactly what is required. Height is now read in millimeters.

To obtain an impression about the error involved in this method, 9 children, whose individual heights varied from 500 to 730 mm, were measured 5 times within one week by two observers who were inexperienced at the beginning of the study. Each observer measured each child independently and did not know the values obtained by the other observer. In this way, each observer obtained 9 groups of 5 values. The range of the values within one group varied for both observers between 3 and 14 mm. It turned out that, for both observers the range was small in children who were easy to measure and large in children who had to be restrained with some force. This indicates that the lack of co-operation in infants constitutes an important factor for the accuracy of the measurements.

The 95 % confidence limits of the means of each group of 5 values — calculated with the aid of the tables for Student's 't' (3) — varied between ± 1.5 and ± 6.9 mm. Thus it appeared that the accuracy could be improved by taking the mean of 5 measurements. This implies, of course, that the small height increment occurring in the period of one week, in which the 5 values were obtained, is neglected. The error, thus produced, especially when growth is fast, can be largely prevented by shortening the period over which measurements are taken.

The means of the group of 5 values obtained by the two observers in each child agreed well. Their difference varied between 0 and 4 mm (average difference: 1.5 mm).

The difference between the values obtained by each observer for a single measurement varied between 0 and 7 mm (average difference: 2.5 mm).

To find out whether the growth rate over short periods of time could be measured with sufficient accuracy, several children were measured twice at an interval of 4 to 6 weeks. The results obtained in 2 of these children are presented in table 1 and fig. 1. It appears that the accuracy of the values obtained for the growth rate may be insufficient to detect small temporary changes. Further longitudinal pilot studies over

Table 1. *Growth-rate in 2 infants calculated from the means of 2 groups of* 5 *values obtained at the intervals indicated. Only the values from one observer are represented.*

Name	First measurement mm (95 % c. l.)	Second measurement mm (95 % c. l.)	Interval days	Growth-rate mm (95 % c. l.) per period
Jrs.	673.0 ± 2.8	682.0 ± 2.4	26	9.0 ± 5.0 in 26 days
Hav.	693.0 ± 5.7	717.0 ± 5.4	34	24.0 ± 1.10 in 34 days

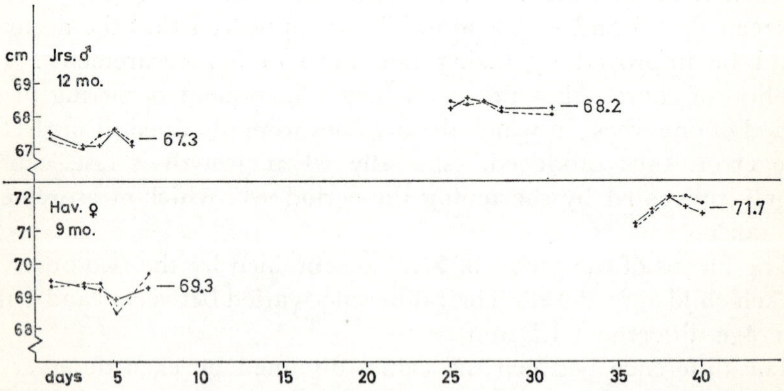

Fig. 1. Graphic representation of the value obtained by two observers in two children (+——+ and o- - -o). The means are also indicated and are identical for each observer. The 95 % confidence limits differed slightly between the observers and are omitted from the figure

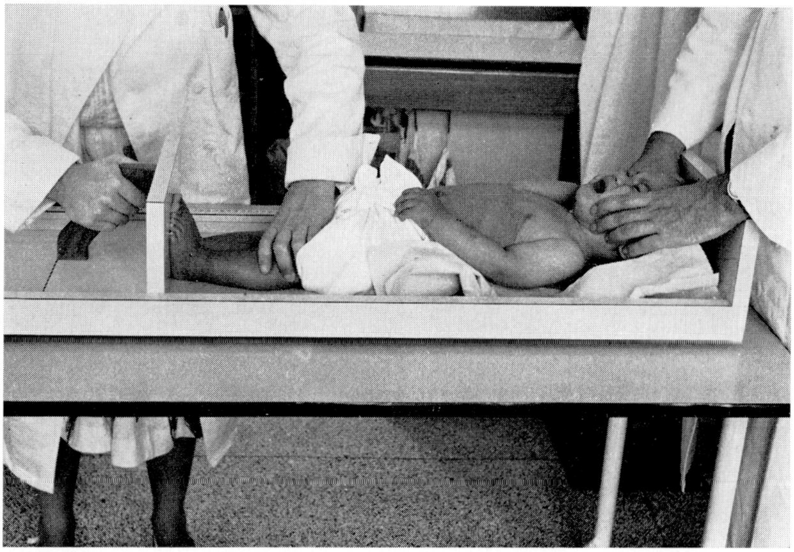

Plate 1. The measuring board

many months, in healthy as well as in sick children, may show whether it will be rewarding to tackle such problems as 'the influence of illness upon growth in infancy' on a large scale. This preliminary study shows that these questions are less easy to answer than one might be inclined to think.

REFERENCES

1. FALKNER, F., Physical growth, in: *Recent advances in Paediatrics*, ed. D. Gairdner, p. 145, D. & A. Churchill, London, 1958.
2. HINDLEY, C. B., Portable measuring board for infants, *Lancet* II: 142, 1953.
3. MORONEY, M. J., *Facts from figures*, Pelican Books, 1957.

LONGITUDINAL AND CROSS-SECTIONAL DATA

W. A. MARSHALL

Any study of growth involves the measurement of individuals at different ages. The usefulness of the data which are collected depends largely on whether the same, or different, individuals are measured at each age. For example, one might wish to determine the average stature of children at each year of age in a particular community and obtain an estimate of the variation about this average in normal children. This problem could be dealt with quite easily in a single year. First one would have to define exactly the population which was to be studied and select a sample of children of each age which would be representative of the children of that age in the whole population. The stature of each child in each sample would then be measured and the mean stature, with its standard deviation, could then be calculated for each age. A study of this type in which a large number of subjects of each age are measured, but any one subject is measured only once, is called a cross-sectional study.

An alternative objective might be to determine how the rate of growth varies as children grow from birth to maturity. This can only be done by measuring the same children repeatedly throughout the whole period of growth. A study in which the same measurement is repeated on the same subjects at different ages is called a longitudinal study.

A cross-sectional study will tell you the mean value and the variance of a measurement at each age, but it will tell you nothing about how much any individual in the sample grows between one age and the next. It is possible to calculate the average increase in the measurement over this period, but the variance about this average cannot be estimated. Cross-sectional studies are therefore useless for the comparison of rates of growth in different groups of subjects and, for many purposes, the rate of growth is a much more useful thing to study

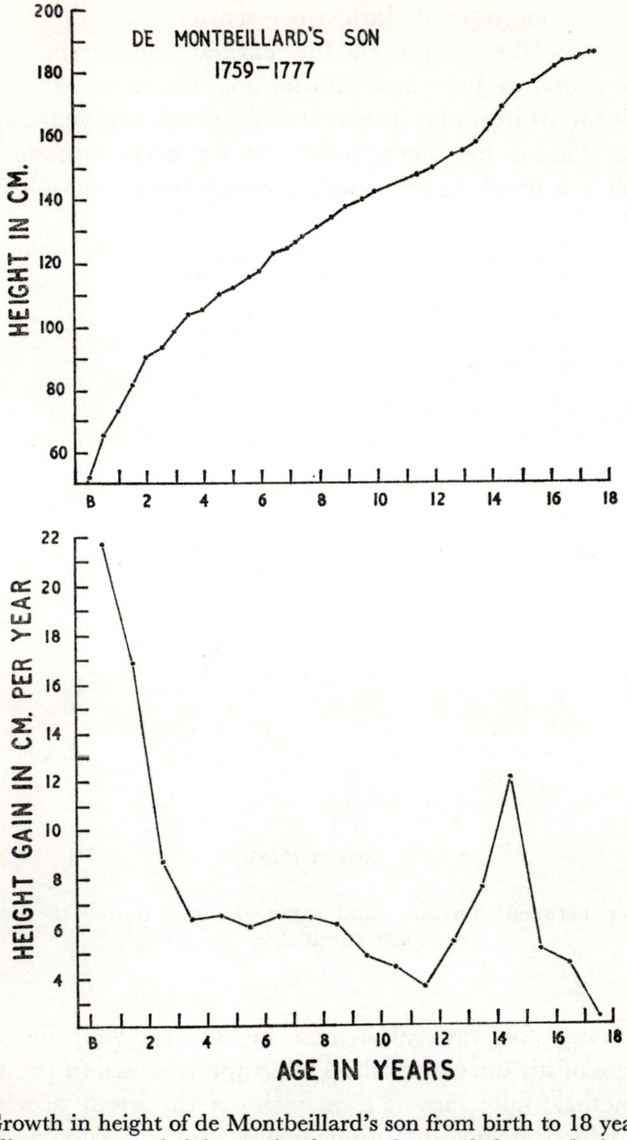

Fig. 1. Growth in height of de Montbeillard's son from birth to 18 years, 1759—77. Above, distance curve, height attained at each age: below, velocity curve, increments in height from year to year (from 2)

than the actual distance which has been grown. In order to study rates of growth longitudinal data are essential.

Figure 1 shows the results of the earliest longitudinal growth study, about which we have any information. Count de Montbeillard measured his son at irregular intervals during eighteen years. Because the same individual has been measured on every occasion, it is possible to tell how much he grew during each interval and so construct

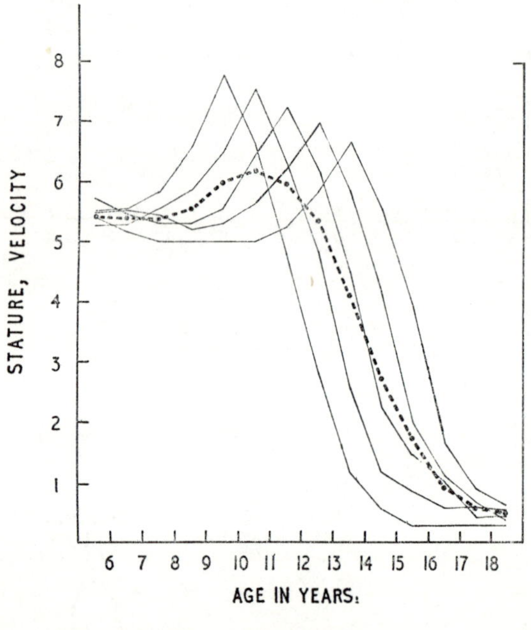

Fig. 2. Relation between individual and mean velocities during the adolescent spurt (from 2)

a graph showing the rate at which he was growing during the different stages of his development. This graph is shown in the bottom half of the picture; note how it clearly shows the great acceleration of growth which occurs at adolescence and is known as the adolescent spurt.

Figure 2 shows how the adolescent growth spurt would be hidden by the use of cross-sectional data. These velocity curves were obtained by the longitudinal study of five boys, each of whom shows a well marked spurt, occurring at a slightly different chronological age in each case. If a crosss-ectional study had yielded exactly the same measurements at each age it would have been possible to calculate only the average velocity for each interval between two sets of measurements so that the dotted curve in the middle would have been obtained and the true nature of the adolescent spurt would not have been detected. Once however, the spurt has been detected by longitudinal study it is possible to show it graphically in the group of individuals by using the time of maximal growth velocity as the datum point from which time measurements are taken.

Obviously then, longitudinal studies are more useful if one wishes to obtain a true picture of the growth process, but they have certain practical disadvantages. A complete study takes a very long time, about 20 years in man, and is therefore very expensive. It may be impossible to retain the whole sample for the duration of the study. Individual subjects may die, move to another part of the world or simply withdraw their co-operation for a variety of reasons. Some aspects of growth of internal organs can only be investigated on post mortem material and this cannot be studied longitudinally. These objections do not apply to cross-sectional studies.

Because it is so difficult to retain a complete sample throughout a longitudinal study, one may be forced to combine data from some individuals who were measured on every occasion, some who were measured on fewer occasions and some who were measured on only one occasion. This is called a mixed longitudinal study and although it is not as useful as a pure longitudinal one, it is certainly better than a cross sectional one provided the results are properly analysed. Even a series of very short longitudinal studies in which for example, some children are measured at age 2 and 3, others at age 3 and 4 and so on, can yield very useful information about rates of growth, provided the statistical treatment is correct.

It is, of course, equally important that the correct statistical treatment should be applied to pure longitudinal studies. It is useless to carry out a longitudinal study and then treat the results as if they had been obtained cross-sectionally. One might as well have saved one's time and money and done a cross-sectional study in the first place. Much valuable information was lost in the earlier growth studies, because longitudinal data were reported in this way.

Cross-sectional data can be dealt with quite easily by working out the mean and deviation of the meassurement at each age. To get the most out of longitudinal data, however, it is necessary to resort to curve fitting.

In principle, curve fitting is not difficult although the arithmetic may be rather complicated. The simplest form of curve is a straight line and is described by the equation $y = bx + c$, b being a constant which indicates the slope of the line and c being another constant which indicates the point at which the line meets the y axis. If growth could be described by a straight line, b would be the rate of growth and c the initial value of the measurement being studied. Unfortunately most growth processes cannot be fitted by straight lines but other equations with more constants can be used to describe curves of various shapes. In dealing with growth, the method is to examine the data and decide what shape of curve will fit them most closely and at the same time be described by an equation, whose constants will have some biological meaning and indicate important characteristics of the growth process. The same type of curve can then be fitted to the data for each child, but the constants will have different numerical values in each case. In order to obtain a curve which characterises the growth of a group of children a curve should be fitted to the data for each child and then the mean value of each constant for the whole group should be determined. For example, if the growth process were so simple that it could be described by a straight line, one would take the mean values of all the b's and the mean of all the c's in the linear equations which had been worked out for each child. This would give you what is called a mean constant curve and must not be confused with the mean curve which would be obtained by taking the mean value of the measurement at each age and fitting a curve to these means. In the case of a straight line the mean curve and the mean constant curve are identical but in the more complicated cases this is not so and the mean curve is less satisfactory than the mean constant curve (see 1). The best procedure is usually to fit a curve to the original measurements. This distance curve can then be converted into a velocity curve by differentiating it.

In order to make the most efficient use of data of the mixed longitudinal type, other statistical techniques may be necessary. These cannot be discussed here but they are clearly and simply described by TANNER (1).

REFERENCES

1. TANNER, J. M., Some notes on the reporting of growth data, *Human Biology* 23: 93, 1951.
2. TANNER, J. M., *Growth and adolescence*, 2nd ed., London, 1962.

ESTIMATION OF AGE AT MENARCHE IN A POPULATION

J. F. DE WIJN

Many of the methods used for the assessment of the mean age at *menarche* are of dubious validity.

VAN 'T LAND and DE HAAS (10) have summarized most of the available literature from 1879 to 1957, including both the first study in the Netherlands by BOLK (2) and the second, carried out 35 years later in the Netherlands Institute of Preventive Medicine, Leiden, in which the author participated. In the same paper methods commonly used for the estimation of the age of menarche are discussed and comparison with other populations is given. This was followed by a paper by RUSBACH, VAN LAAR and DE HAAS (15) on the statistical approach of two different methods used for the evaluation of a single set of data, and by four more studies in the Netherlands (6, 7, 18, 9).

Though numerous authors in various countries have given their contributions to the methodology of the assessment of the menarcheal age, confusion about the validity of the method of choice for population surveys still exists all over the world. This paper deals with the pros and cons of three methods often used:

a. prospective method, recording onset of periods in a longitudinal study;

b. retrospective method, recording age at menarche as stated when interrogated;

c. status quo method, recording whether or not periods have started at the time of investigation.

a. PROSPECTIVE METHOD

The only way to learn the exact time of onset of menstrual periods is through a longitudinal study, by keeping careful records of each girl from some time before menstruation. This method eliminates inaccuracies when performed: (1) with trained personnel, (2) in a closed population, in which every member is prepubertal at the beginning of the study and is followed until every member has attained menarche, (3) with girls who have approximately the same age at the beginning of the study. (Ad 1) Since the onset of menstrual periods is often accompanied bij emotional feelings which may prevent straight answers when girls are interrogated by strangers, trained personnel is necessary. (Ad 2 and 3) The age at onset of menstrual periods in healthy European girls now varies from 10 to 16 years. Longitudinal studies will therefore require at least six years. Because menarche tends to occur earlier in prosperous countries, with an acceleration of 4—6 months per decade (11, 16) girls must be of approximately the same age when the longitudinal study commences. When girls still prepubertal at age 15 are mixed with girls of 10 years, the mean age at menarche of the whole group will be influenced by the secular acceleration which occurs during the 5 years which separate the times of birth of the two groups of girls.

Longitudinal studies are difficult to perform, expensive and rather tedious for the investigator who wants results quickly. Such studies are often part of a more elaborate growth study.

Longitudinal data are only available for the USA (5, 13, 14, 17). The mean age at menarche thus found for small groups of American white girls in these studies is about $12^3/_4$ year, which is half a year to one year earlier than the figure obtained in non longitudinal studies in most of the European countries. A number of longitudinal studies are now in progress, in various parts of the world, which are co-ordinated by the Centre International de l'Enfance in Paris.

In conclusion the advantages of the prospective method are that this method eliminates inaccuracy, and that relatively small groups are needed. The drawbacks are that it takes at least six years and therefore is expensive and tedious, unless it forms part of an overall growth study.

b. RETROSPECTIVE METHOD

This method entails false information because of poor memory and other sources of bias. Nevertheless, this type of study has been the most frequently used in earlier work and in many recent studies. In the

Netherlands BOLK (2) found that adult women, when interviewed, gave menarcheal ages which averaged $13^{9}/_{12}$ years. Retrospective studies based on statements by adult women always measure, however accurately, a past event. Thus the average age at menarche which BOLK calculated in 1923 related to the situation in the Netherlands of 15—20 years earlier, and yet his average was the same as was obtained again in the Netherlands 35 years later. BOLK did not state the social classes to which his subjects belonged. In his study young women were found to state an earlier age than the elderly, and the difference may be due to either a secular trend, or a greater degree of inaccuracy of the older women. In 1960 BENJAMIN (1) described a mean age at menarche of 14.6 years for 1444 postmenopausal white women of the Cape Province; in view of the age of these women at the time of investigation this figure applies to the South African situation at least 35 years earlier.

Retrospective surveys should be undertaken only when the entire 'population' has attained menarche before the interviews take place, otherwise the younger the group which is investigated, the lower will be the figure obtained for age at menarche. This may be so for two reasons. First because of greater inaccuracy of the statements by older girls. In KARK's study (8) from rural districts in the Northern Transvaal and in the Cape Province, girls of 18 to 20 gave 15 to 16 years as their age of onset of menses, whereas those of 15 to 17 gave an age of 13 to 14 years. Similar experiences have been described by ELLIS (4) in Africa, BOJLÈN (3) in Denmark, and RUSBACH e.a. (15) and KOLK (9) in the Netherlands. All subjects who cannot remember the month during which the first menstruation occurred, should be rejected. In the adolescent survey among schoolchildren in the west of the Netherlands (table 1) 25 % of 16-year-old girls could not remember the exact month! From the girls aged 12 to 19 years 18 % had to be rejected for this reason. This percentage varies with differences in cultural and educational background. HORDIJK (6) in the south of the Netherlands rejected 30 %, MICHELSON (12) rejected 50 % of Negrogirls. Moreover, there is no evidence to show that the information from girls who are prepared to state the month of their first menstruation is accurate, unless girls are asked why this date was remembered. Even girls who have not yet menstruated, may tell the investigator that they have, from a desire to be regarded as an adolescent rather than a child. The omission of a

Table 1. *Percentage of girls unable to recollect the month in which menarche occurred (15).*

Age at first inquiry	Total number of menstruating girls	Month of menarche unknown	
		number	%
12	39	—	0
13	183	7	4
14	280	26	9
15	225	37	16
16	186	48	26
17	151	52	34
18	65	35	54
total	1129	205	18

section of the population because of poor memory regarding the time of onset of menstruation introduces another possible source of bias.

The second reason why girls in retrospective surveys have to be postpubertal is that the inclusion of prepubertal girls will lower the average age at menarche for the group. Thus the difference found by WILSON and SUTHERLAND (19) between two groups of children in the South of England (13.4 years in Oxford, 13.09 years in Oxfordshire) was solely due to the younger age of Oxfordshire girls. By probit analysis on both sets of data a mean age of 13.6 was obtained for both groups. HORDIJK (6) has published figures of menarcheal age of 3129 girls 12—15 years old, including those who were still prepubertal, and he suggested that menarche occurred at an average age of $12^1/_4$ years in 12-year-olds, $12^1/_3$ years in 13-year-olds, $13^2/_5$ years in 14-year-olds and $13^4/_5$ years in 15-year-olds. For the group of girls 12—15 years old he thus obtained the incorrect average age at menarche of $13^1/_4$ years.

Yet this method of retrospective statements may be the method of choice when the investigator wants to compare menarcheal age of small groups within the same age range, but different by social class, race, nutritive state and so on. When all girls of the group are over

15 years of age, this will include a fairly low percentage of about 10 % pre-menarcheal girls, and the average thus obtained may be less erroneous, though still below the correct figure. When the *median age* is estimated instead of the average age, those who have not yet menstruated will not influence the outcome, because the median age is always less than 15 years, and for most European populations even less than 14 years. For the evaluation of the significance of differences

Table 2. *Median age at menarche (M) compared for 15—17 year old girls from medium (A) and high (B) social classes.*

Age at menarche	A			B		
	M+		M—	M+		M—
$10^1/_2$	—		—	—		—
$10^3/_4$	—		—	—		—
11	2		—	3		—
$11^1/_4$	—		—	1		—
$11^1/_2$	2		—	4		—
$11^3/_4$	3		—	3		—
12	7		—	7		—
$12^1/_4$	4		—	3		—
$12^1/_2$	6		—	5		—
$12^3/_4$	7		—	7		—
13	11		—	13		—
$13^1/_4$	6		—	3		—
$13^1/_2$	10		—	9		—
$13^3/_4$	7		—	7		—
14	7		—	8		—
$14^1/_4$	10		—	8		—
$14^1/_2$	9		—	4		—
$14^3/_4$	6		1	1		4
15	4		7	3		3
$15^1/_4$	1		2	1		—
$15^1/_2$	—		1	—		1
$15^3/_4$	—		—	—		1
16	3		—	3		—
$16^1/_4$	—		—	—		—
$16^1/_2$	—		—	—		—
$16^3/_4$	—		—	—		—
n	105	+	11	93	+	9
$^1/_2$ n		58			51	
median		13.8			13.5	

in median ages appropriate statistical tests are available. Even in our prosperous industrialized country figures of median age so compared for two groups of elderly schoolchildren were 13.8 years for group A, girls from a school for domestic training in a small town of the Western Netherlands, where 70 % of the girls' fathers belong to the lower or medium social classes including skilled and semiskilled labourers, and 13.5 years for group B, grammar school girls of whom 70 % belong to social classes I and II (table 2). The difference in height between the two groups, plotted in fig. 1 from cross-sectional data, corresponds to a difference in development of about one year.

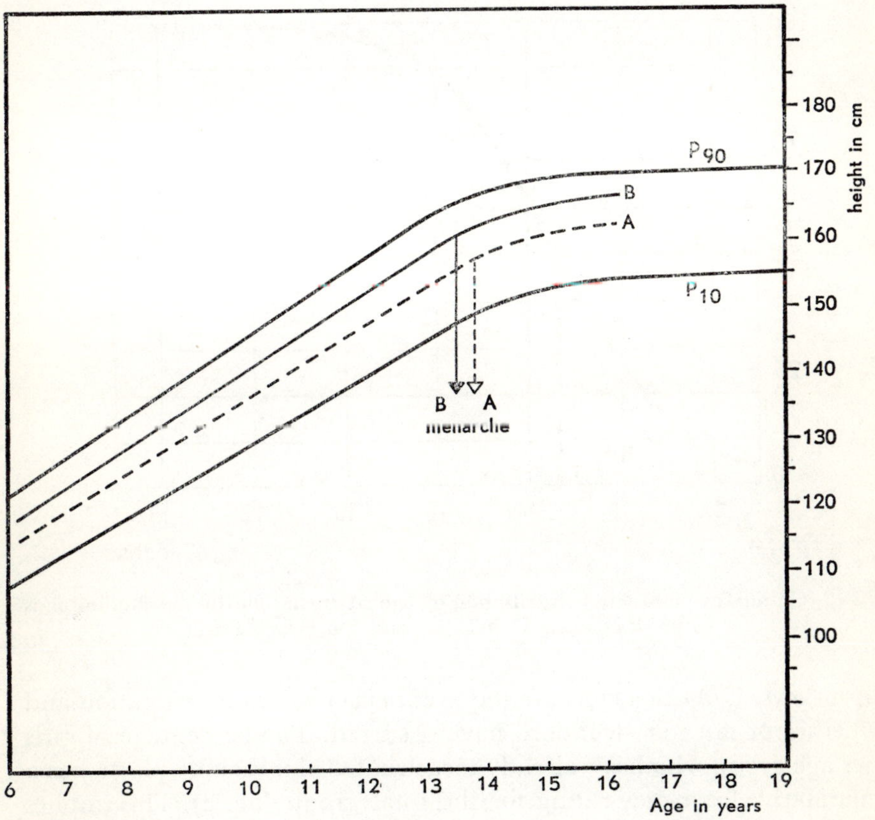

Fig. 1. Cross-sectional growth curves for height of two groups of girls of different social status in the Netherlands, of which the average ages at menarche was estimated to be 13.8 years (group A) and 13.5 years (group B)

In conclusion the only advantage of the retrospective method is that it may be used for comparison of median age at menarche in relatively small groups, while the disadvantages are the poor memory and the tendency of older girls to state higher ages.

c. STATUS QUO METHOD

When the prospective method cannot be used, the simple information whether or not mentruation has started (status quo) is the most suitable technique for the estimation of the mean age at menarche

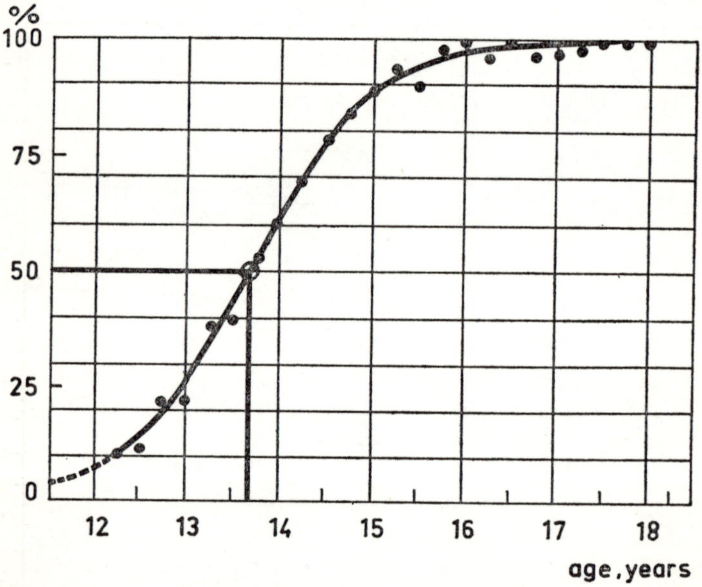

Fig. 2. Cumulative frequency distribution of age at menarche in the Netherlands (from Rusbach, Van Laar and De Haas, 1961)

in surveys. Only two facts are required: exact age at investigation and whether or not menstruations have occurred. The percentage of girls per age group who have already menstruated can then be plotted as a cumulative frequency rating for the total group (fig. 2). This implies that both pre-menarcheal and post-menarcheal girls of at least 12 years of age must be included. To learn the exact range girls from age 9 or 10 up to 18 must be included, in order to calculate the lower and higher percentile levels. The only drawback of this method is that it requires a large number of girls. Advantages are the little information required and the fact that the figures obtained represent the actual situation.

When the retrospective method is applied to girls not younger than 15 years, it may happen that the results correspond with those of the status quo method (15) in spite of the fact that about 10 % of these girls do not menstruate. The lowering of the average figure caused by the latter circumstance is possibly compensated by the tendency of older girls to overestimate the age at menarche and by the lesser influence of the secular trend on older than on younger girls.

Investigations in the Netherlands between 1955 and 1960 have yielded average ages at menarche of $13^{2}/_{3}$ years (status quo method: 10), of $13^{4}/_{5}$ years (status quo method 9) and of $13^{1}/_{5}$ years (retrospective method: 18). In these studies 96.5 % of girls attained menarche before age 17, 7.5 % before age 12.

In the evaluation of the mean age at menarche many views have been put forward to explain menarcheal variation between groups different in race, type, social class, rate of growth, climatic conditions etc. Genetic factors are evident, particularly in individual cases. In tropical regions age at menarche is later, which few would consider the effect of temperature. Tropical diseases and undernutrition inhibit both growth and maturation. When social classes are compared within a racially homogeneous population, the poorer nutritional status show a later age at menarche. Endocrine activity is somehow related to overall nutritional health rather than to metabolic processes of specific nutrients. This relationship, however, is far from completely understood and wants further studies.

REFERENCES

1. Benjamin, F., The age of the menarche and of the menopause in white South African women and certain factors influencing these times, *S. Afr. Med. J.* 34: 316, 1960.
2. Bolk, L., The menarche in Dutch women and its precipitated appearance in the youngest generation, *Proc. Kon. Akad. Wetensch. Amst.* 26: 650, 1923.
3. Bojlèn, K., G. Rasch and M. W. Benzon, The age incidence of the menarche in Copenhagen, *Acta Obstet. Gynec. Scand.* 33: 405, 1954.
4. Ellis, R. W. B., Age of puberty in the tropics, *Brit. Med. J.* I: 85, 1950.
5. Engle, E. T. and M. C. Shelesnyak, First menstruation and subsequent menstrual cycles of pubertal girls, *Human Biol.* 6: 431, 1934.
6. Hordijk, W., *Groei en ontwikkeling in de puberteit en de adolescentie,* Thesis, Utrecht, 1961.
7. *Onderzoek naar de lichamelijke conditie van leerlingen van de primaire opleiding aan nijverheidsscholen voor meisjes,* Rapport van de Commissie tot bevordering van goede onderwijsmethoden etc., subcommissie voor de lichamelijke opvoeding, 1958.
8. Kark, E., Menarche in South African girls, *S. Afr. J. Med. Sci.* 8: 35, 1943.
9. Kolk, J. J., De menarche leeftijd, *Tijdschr. v. Soc. Geneesk.* 40: 645, 1962.
10. Land, G. M. van 't and J. H. de Haas, Menarche leeftijd in Nederland, *Ned. Tijdschr. Geneesk.* 101: 1425, 1957.
11. Letting, O., Menarchealderem hos skolepiker i Oslo og dens forhold til fysisk utvikling, *12. Nordiske Kongres for legemlig opdragelse, Børneog Ungdomshygiejne,* 4—9 aug., 1953, p. 105.
12. Michelson, N., Studies on the physical development of Negroes. IV. Onset of puberty, *Amer. J. Phys. Antrop.* 2: 151, 1944.
13. Nicolson, A. B. and C. Hanley, Indices of physiological maturity: derivation and inter-relationship, *Child. Developm.* 24: 3, 1953.
14. Reynolds, E. L. and J. V. Wines, Individual differences in physical changes associated with adolescence in girls, *Amer. J. Dis. Child,* 75: 329, 1948.
15. Rusbach, H. W., F. van Laar and J. H. de Haas, Menarche leeftijd, *Tijdschr. v. Soc. Geneesk. 39*: 411, 1961.
16. Simell, G., Ueber das Menarche-alter in Finnland, *Acta Pediat.* (Uppsala), Suppl. no. 84, 1952.
17. Simmons, K. and W. W. Greulich, Menarcheal age and the height, weight and skeletal age of girls age 7 to 17 years, *J. Pediat. 22*, 518, 1943.
18. Swaak, A. J., Een geneeskundig onderzoek naar de voeding en voedingstoestand van meisjes van 14—24 jaar in Maastricht en omstreken, *Voeding* 22: 513, 1961.
19. Wilson, D. C. and I. Sutherland, The age of the menarche, *Brit. Med. J.* II: 130, 1949.

DISCUSSION

Steendijk: I should like to ask Dr. MARSHALL whether he has any experience with the measurement of babies.

Marshall: Measurements of this type have been done in our big London growth study, but I unfortunately had no experience of it at the time, because I joined the group after the children had grown beyond this stage. I have, however, met the problem as a clinical one in our growth clinic and it is certainly true that if the child does not co-operate, one can get very strange results sometimes. We have no very good answer to this, except to hope that one can eventually calm the child down, and repeat the measurement perhaps later on in the afternoon. I think that if you decide that the child is not co-operating, you are much better to neglect the measurement entirely, and hope that on a later occasion you can repeat it satisfactorily.

Laron: I should like to ask Dr. MARSHALL what he thinks about measuring the length in all children. We sometimes see differences of up to $1^{1}/_{2}$ cm between the height and the length in children of any age, which is due to the curvature of the spine.

Marshall: In the study we do in fact measure the lying down length of all our children as well as the height, and we sometimes do find this difference. This, I agree, is probably a matter of curvature of the spine which one does not eliminate fully by the stretching technique on the standing measurement, but when the child is lying down on a hard, flat surface, he automatically eliminates this, I think, for his own comfort.

Laron: Would you agree that if one measurement only is taken, length might be better than height?

Marshall: Speaking purely scientifically, I think it would probably be a better measurement. Speaking practically this might not be so as the apparatus has to be slightly more complicated. It has to be designed so that both the head-end and the foot-end are at right angles to the base. It is less easy to make an accurate apparatus although it can perfectly well be done, but is is more expensive. It also takes up more space so it is probably more difficult to use it on a wide scale in schools.

Laron: I should like to raise the general problem of measuring the new-born. In our country the orthopaedic people are very much against measuring the new-born. They think that stretching the legs might influence the hip joint, and they persuaded the Ministry of Health to issue an order, not only an advice but an order, to the hospitals, not to measure the length of the new-born. We disregard this order in our hospital, and continue to measure new-borns, but I should be very interested to hear what happens in other countries and what is considered the right thing to do.

Steendijk: In our experience the hip joint is not endangered by this method. Stretching is done gently and the knees are not kept rigid to the board. I consider that measuring new-borns is of the utmost importance and much more important than getting the birth weight.

Van der Werff ten Bosch: Is the fear of the orthopaedic surgeons based on experience?

Laron: They seem to have some evidence, that I am not completely convinced by.

Sobel: I should like to ask both, Dr. MARSHALL and Dr. STEENDIJK about the measurement of leg-length or sitting height, which may be very useful for evaluating the growth and the development of the child. In what way would one best find out if the legs are indeed growing in appropriate proportion to the linear growth of the child at his particular age? Dr. LARON has already raised the question of the possible advantages of measuring length only in both infants and older children if one cannot have equipment for obtaining both standing height and length. It can be as difficult for a short paediatrician to stretch a tall child to obtain an accurate standing height as for the young child to co-operate while that same measurement is being taken.

Marshall: I feel that sitting height is an extremely useful measurement in that it does reveal something at least of the proportional growth of the child, and the more we know about this, the better. The measurement can be very simply used as an index of normality of growth in proportion by the simple procedure of drawing a graph in which the total stature is plotted against the sitting height and there are normal standards published in England by TANNER and WHITEHOUSE, showing this relationship, and for clinical purposes we do find them very useful. It is scarcely the time to go into the technique in detail at the moment, but is it quite a simple one. The measurement is taken more or less the same way as stature, using a similar apparatus, although it can be done with an ordinary anthropometer. We use an apparatus rather like the stature apparatus, but with provision for the child to be sitting, while the measurement is taken. And the general principles of the technique are the same.

Thomson: I just like to make one comment to possibly redress a point of balance. Dr. MARSHALL's insistence upon accurate measuring technique is of course quite essential in intensive research studies. But there may be numbers of people here who are concerned with routine measurements in schools, who may be rather depressed; is their work worth while at all, when precision is difficult? It has been shown that routine measurements of school children are perfectly capable of showing such phenomena as secular trends, and differences between different areas of a country. Routine measurements done with ordinary care are certainly worth while.

CHAPTER II

SKELETAL MATURATION

ASSESSMENT OF SKELETAL MATURITY

W. A. MARSHALL

If any one were to tell us that a girl whom we had never seen was 12 years old we would have no idea as to whether we were discussing a small child who had not yet entered into puberty and who had a considerable amount of growth ahead of her, or someone who in physiological terms at least, was a woman and had completed adolescence, begun to menstruate and nearly reached her maximum stature. There are many twelve year old girls who fit either of these descriptions and the same variation in maturity can be found among boys of about 14 years of age. Although the differences between individuals of the same age are most striking at adolescence there are differences in the degree of advancement in growth and development of different children at all chronological ages throughout the whole period of childhood. Thus the chronological age of a child gives us no indication of his or her physiological maturity. There is clearly a need for some measure which will indicate what proportion of a child's total potential growth has been completed and what stage of physiological maturity a child has reached. In order to be of real value the measurement of physiological maturity must be such that it reaches ultimately the same maximum value in all children and preferably it should be possible to apply the same method of assessing it throughout the whole period of childhood.

PRYOR showed that the x-ray appearances of the bones of the hand and wrist of children of the same chronological age showed considerable individual differences. These differences were apparent at all ages from birth onwards and on the average girls presented a more advanced picture of calcification than did boys (15, 16, 17). PRYOR's observations led to the concept of skeletal age which has since been far the most commonly used indicator of physiological maturity. Dental age, assessed by counting the number of teeth present is also used sometimes, but bears little relationship to other aspects of development and is only applicable throughout part of the age range. The value of dental age can be greatly increased by more complicated techniques which take into account the different stages in the development of individual teeth. Morphological age, based on the assessment of height, weight or other anthropometric measurements in relation to the average value for children of different ages is also used, but is a most unsatisfactory index, because if one finds that a child has an advanced height age one cannot tell whether his size is due to the fact that he is advanced in development or only to his being a genetically large child who will ultimately become a large adult. As assessment based on the secondary sex characteristics is useful for the period of puberty and adolescence. The age at which a child reached his maximum velocity of gain in heigth or the age at which he reached 90 % of his final adult heigth are useful measurements for relating physiological maturity to chronological age in retrospective data.

The concept of skeletal age is based on the fact that each bone begins as a primary centre of ossification which passes through various stages of enlargement and change of shape. Some bones may also have secondary centres or epiphyses which have their own patterns of enlargement and shape change. The skeleton only reaches its adult form when all the bones are fully calcified and the epiphyses have fused with their diaphyses. This final stage of skeletal maturity is the same in all individuals. The stages through which each bone develops vary very little between individuals. It is therefore possible to estimate the maturity of the skeleton by studying the x-ray appearances of the bones. It is not necessary to x-ray the whole body for this purpose as sufficiently accurate information can be obtained by studying x-rays of certain small areas. The hand and wrist form the most convenient area as it is easily x-rayed without exposing the gonads to radiation and it includes a large number of bones, both round and long, with at least some degree of differentiation in progress at every age from birth to maturity. The knee may also be used as described by Pyle and Hoerr (18). Acheson (2) and Speijer (20) have described the development of the hip in such a way as to be useful in the assessment of skeletal maturity, but it is impossible to shield the ovaries from radiation while x-raying the hip and this region is therefore unsuitable for routine work in girls, although protective clothing is available for boys. All these authors have used in some form the method of dividing the development of each bone into a series of stages and assessing the skeletal maturity of a particular child by examining his x-ray and determining which of these stages has been reached by each bone. Not all the stages are equally recognisable, however, and a certain amount of observer error enters into all the assessments. This method can however be quite satisfactory provided the stages are carefully chosen so as to be easily recognisable and are well illustrated, as well as being accompanied by clear verbal descriptions, in the key book in which the method is described.

Some authors have tried to minimise observer error by eliminating intermediate stages entirely from the assessment and using only the appearance and disappearance of centres and the fusion and nonfusion of epiphyses (6, 7, 8, 9, 12, 14). PYLE and SONTAG (19) have estimated directly the mean and standard deviation of the time of appearance of 61 centres from birth to the age of nine, using data from the Fels longitudinal study. HARDING (11) gave incidence curves of the appearance of 43 centres and fusions at 11 sites throughout the age range of 0—4 in Boston children. Standards based on these data were published but they are unsuitable for giving any exact statement of the skeletal maturity of a particular child, it being possible only to classify a child as advanced, average or retarded. The method using only appearance of centres and fusion of epiphyses neglects a good deal of information which might be obtained by studying also intermediate stages in the development of bones and in order to obtain an accurate assessment of skeletal age a great many more x-rays are necessary. If intermediate stages in the development of bone are studied it is only necessary to study one or at the most two areas as, in normal children, the development of bone throughout the whole skeleton is very closely co-ordinated. For example, a correlation of Todd skeletal ages on the hand and knee, as calculated within 6 month chronological age groups for adolescent boys and girls, is of the order of 0.87 (5). When one allows for the unreliability of this method of assessment in both regions this must be regarded as a very high degree of correlation.

For practical purposes nowadays radiographs of the wrist and hand are used almost exclusively in the assessment of skeletal development. Three different methods of making this assessment have been suggested.

The first involves measurement of the ossified area, either alone or taken in comparison with the area of the wrist and hand. Methods of this type are in fact of little value as the area of the bone is related to the size of hand as well as to the degree of skeletal development. The hand may be large because the child is advanced on the way to maturity but it may also be large because the child is simply a large child growing into a large adult. The method is therefore open to the same objections as morphological age as an estimate of physiological maturity.

The second method involves the matching of a given radiograph with one of a series of standard radiographs representing successive years of skeletal age and collected in an atlas. This method was developed by TODD (23) in his 'Atlas of Skeletal Maturation of the Hand' and was further revised by GREULICH and PYLE in their 'Radiographic atlas of skeletal development of the hand and wrist' (10). These atlases have been the most commonly used bases for assessing skeletal ages during the past 20 years. They are both based on children from professional class homes and do not represent an average standard for the development even of American children. The development of most children is somewhat retarded in relation to these standards, more so in the case of the Greulich and Pyle ones than Todd's, which are a little less advanced. Certainly average Dutch children (20) and English children (3) are less mature for a given chronological age than the children on which the American standards are based. On the other hand the secular trend towards earlier maturation brings European children closer to the published American standards. Standards should be revised approximately every ten years, so that the effect of the secular trend may be taken into account. In using an atlas the procedure is to compare the x-ray to be assessed with each of the standards. Having found the standard which superficially most resembles the unknown, the two are then compared in detail, proceeding in an orderly fashion from bone to bone. If the unknown is found to match the standard exactly, it is given the same skeletal age as the standard. If the unknown is found to be either retarded or advanced in relation to its nearest standard it is given a suitable intermediate age. Agreement between trained observers, using the atlas method is relatively good, but systematic errors of the order of 3 or even 6 months do occur between one observer and another. The consistency of even a single observer when continually in practice is only such that two thirds of a duplicate assessment fall with plus or minus 3 months of the previous reading, 95 % with ± 6 months (13). There is also slight individual variation in the relative maturities of different bones, so that some bones of the wrist may show different skeletal ages in relation to the standards and the question of what weight should be given to each bone for the overall assessment in atlases has not been settled.

This difficulty is largely overcome by the third method of assessment in which each bone is assigned a rating on a scale of development by matching its appearance with a series of standards. The ratings for each bone are then added up to produce a maturity score which can be compared with the score normally expected for the sex and chronological age of the child in question. This method depends on the fact that for each bone there is an invariable order in the successive steps whereby the joint surface is shaped. No known factor alters this succession. If growth of the cartilage plates is disturbed the modelling of the joint is delayed but when conditions return to normal, development continues as before. Any abnormal growth which occurs during the period of interruption is incorporated as a permanent feature of the bone, as in rickets. The basic problem in making standards for a rating system is to recognise those steps of development which are of universal occurrence and to distinguish them from individual idiosyncrasies of shape and moulding. A further advantage of the progressive rating method over the atlas method is that the same stages occur in the same order in both sexes, although the rate at which they are passed may differ. Thus a single series of standards can be used for both boys and girls, the allowance for the girls' advancement being made in the next step of the procedure, which is to compare the maturity indicator score with the score for the standard group.

Drawings of the individual stages distinguishable in the development of each hand and wrist bone, were first published in the 1950 edition of GREULICH and PYLE's atlas, revised drawings in the 1959 edition of the atlas are very similar to another series of drawings produced independently by TANNER and WHITEHOUSE (21). ACHESON (1), ACHESON, KEMP and PARFITT (4) suggested that skeletal maturity should be assessed by assigning scores for each illustrated stage for each bone and adding together the scores achieved by each bone with or without differential weighting (2) thus reaching a total maturity score for the whole wrist for comparison with the mean score for the standard series.

The new Tanner, Whitehouse and Healy standards (22) also adopt this approach. In these standards eight stages are described for each bone, except the radius which has nine, and verbal descriptions of the criteria for assigning a particular stage are given. These descriptions are so clear and precise that it is relatively seldom that disagreement occurs between observers as to whether a stage has been reached or not. If a bone happens to be midway between two of the stages, then it does not fulfill the criteria of the later one and should be assigned to the earlier. Two observers should virtually never assign ratings differing by more than one stage to any bone on any film. Differences between total score for the whole film as obtained by different observers are therefore usually very small indeed. Tanner, Whitehouse and Healy have assessed the weighting which should be given to each bone in estimating the total score and have given scores to each stage of development in each bone in accordance with this weighting. When using their system it is customary to express the final result as a simple maturity score instead of a skeletal age. The distribution of scores at each chronological age has been published in the form of percentile charts from which bone ages can be obtained if required. The bone age of a particular child being that at which his bone score lies on the 50th percentile. These percentile charts are based on a survey of 2.600 British children and the distribution of scores at various ages in other populations must be determined, but the basic standards and scoring system are equally applicable to all communities. In view of its high accuracy and universal validity, it must be expected that this and similar methods will replace the atlas methods for most research and clinical purposes.

REFERENCES

1. Acheson, R. M., A method of assessing maturity from radiographs: A report from the Oxford Child Health Survey, *J. Anat.* (Lond.) 88: 498—508, 1954.
2. Acheson, R. M., The Oxford method of assessing skeletal maturity, *Clin. Orthop.* 10: 19—39, 1957.
3. Acheson, R. M. and D. Hewitt, Oxford Child Health Survey: Stature and skeletal maturity in the pre-school child, *Brit. J. prev. Soc. Med.* 8: 59—65, 1954.

4. Acheson, R. M., F. H. Kemp and J. Parfit, Height, weight and skelleta maturity in the first five years of life, *Lancet* 1: 691—2, 1955.
5. Bayley, N. V., Skeletal maturing in adolescence as a basis for determining percentage of completed growth, *Child Develpm.* 14: 1—46, 1943.
6. Buehl, C. C. and S. I. Pyle, The use of age at first appearance of three ossification centres in determining the skeletal status of children, *J. Pediat.* 21: 335—42, 1942.
7. Elgenmark, O., The normal development of the ossific centres during infancy and childhood. A clinical, roentgenologic and statistical study, *Acta Paediat.* (Uppsala) 33: suppl. 1, 79 pp., 1946.
8. Francis, C. C., The appearance of centres of ossification from 6—15 years, *Amer. J. phys. Anthrop.* 27: 127—138, 1940.
9. Francis, C. C. and P. P. Werle, The appearance of centres of ossification from birth to five years, *Amer. J. phys. Anthrop.* 24: 273—99, 1939.
10. Greulich, W. W. and S. I. Pyle, *Radiographic atlas of skeletal development of the hand and wrist,* Stanford, California, Stanford University Press, 190 pp., 1950.
11. Harding, V. S. V., A method for evaluating osseous development from birth to fourteen years, *Child Develpm.* 23: 247—71, 1952.
12. Lurie, L. A., S. Levy and M. L. Lurie, Determination of bone age in children. A method based on a study of 1129 white children, *J. Pediat.* 23: 131—40, 1943.
13. Mainland, D., Evaluating of the skeletal age method of estimating children's development. I. Systematic errors in the assessment of roentgenograms, *Pediatrics* 13: 165—73, 1953.
14. Milman, D. H. and H. Bakwin, Ossification of the metacarpal-metatarsal centres as a measure of maturation, *J. Pediat.* 36: 617—20, 1950.
15. Pryor, J. W., *Development of the bone of the hand as shown by the x-ray method,* Bull. State Coll. Kentucky, series 2, no. 5, 1905.
16. Pryor, J. W., Differences in the time of development of the centres of ossification in the male and female skeleton, *Anat. Rec.* 25: 257—73, 1923.
17. Pryor, J. W., Time of ossification of the bones of the hand of the male and female, and union of the epiphyses with the diaphyses, *Amer. J. phys. Anthrop.* 8: 401—10, 1925.
18. Pyle, S. I. and N. L. Hoerr, *Radiographic atlas of skeletal development of the knee,* Thomas, Springfield, Ill., 82 pp. 1955.
19. Pyle, S. I. and L. W. Sontag, Variability in onset of ossification in epiphyses and short bones of the extremities, *Amer. J. Roentgenol.* 49: 795—8, 1943.
20. Speijer, B., Betekenis en bepaling van de skeletleeftijd. With a summary and atlas in English, Leiden, Sijthoff, 153 pp., 1950.
21. Tanner, J. M. and R. H. Whitehouse, *Standards for skeletal age,* Centre International de l'Enfance (Paris), 1959.
22. Tanner, J. M., R. H. Whitehouse and M. J. R. Healy, *A new system for estimating skeletal maturity from the hand and wrist, with standards derived from a study of* 2,600 *healthy British children. Part II. The scoring system,* Centre International de l'Enfance (Paris), 1962.
23. Todd, J. W., *Atlas of Skeletal Maturation* (Part I: Hand), London, Kimpton, 1937.

FACTORS THAT CONTROL OR INFLUENCE SKELETAL MATURATION

J. J. VAN DER WERFF TEN BOSCH

If the bone age or the degree of skeletal maturity is to be used in clinical studies, it is essential to know by which factors skeletal maturation is controlled or may be affected. Three main categories are: sex chromosomes, hormones and a vaguely delimited group of nonspecific factors.

There is a marked difference in skeletal maturity at all ages between boys and girls, girls being constantly ahead of boys by almost all criteria which have been studied (see e.g. table 1 in 6). It is possible that sex hormones secreted before birth and during infancy influence skeletal maturation, and that the girl's secretions are more effective than those of the boy. However, girls with gonadal dysgenesis, who often possess only barely detectable amounts of gonad tissue, usually of an undifferentiated nature, follow the same pattern of skeletal maturation as normal girls until the approach of puberty (17, 4). When such girls are sex chromatin-negative, they possess only one, the X-, sex-chromosome. They differ from boys in that the latter have a Y-chromosome besides a single X-chromosome, so that it seems that the Y-chromosome has an inhibiting influence on skeletal maturation (14). It is of interest that extraneous factors such as malnutrition cause a greater degree of retardation in the skeletal maturation of boys than of girls (3). It seems possible that the Y-chromosome renders the skeleton more vulnerable to disturbing factors. There is no indication as to whether the Y-chromosome operates locally, in the centres of bone formation, or through other regulating factors. The sex difference just described exists before puberty. From the age of about 10 years the rate of skeletal maturation is largely determined by the sex steroids. A distinct divergence can be observed between skeletal maturation in normal girls, who enter puberty, and girls with gonadal dysgenesis, who for the lack of normal ovaries fail to become sexually mature (fig. 1).

The hormones that are clearly involved in the control of skeletal maturation are thyroid and sex hormones. For both of these classes of hormones it has been amply shown that they accelerate skeletal maturation when present in excess, and that deficiency causes retardation in skeletal maturation. No clearcut evidence is available for a role, permissive or otherwise, of any other hormone. There are some arguments in favour of the view that *pituitary growth hormone* does not stimulate skeletal maturation. (1) Children with excessive amounts of endogenous growth hormone (from an eosinophilic pituitary tumour)

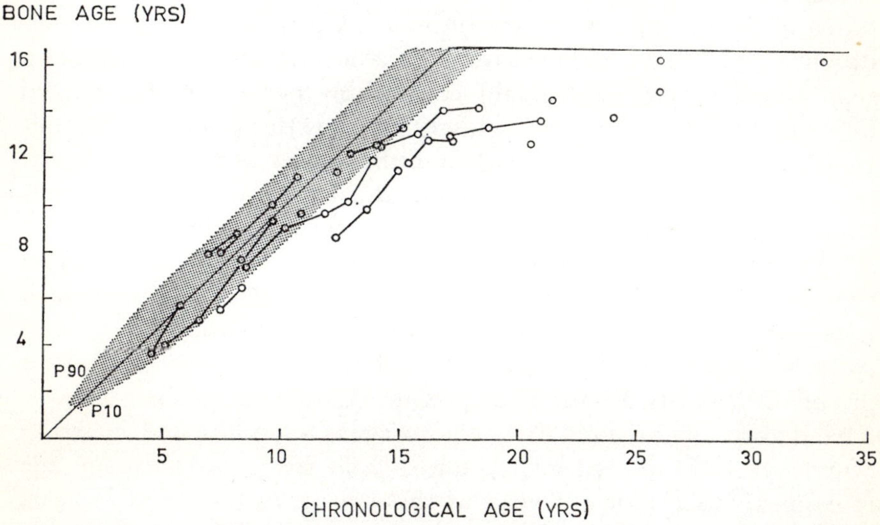

Fig. 1. Skeletal maturation of 20 cases of gonadal dysgenesis. Lines connect multiple observations on a single individual (from 4)

may grow to an enormous height (230—240 cm in classical instances of giantism). While it may be argued that in such cases the growth period is unduly prolonged by hypogonadism, in consequence of destruction of pituitary gonadotrophic cells, the fact remains that there is an enormous discrepancy between the stimulating effect of growth hormone on linear growth and the possible influence of growth hormone on the *final stages* of skeletal maturation. The case of a girl who developed signs of an eosinophilic pituitary tumour at the age of 5 years indicates that growth hormone is also ineffective in promoting skeletal maturation during the *first decade* of life. At $8^1/_2$ years the girl had a bone age of $8^1/_2$ years and the great height of 152.5 cm (11). (2) Children with pituitary insufficiency and stunted growth who are treated with growth hormone preparations from human pituitary glands have not shown an increase in skeletal maturity above that which could have been caused by the simultaneously administered thyroid or sex hormone. (3) The skeleton of hypophysectomized children can be brought to full maturity by the administration of sex hormones, presumably in the complete absence of growth hormone. These facts permit the inference that dwarfism which is associated with retarded skeletal maturation cannot be attributed to the sole lack of growth hormone. On the other hand, a condition characterized by dwarfism with normal skeletal maturation (e.g. gonadal dysgenesis) might conceivably be due to the isolated deficiency of, or skeletal insensitivity to, growth hormone (15); this view has recently gained support from the finding of high blood levels of apparently normal growth hormone in cases of gonadal dysgenesis, which suggests that the skeleton is relatively insensitive (1).

The role of *thyroid hormones* can be deduced from the common experience that skeletal maturation is retarded in children with hypothyroidism. The most severe degrees of retardation are seen in cases of congenital athyroidism. Plate 1 shows the photograph of a girl of $12^{10}/_{12}$ years, height 63 cm, serum PBI 0.5 μg %. Plate 2 shows a hand x-ray of this child, with a bone age of 6 months, and an x-ray of a 13-year-old normal girl. Upon thyroid treatment the bone age rose quickly to a value of 8 years at $15^7/_{12}$ years. At the age of 20 years the child had breast development, a bone age of 15 years, and a height of 102 cm. While there is no doubt that thyroid hormone is necessary for maturation of the skeleton (by the current arbitrary standards!) up to a bone age of 10—12 years, its role during later stages of skeletal development is uncertain. During the second decade skeletal maturation is retarded in individuals who do not mature sexually, as in gonadal dysgenesis (fig. 1) or hypogonadotrophic hypogonadism, although they have normal thyroid gland activity in terms of serum PBI-levels and radioiodine studies. In patients with hypopituitarism (including gonadotrophin deficiency) and dwarfism, treatment with thyroid hormone without the addition of sex steroids does not result in complete skeletal maturation (16).

In the normal boy and girl the *sex steroids* secreted during puberty

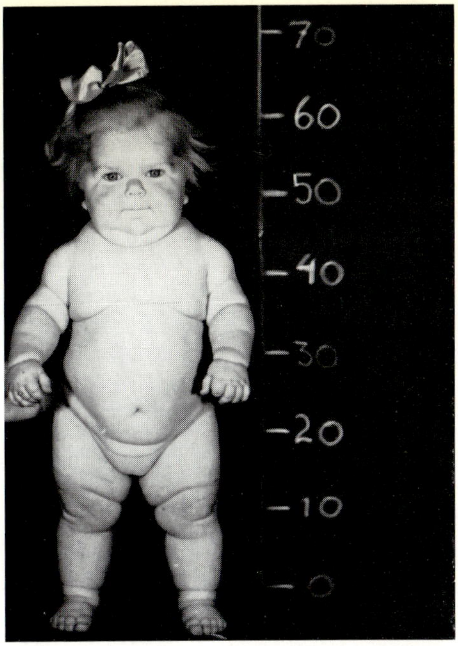

Plate 1. Girl of $12^{10}/_{12}$ years, with untreated congenital hypothyroidism

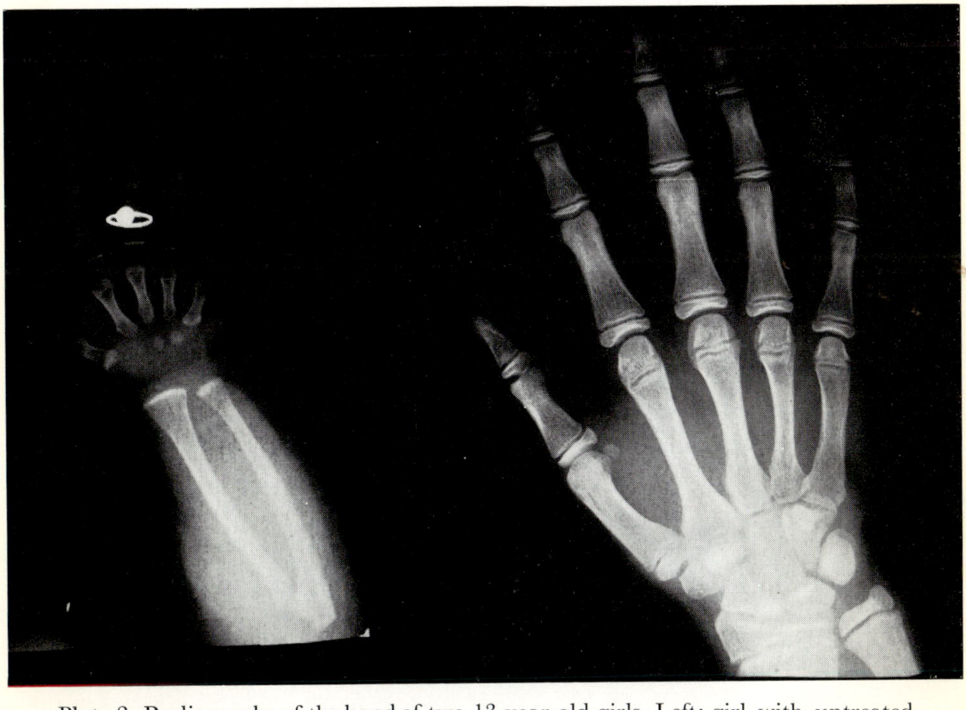

Plate 2. Radiographs of the hand of two 13-year-old girls. Left: girl with untreated congenital hypothyroidism (see Plate 1); right: normal girl

induce the completion of skeletal maturation. Skeletal sensitivity to sex steroids is not confined, however, to the pubertal age period. It is clear from numerous records of children with true sexual precocity (e.g. 10) or precocious pseudopuberty (due to gonadal, adrenal or administered sex steroids) that sex steroids can accelerate skeletal maturation at any time during infancy, that is, well before pubertal changes would normally set in. It is not certain whether the presence of thyroid hormone is necessary for the skeletal action of sex steroids during infancy, when these steroids are possibly not involved in the physiological maturation processes of the skeleton. There is some doubt as to the role of sex steroids before puberty. Several authors have shown that skeletal maturity during infancy is more advanced in normal children who later come in puberty relatively early than in children in whom puberty sets in later (13, 12, 7). The time of onset of puberty is related more to skeletal age than to chronological age, and, conversely, skeletal age is related more to the stage of sexual maturity than to chronological age (page 78, fig. 2). The nature of the possible causal relationship between age of onset of puberty and skeletal maturation prior to the onset of puberty is not known. There is no doubt, however, that the skeletal changes in linear growth rate and in rate of skeletal maturation which take place during puberty are caused by the gonadal sex steroids. It is possible to induce alterations similar to these physiological changes by the administration of sex steroids to children who do not come in puberty spontaneously (fig. 2, B) and in a like fashion such changes are brought about at an excessively early age in children with true sexual precocity (fig. 2, A).

In almost all types of dwarfism there is delayed skeletal maturation. Such a delay seems unrelated to thyroid gland activity. An example appears in fig. 3, which shows the curves for height and skeletal maturation of a girl with coeliac disease. At the age of $10^{8}/_{12}$ years the child had a bone age of 5 years, while thyroid function assessed by radioiodine studies and serum PBI level was normal. During a regimen which was free of wheat gluten there occurred a marked acceleration in both the growth in height and in skeletal maturation. The retarding influence of undernutrition or malnutrition, and of acute childhood illnesses, on skeletal maturation has been demonstrated on many occasions (e.g. 5, 8, 3, 9). The pathogenesis of the reduction in skeletal maturation rate is not known. An interpretation in terms of known

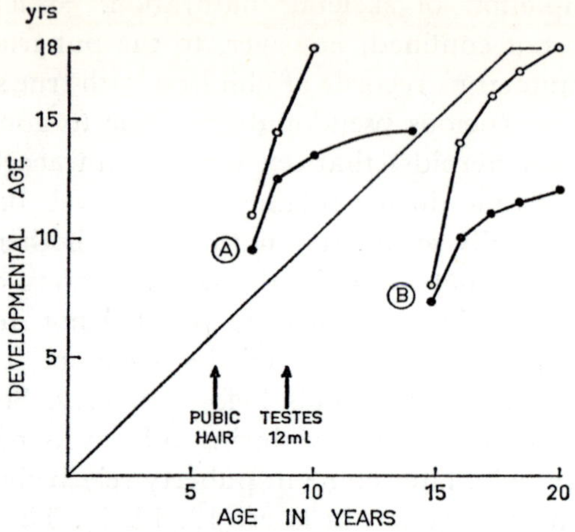

Fig. 2. Curves for height age (•) and bone age (o) of two boys during a steroid-induced growth spurt. A. Case of true sexual precocity. B. Case of hypopituitarism and dwarfism during androgen treatment

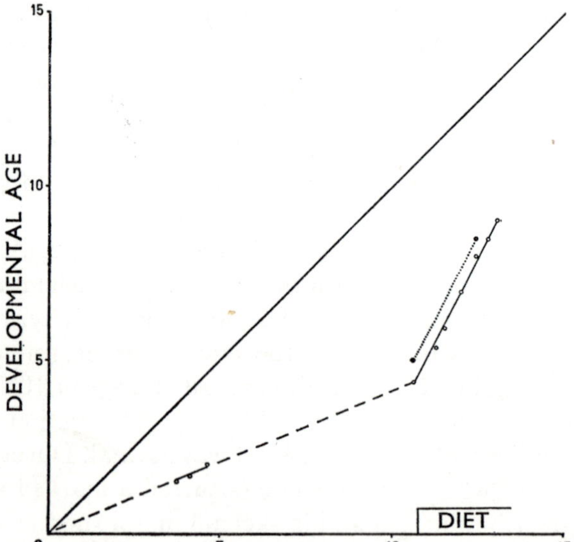

Fig. 3. Curves for height age (o——o) and bone age (• - - - •) of a girl with coeliac disease, before and during treatment with a gluten-free diet (patient of the Department of Paediatrics, Leiden University Hospital)

effects of hormones is difficult. Although it is tempting to compare the effects of malnutrition and non-specific diseases with the effects that can be obtained during cortisone administration (retardation of linear growth and skeletal maturation), it seems unlikely that the former conditions act through increased corticosteroid secretion. BLODGETT et al. (2) studied the effects of a range of doses of cortisone, and concluded that dosages sufficient to cause a reduction in growth rate to subnormal levels were apt to produce facial changes and obesity of the type seen in patients with Cushing's syndrome.

REFERENCES

1. ALMQVIST, S., K. HALL, S. LINDSTEDT, J. LINDSTEN, R. LUFT and H. E. SJÖBERG, Effects of short term administration of physiological doses of human growth hormone in three patients with Turner's syndrome, *Acta endocr.* 46: 451, 1964.
2. BLODGETT, F. M., L. BURGIN, D. IEZZONI, D. GRIBETZ and N. B. TALBOT, Effects of prolonged cortisone therapy on the statural growth, skeletal maturation and metabolic status of children, *New Engl. J. Med.* 254: 636, 1956.
3. DREIZEN, S., R. M. SNODGRASSE, H. WEBB-PEPLOE, T. D. SPIES, The retarding effect of protracted undernutrition on the appearance of the postnatal ossification centers in the hand and wrist, *Hum. Biol.* 30; 253, 1958.
4. ENTHOVEN, R. and J. J. VAN DER WERFF TEN BOSCH, Lengte, skelet en gonadotrofinen by chromatine-negatieve gonadale dysgenesie, *Maandschrift voor Kindergeneesk.* 32: 466, 1964.
5. GREULICH, W. W., The growth and developmental status of Guamanian school children in 1947, *Amer. J. Phys. Anthropol.* (*N.S.*) 9: 55, 1951.
6. GREULICH, W. W. and S. I. PYLE, *Radiographic atlas of skeletal development of the hand and wrist*, 2nd ed., Oxford University Press, London, 1959.
7. HEWITT, D. and R. M. ACHESON, Some aspects of skeletal development through adolescence. I. Variations in the rate and pattern of skeletal maturation at puberty, *Amer. J. Phys. Anthropol.* (*N.S.*) 19: 321, 1961.
8. HEWITT, D., C. K. WESTROPP and R. M. ACHESON, Oxford child health survey. Effect of childish ailments on skeletal development, *Brit. J. Prevent. Social Med.* 9: 179, 1955.
9. JONES, P. R. M. and R. F. A. DEAN, The effects of kwashiorkor on the development of the bones of the knee, *J. Pediat.* 54: 176, 1959.
10. LENZ, J., Vorzeitige Menstruation, Geschlechtsreife und Entwicklung, *Arch. Gynaekol.* 99: 67, 1913.
11. MCLAREN TODD, R., Acromegaly in a girl of 8 years, *Arch. Disease Childhood*, 33: 49, 1958.
12. NICOLSON, A. B. and C. HANLEY, Indices of physiological maturity: derivation and interrelationships, *Child Developm.* 24: 1, 1953.
13. SIMMONS, K. and W. W. GREULICH, Menarcheal age and the height, weight and skeletal age of girls age 7—17 years. *J. Pediat.* 22: 518, 1943.

14. TANNER, J. M., A. PRADER, H. HABICH and M. A. FERGUSON-SMITH, Genes on the Y chromosome influencing rate of maturation in man. Skeletal age studies in children with Klinefelter's (XXY) and Turner's (XO) syndromes, *Lancet* II: 141, 1959.
15. WERFF TEN BOSCH, J. J. VAN DER, The syndrome of brachymetacarpal dwarfism ('pseudo-pseudohypoparathyroidism') with and without gonadal dysgenesis, *Lancet* I: 69, 1959.
16. WERFF TEN BOSCH, J. J. VAN DER, Hypofysaire dwerggroei, *Ned. T. Geneesk.* 106: 1282, 1962.
17. WERFF TEN BOSCH, J. J. VAN DER and J. C. CHOUFOER, The growth pattern in gonadal dysgenesis, *Acta endocr.* Suppl. 38: 66, 1958.

DISCUSSION

Van Gemund: Dr. MARSHALL, the concept of dental age comprises not only the eruption number, but also the calcification rates of crown-formation and root-formation. Next year an atlas will be published with standard radiographs of tooth development.

Marshall: I agree there are extremely accurate measures of dental ageing, some are available, some more are coming, but they still are limited in their application. I did not mean in any way to decry the accuracy of dental ageing within its scope and I know it is very important and useful from the dental point of view. But as an index of general physiological maturity, I think, it still has severe limitations.

Sobel: Could Dr. VAN DER WERFF TEN BOSCH comment on two problems which cause me some difficulty in accepting such a sharp separation of the influences of hormones on skeletal maturation at different stages of its development. Recently it has been shown that there is an increased incidence of thyroiditis, with various degrees of hypothyroidism, in girls with gonadal dysgenesis (WILLIAMS, E. D., E. ENGEL, A. P. FORBES, *New Engl. J. Med.* 270: 805, 1964). These observations have made me wonder whether it is possible that in some such patients the delayed skeletal maturation could be partly due to hypothyroidism. With regard to the role of thyroid hormone in skeletal maturation after the beginning of puberty, I wonder about a hypothyroid girl whom I saw many years ago in the Department of Medicine of the Massachusetts General Hospital. She was about 18 years of age, pregnant and had retarded skeletal maturation.

Van der Werff ten Bosch: There are several answers to your first question. It is difficult to decide when thyroid function is normal, but if we look at the protein bound iodine levels in the blood of cases of gonadal dysgenesis, these are nearly always well within the normal limits. There is another example, however, and that is the syndrome of hypogonadotrophic hypogonadism in males, who do not mature sexually, have small testes, the normal complement of sex chromosomes and absence of gonadotrophins from the urine. Such men may have a greatly retarded bone age, which remains at 13—15 years in the 2nd and 3rd decade. These men also have normal thyroid function, again in terms of P.B.I. and radioiodine studies.

Your second question concerns bone age when puberty occurs in untreated hypothyroidism. I think what probably happens, is that in hypothyroidism there is such a delay that when puberty sets in, it takes some time before skeletal maturation has caught up.

Sobel: Of course I would not question the very important effect of sex steroids on skeletal maturation. The patient had been hypothyroid for some time; at the age of 17 she was only 142 centimeters tall (height-age $10^6/_{12}$). She failed to take the prescribed treatment and at age $18^9/_{12}$, when she was 3 months pregnant, her bone-age was approximately 14 years. An entirely normal baby was delivered by Caesarean section 6 months after treatment was begun. She must have produced a lot of sex steroids during the pregnancy, and yet had retarded skeletal maturation. Perhaps the gonadal steroids were not able to influence skeletal maturation in the presence of co-existing hypothyroidism.

Evaluation of the effect of adrenal cortical androgens on the skeletal maturation of normal children is difficult. In adolescent boys with adrenal insufficiency one would expect the testicular androgens to be as successful in maintaining normal skeletal maturation as they are in maintaining normal rate of growth and of masculinization. As you pointed out, boys with eunuchoidism show a delay in skeletal maturation after the age at which adolescence should have begun. Talbot et al (p. 432 in: *Functional endocrinology from birth through adolescence*, Harvard University Press, Cambridge, Mass., 1952) mention a boy with testicular atrophy whose bone-age was 12 years when he was $12^6/_{12}$ years old. No therapy was given at that time, and at the age of 15 years the skeletal maturity was only $13^6/_{12}$.

Couldn't one interpret these relationships as indicating that adrenal androgens normally play very little role in the rate of skeletal maturation, just as they are not able to induce masculinization in a boy with eunuchoidism?

Unfortunately I do not seem to have useful information about skeletal maturation in a girl with adrenal insufficiency, but normal ovarian function. The only such patient in my own experience had been given excessive amounts of cortisone, although she had not received DOC.

Laron: I wonder if Dr. VAN DER WERFF TEN BOSCH, or any other member could answer the following question.

We know that there are children with hypothyroidism with precocious puberty; what is the bone-age in these patients, compared to the hypothyroid patients who do not show precocious puberty. One remark also concerning the role of growth hormone in bone maturation. I am not so sure that we can state in a definite manner that growth hormone has no influence whatsoever on skeletal maturation.

Van der Werff ten Bosch: As in any developmental process, the bone age of such patients depends on the time at which you study the phenomenon.

The bone age in a child with precocious puberty and hypothyroidism is retarded at first and may catch up later (see: WIJK, J. J. VAN, M. M. GRUMBACH, *J. Pediat.* 57: 416, 1960; VAN GELDEREN, H. H., *Arch. Dis. Childh.* 37: 337, 1962; FRANKS, R. C. and R. S. STEMPFEL, *J. Clin. Endocr.* 23: 802, 1963). Menarche may occur in such cases at a time when bone age is well below 10 years.

Prader: I should like to comment on bone age and skeletal maturity. Dr. MARSHALL has not mentioned one very important aspect for the clinician and that is to predict adult height, with the aid of bone age and actual height, and this can be done so far with the Greulich and Pyle method but not yet with the Tanner, Whitehouse and Healy method. I am sure all clinicians look forward with anticipation to such a paper from your group. Till then, we do not really know which is the best method to evaluate bone age with. From the point of view of the clinician, the best system to assess bone age will be the one which gives the most exact prediction of adult height.

Not until this has been studied shall we know how much weight we should give to the different bone centres. Some bone centres may give much more information about the final height than others, and it may be that in the future we can greatly simplify the assessment of bone age. The system of TANNER and his collaborators is still rather complicated, it needs some training, you can't just take the tables and do it.

CHAPTER III

HISTOLOGY OF GROWING BONE

EPIPHYSEAL GROWTH IN THE RAT

J. VAN DER SLUYS VEER D. SMEENK J. C. BIRKENHÄGER
R. O. VAN DER HEUL

HISTOLOGY OF THE EPIPHYSEAL 'GROWTH APPARATUS'

Linear growth is the result of an increase in the number and the size of the epiphyseal cartilage cells in conjunction with endochondral formation of bone. Skeletal maturation may be defined as the appearance of centres of ossification and their subsequent fusion. Normally the ossification centre within the epiphysis develops sufficiently to establish an epiphyseal disc.

Plate 1 shows the proximal epiphyseal and metaphyseal region that constitutes the 'growth apparatus' of the normal rat tibia. Detailed descriptions of the histological pictures may be found in textbooks of histology. The cartilage cells in the epiphyseal disc are arranged in longitudinal rows. In these columns the cartilage cells proliferate, hypertrophy and degenerate (burst). Cell divisions occur at the epiphyseal side of the disc. KEMBER (9) showed with the aid of tritiated thymidine that in cartilage columns of about 25 cells, mitosis mainly occurs in cells at positions from 12 to 22 (1 being the first intact hypertrophic cartilage cell at the metaphyseal side). In the top of the columns (cells 23—25) mitosis takes place at a much lower rate, and these cells constitute the 'reserve layer'. Replacement of the cartilage cells by bone occurs at the diaphyseal side of the cartilage disc. The proliferating cartilage cells are displaced by the tissue advancing from the bone marrow. In this way the epiphysis grows 'away' from the fixed bony diaphysis. As the net result of this process the cartilage disc remains at an approximately constant thickness. The metaphysis that unites the epiphyseal cartilage plate and the diaphysis consists of columns of spongious calcified tissue of which the primary spongiosa is a continuation of the rows of cartilage cells that have burst and of which the plasma has been replaced by vascular connective tissue between cores of calcified intercolumnar substance.

Little or no bone is deposited on the calcified intercolumnar substance of the primary spongiosa, contrary to the secondary spongiosa, where deposition of new bone on the cores of calcified cartilage matrix is prominent. Most of the calcified cartilage matrix disappears during this reconstruction. With the exception of a small lateral part which is involved in the remodelling of the shaft, most of the trabeculae of the secondary spongiosa are resorbed as linear growth continues.

Factors which control normal growth are *age*, and *endocrine* and *dietary factors.*

Age

Variations in the rate of linear growth are associated with characteristic features in the histological picture of epiphyseal disc and metaphysis. The young and rapidly growing animal shows all the histological features of active growth of which the presence of a wide epiphyseal cartilage disc is the most obvious (plate 1). The cartilage disc decreases in width when the growth rate slows down. The reduction in width of the disc is the result of a reduction both in cell size and in number of cell layers in the proliferating and hypertrophying zones. The trabeculae of the primary spongiosa, delicate, numerous and close together in the young animal, decrease in number and become coarser and more irregular in shape (plate 2). With advanced age the cartilage plate becomes 'sealed off' almost completely from the marrow by calcification of the marginal cartilage matrix and cellular capsules, on which lamellar bone is laid down.

The proximal tibial epiphyseal cartilage plate persists in the rat until old age but other epiphyseal discs continue to be eroded from the diaphyseal aspect of the plate.

The cartilage finally disappears completely, initially with bone and subsequently with marrow between the medullary cavities of diaphysis and epiphysis. Epiphyseal fusion is then complete and further linear growth impossible.

Pituitary and thyroid gland

Both hypophysectomy (2, 10, 16) and thyroidectomy (14) of growing rats cause retardation of skeletal maturation and linear growth. The nature of the histological changes in the growth apparatus

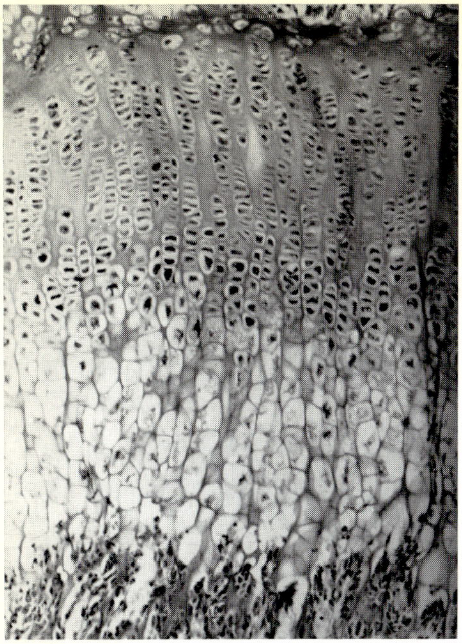

Plate 1. 'Growth apparatus' of proximal tibial epiphysis of a rat twenty five days of age (140 x)
a. epiphysis; b. uncalcified epiphyseal cartilage; c. metaphyseal primary spongiosa

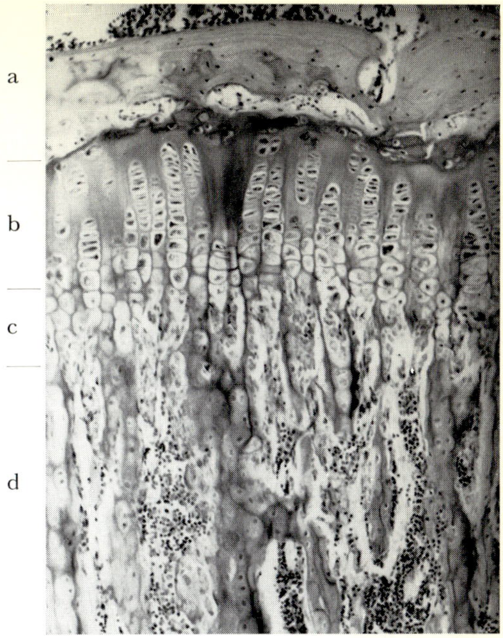

Plate 2. Proximal tibial epiphyseal plate of a rat 90 days old (140 x)
a. epiphysis; b. uncalcified epiphyseal cartilage; c. metaphyseal primary spongiosa; d. metaphyseal sec. spongiosa

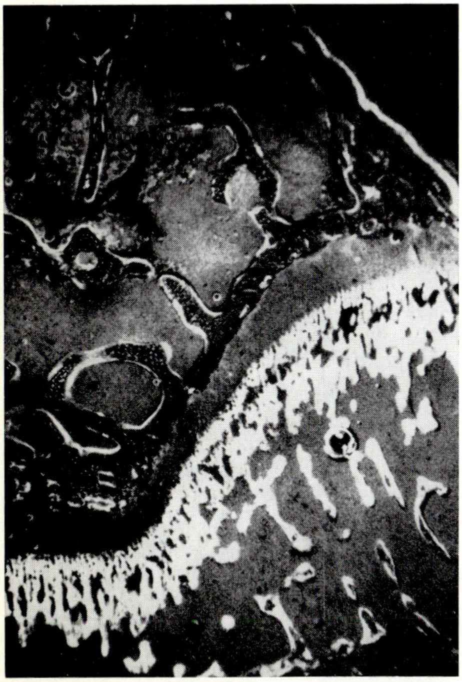

Plate 3A. Tetracycline labelling of the proximal tibial epiphysis of a rat, killed twenty four hours after administration of a single dose (20 mg/kg). Undecalcified section (30 x)

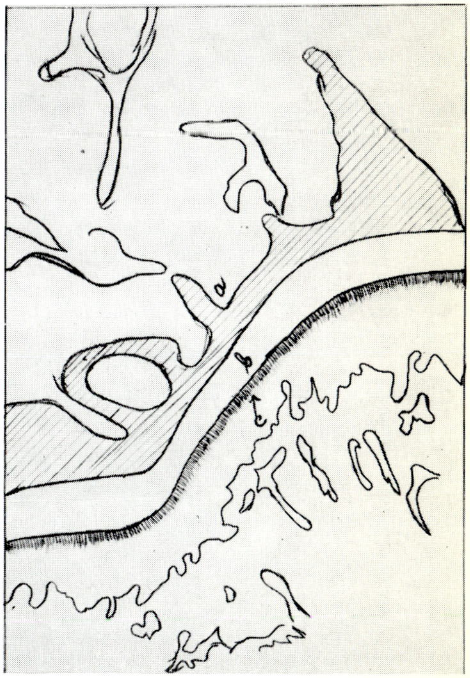

Plate 3B. Schematic presentation of plate 3A
a. epiphyseal spongiosa; b. uncalcified epiphyseal cartilage; c. proximal limit of tetracycline label

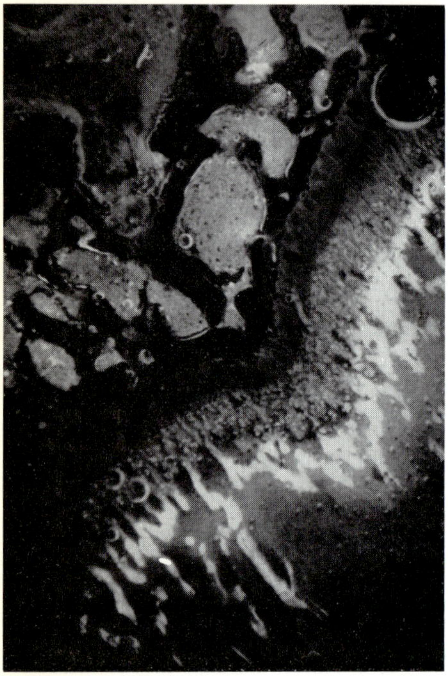

Plate 4A. Tetracycline labelling of the proximal tibial epiphysis of a rat, killed four days after the administration of tetracycline (single dose, 20 mg/kg). Undecalcified section 30 x

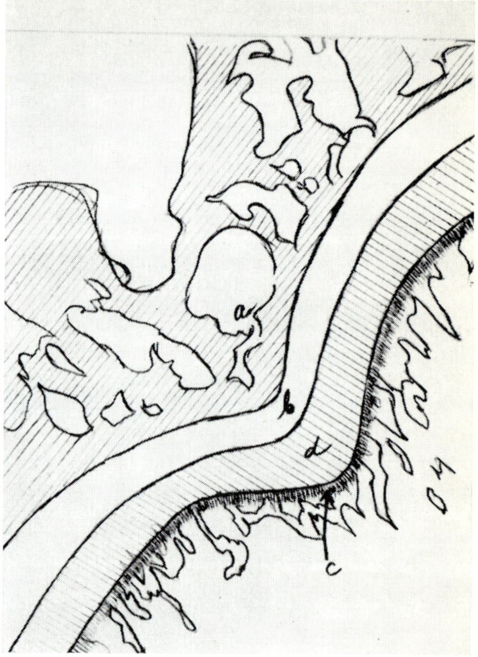

Plate 4B. Schematic presentation of plate 4A
a. epiphyseal spongiosa; b. uncalcified epiphyseal cartilage; c. proximal limit of tetracycline label; d. 'calcified zone', not labelled shift of the tetracycline label (c) in diaphyseal direction

depends upon the age at which operations are carried out. When animals are operated at an early age, the histological changes following hypophysectomy and those following thyroidectomy are indistinguishable (14).

After hypophysectomy at the age of six days (16), ossification centres do not develop properly and fusion of epiphysis and diaphysis is retarded. The epiphysis retains relatively large amounts of cartilage, so that the cartilage discs appear to be very wide. However, the cartilage cells are not arranged in rows, as they are in normal growing bones.

Hypophysectomy at the age of 26 days (2), when ossification centres and epiphyseal cartilage discs are already present, causes retrogressive changes in the epiphyseal-metaphyseal region. The cartilage plate becomes narrower in consequence of a decrease in the number and, more particularly, the size of the cells. The latter changes may be seen as early as four days after operation. In the metaphyseal cartilage the trabeculae become rare, bone formation stops, and the marginal cartilage calcifies, thus 'sealing off' the cartilage from the marrow.

The effects of thyroidectomy can be prevented or, partially, reversed by administration of thyroid hormone alone (1, 3). In hypophysectomized rats administered thyroid hormone can restore skeletal maturation. To reinstate normal growth in the absence of the pituitary gland, growth hormone is necessary; even after long post-operative intervals linear growth may be restored to a rate equal to or exceeding the normal. Growth hormone alone does not promote skeletal maturation of hypophysectomized rats, but may rapidly repair degenerative changes in the epiphysis and metaphysis of rats hypophysectomized at 20—30 days of age. The Li-Evans-Greenspan test for the bioassay of growth hormone is based on the fact that growth hormone causes an increase in the width of the cartilage plate of the proximal tibial epiphysis of hypophysectomized rats, that is proportional to the dose of hormone given (8). The effects of growth hormone may be augmented by simultaneous administration of thyroid hormone (1, 3). In order to normalize skeletal maturation and growth of rats thyroidectomized at birth and hypophysectomized three weeks later, the combined administration of growth hormone and thyroid hormone is essential (14).

Histological changes and growth rate

The histological appearance of the growth apparatus gives a static view of the dynamic process of growth. Under normal conditions a high rate of growth is associated with a thick epiphyseal plate, while the plate is thin when growth is slow. This rule does not always apply in abnormal conditions. In hypothyroidism the epiphyseal plates are thick although there is little or no growth.

Methods other than the measurement of epiphyseal plate thickness have to be used for evaluation of the growth rate. Such methods require that significant alterations occur in the measured dimension within the period of time available for the investigation. In the next part of this paper a method will be described, by which the rate of calcification of the cartilage is estimated following administration of tetracycline. This drug induces fluorescence of calcifying tissues. Results obtained with this technique may give important information on the growth rate.

MEASUREMENT OF EPIPHYSEAL GROWTH

It was first shown by MILCH et al. (12) that tetracycline becomes fixed in calcified tissue during mineralisation.

The fluorescent properties of this antibiotic enable its localization in non-decalcified bone sections. Tetracycline label not only surfaces of new bone growth but all sites of calcification, including calcifying cartilage matrix. This occurs in the zone of provisional calcification, two or three cells up in the columns of hypertrophying cartilage cells (plate 3A and 3B). Calcifying tissue is labelled only during the presence of a sufficiently high tetracycline level in the blood. The period between injection and completion of labelling is called labelling time.

As linear growth continues, an apparent shift of the label occurs towards the diaphysis until it disappears during resorption of the spongious bone of the metaphysis. The non-labelled zone of cartilage that became calcified later (here arbitrarily named 'calcified zone') can be recognised in the fluorescence micrograph by its autofluorescence distinguishable from the bright tetracycline-labelled zone and the non-fluorescent uncalcified epiphyseal cartilage (plate 4A and 4B).

The 'calcified zone' is formed within a known period of time, its width can be measured, and it is thus possible to calculate a 'calcification rate'. Since calcification of the cartilage cells is an integrated part of the process of growth, its rate must be correlated with the rate of linear growth. The magnitude of the calcification rate is such that alterations are demonstrable in experiments of two days' duration. This technique may be helpful in growth studies, and has been used in an investigation on the influence of fasting and re-feeding upon growth. A detailed description of the method has been given elsewhere, and it has been shown that the growth rate is not affected by tetracycline in these studies (15). In these experiments, tetracycline hydrochloride, in a dose of 20 mg per kg body weight, was administered by single intraperitoneal injection. For every determination of average

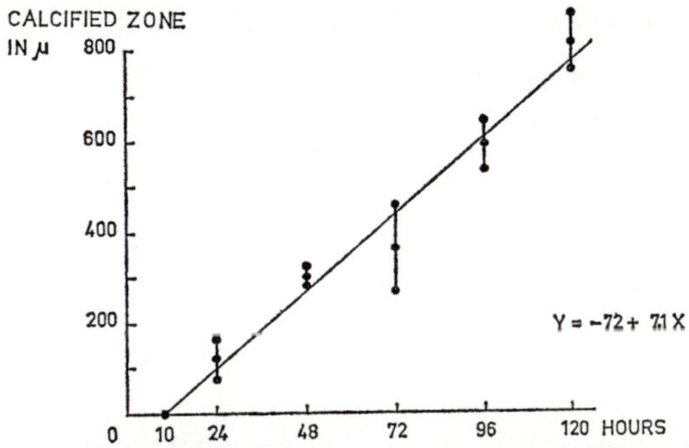

Fig. 1. Labelling time in 42-days-old female rats after a single dose of tetracycline (20 mg/kg). For explanation, see text

epiphyseal plate width and calcification rate a group of 5—6 rats was used. The animals were usually killed four days after the injection. The proximal part of each tibia was excised and divided in the parasagittal plane. The width of the decalcified proximal epiphyseal plate was measured using microscopic projection with incident U.V.-light illumination. Along each epiphyseal plate about twenty measurements were made, from which an average figure was calculated. Thereafter the halved tibiae were embedded in methacrylate and cut non-decalcified by a heavy sledge microtome (Jung) or a rotating bone saw. The sections were ground to a thickness of 25 micra. Using microscopic projection with transmitted U.V.-light, the width of the zone of calcified tissue between the decalcified cartilage and the tetracycline label was measured. The 'calcification rate' for each animal was calculated by dividing the average width of this 'calcified zone' in micra by the number of days elapsed after the injection of tetracycline. The result was corrected for a labelling time of 10 hours (vide infra) and recorded in micra per day.

The labelling time was calculated from measurements of the width of the 'calcified zone' of groups of rats sacrificed at intervals of 24 hours up to 5 days after a single injection of tetracycline (fig. 1). The regression line in the figure intercepts the abscissa at a point ten hours following the injection of tetracycline. It was therefore assumed that labelling stopped ten hours after injection.

EFFECTS OF FASTING AND RE-FEEDING

Fasting for four days resulted in remarkable changes in the histological picture of the epiphyseal plate and adjacent metaphyseal structures. The width of the epiphyseal cartilage plate decreased, the number of cartilage cell rows and that of the cells in the columns

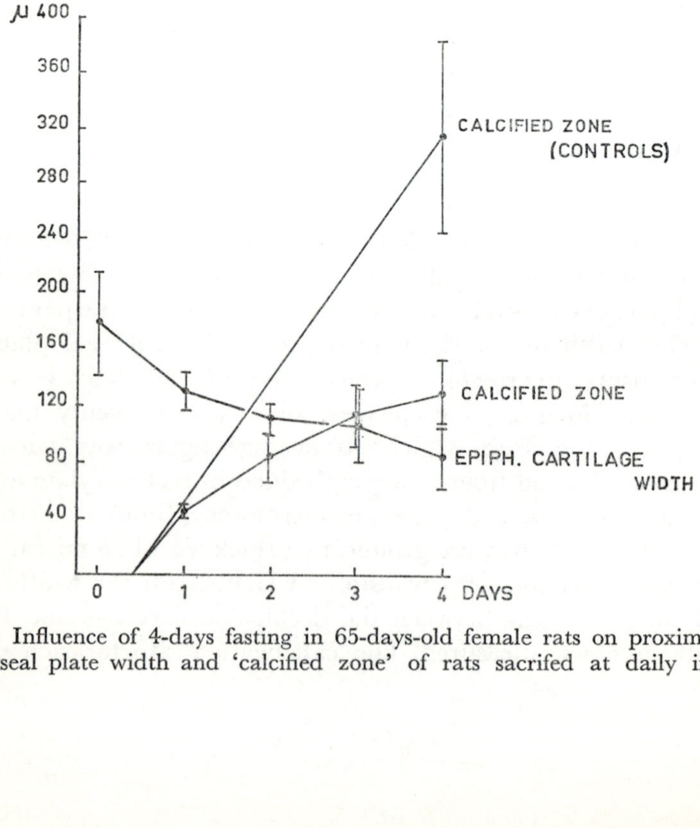

Fig. 2. Influence of 4-days fasting in 65-days-old female rats on proximal tibial epiphyseal plate width and 'calcified zone' of rats sacrifed at daily intervals.

diminished, and the trabeculae in the metaphysis became more irregular and reduced in number. These changes are identical to those which occur after hypophysectomy and during ageing. The influence of fasting on the width of the epiphyseal plate and of the 'calcified zone' measured after tetracycline labelling is demonstrated in figure 2. After one day of fasting the decalcified cartilage plate decreased in width considerably, but the width of the 'calcified zone' was the same as that of the controls. Rats killed at further intervals of one day showed further thinning of the epiphyseal plate. From the second day of fasting the 'calcified zone' lagged behind that of the control rats.

Table 1. *Tibial epiphyseal width and calcification rate of groups of 5—6 female rats with normal food intake compared with those obtained after fasting for four days.*

			Calcification rate			Epiphyseal cartilage width		
Exp. no	age in days	spayed	normal μ	fasting 4 days μ	reduction %	normal μ	fasting 4 days μ	reduction %
513	46	+	180	110	39	405	192	53
469	49	+	118	59	50	263	110	58
458	53	+	140	58	59	286	134	53
508	66	+	116	64	45	276	140	49
483	71	+	87	41	53	196	114	42
485	72	+	117	59	50	332	212	37
487	76	+	94	50	47	225	153	32
513	46	—	196	94	52	323	165	49
511	52	—	151	63	59	269	119	56
510	54	—	116	56	52	242	137	44
500	65	—	78	32	59	179	85	53
505	70	—	62	33	47	187	86	54

Data in table 1 show the influence of fasting for four days, on the epiphyseal plate width and the calcification rate of intact and spayed rats of various ages. There was an average thinning of the epiphyseal plate to 48 % and a reduction of the calcification rate to 51 % of the control values. The magnitude of the reduction in calcification rate caused by fasting was not correlated with the calcification rate of the controls or with the age of the animals. Methyl-testosterone (300 micrograms daily) and bovine growth hormone (500 micrograms daily) failed to prevent the narrowing of the epiphyseal cartilage plate and the reduction of the calcification rate, caused by 4-days' starvation in spayed female rats (figure 3). Spaying in these experiments

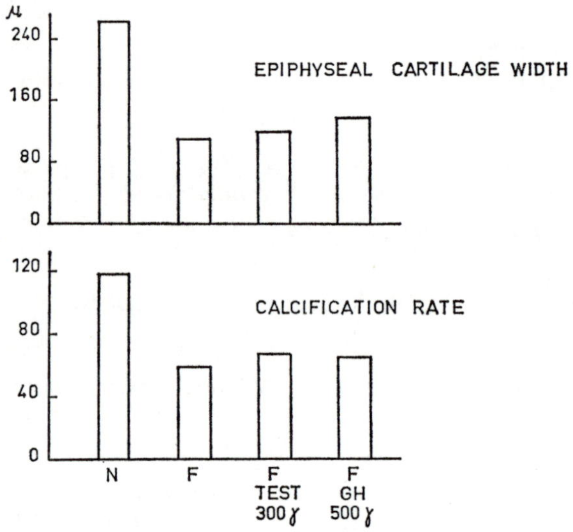

Fig. 3. Influence of bovine growth hormone and testosterone on reduction of epiphyseal cartilage width and calcification rate of 49-days-old spayed female rats caused by four days fasting

was done 2—3 weeks before administration of tetracycline. The results of *re-feeding* after a four days' fast, on epiphyseal cartilage width and calcification rate of female rats are shown in figures 4 and 5. The width of the epiphyseal cartilage plate started to increase rapidly before the calcification rate started to recover. The epiphyseal cartilage width and calcification rate reached normal levels after seven to eight days of re-feeding. Later still, both showed an increase to a slightly higher than normal level, and it is possible that this might compensate for the retardation caused by fasting.

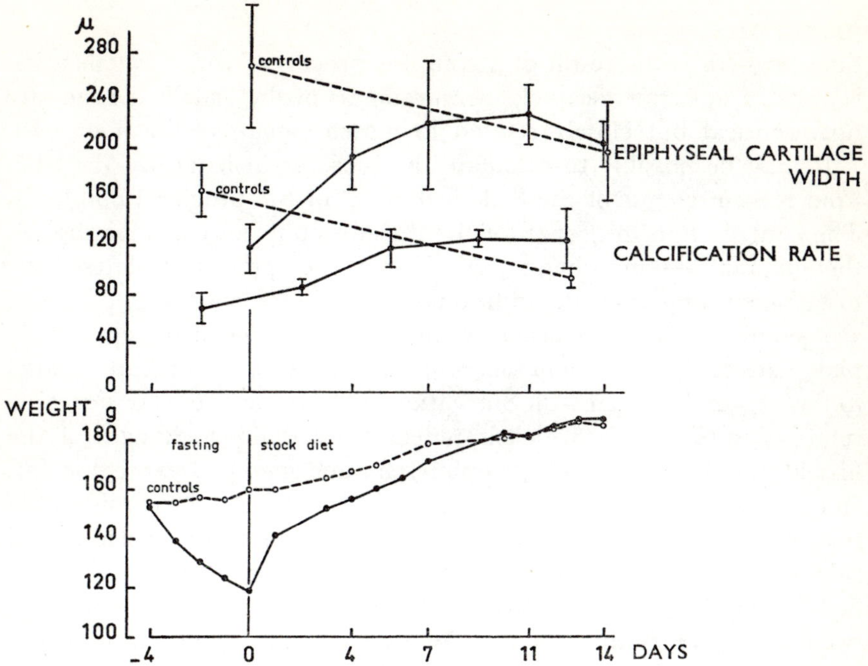

Fig. 4. Influence of fasting and subsequent refeeding on calcification rate and width of the uncalcified epiphyseal cartilage of 52-days-old female rats, measured at intervals of three to four days

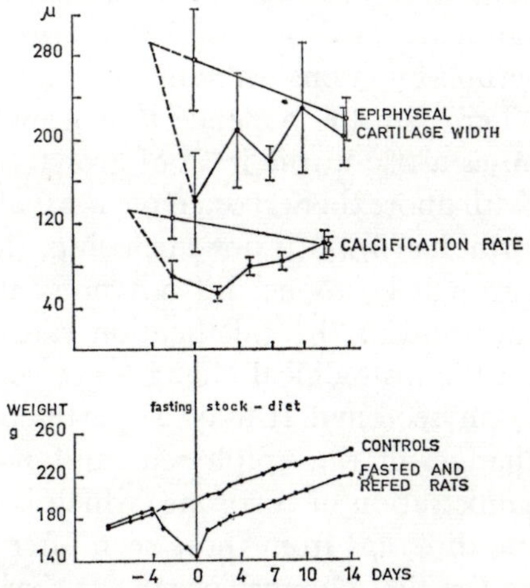

Fig. 5. Influence of fasting and subsequent refeeding on calcification rate and width of the uncalcified epiphyseal cartilage of 66-days-old female rats, measured at intervals of three to four days

DISCUSSION

Since growth is the result of a complex process of which calcification is only an integrated sequel, measurements of the 'calcified zone' are not identical but closely related to measurements of linear growth.

It may be possible to calculate the increase in length of the tibia from measurements of the 'calcified zone' of the proximal epiphysis. The contribution to growth of the distal epiphyseal cartilage disc — though small — and changes in width of the epiphyseal plates, have to be taken into account. Additional factors complicating calculations are geometrical errors caused by the slight V-shape of the epiphyseal plate, and the possibility of sectioning the tibia in a plane not parallel to the axis of linear growth. Starvation is known to cause considerable retardation of growth, which is reflected by striking changes of the histological appearance of the epiphyseal and metaphyseal region (5). In the present study the calcification rate was found to be considerably reduced by fasting. Measurements of epiphyseal cartilage width and calcification rate indicate that the first changes occur in the uncalcified epiphyseal cartilage, and that after a latent period of at least twenty-four hours the calcification rate changes. The width of the uncalcified cartilage plate and the calcification rate are reduced to about fifty percent of normal after four days of fasting. The mechanisms through which fasting causes these changes are not known.

Inanition is sometimes considered to cause functional hypopituitarism (13). Arguments against this view are to be found in investigations of endocrine functions in clinical conditions as anorexia nervosa (4, 11). There is little evidence that growth hormone is involved. Fasting causes a rise in the level of growth hormone in blood (7) while patients with anorexia nervosa have normal or elevated blood levels of growth hormone (6). It is not surprising, therefore, that high doses of (bovine) growth hormone did not prevent the reduction of cartilage plate width and of the calcification rate caused by fasting (figure 3), although the histological changes are very similar to those observed after hypophysectomy. It may be pertinent here to mention that histological changes of the epiphyseal and metaphyseal region caused by the administration of cortisone, which is a potent inhibitor of growth, are quite different from those seen after hypophysectomy.

During refeeding the first changes occur (as during fasting) in the uncalcified part of the epiphyseal cartilage, which rapidly regains its original dimension. The calcification rate does not increase, or increases so slowly that the average rate after four days of feeding is equal to or lower than that during fasting (figures 4 and 5). It takes at least seven days for the calcification rate and epiphyseal cartilage width to reach the level of the control animals. This period of recovery is twice as long as the period of starvation. Food consumption was not measured during the re-feeding experiments, but the rapid gain in weight indicates that the food intake was probably adaequate.

From the reduction in calcification rate it is clear that short periods of fasting may cause a considerable fall in the growth rate, and that resumption of a normal growth rate begins relatively late. This delayed recovery may not be restricted to the reaction of the epiphyseal cartilage to fasting, but may also complicate the assessment of hormonal control of epiphyseal growth.

ACKNOWLEDGEMENTS

The experiments reported here were carried out with technical assistance of Miss Ingeborg B. A. M. van den Brand. Plates and figures for this paper were made by Mr. W. Zuidervaart.

REFERENCES

1. Asling, C. W. and H. M. Evans, in: *The biochemistry and physiology of bone*, ed. by G. H. Bourne, New York, 1956.
2. Becks, H., M. E. Simpson and H. M. Evans, Ossification at the proximal tibial epiphysis in the rat, *Anat. Rec.* 92: 121, 1945.
3. Becks, H., M. E. Simpson, H. M. Evans, R. D. Ray, C. H. Li and C. W. Asling, Response to pituitary growth hormone and thryroxin of the tibias of hypophysectomized rats after long postoperative intervals, *Anat. Rec.* 94: 631, 1946.
4. Van Beugen, L., E. Kropveld, J. de Graeff, D. Smeenk and A. Querido, Anorexia nervosa, *Ned. T. Geneesk.* 105: 464, 1961.
5. Follis, R. H., A survey of bone disease, *Am. J. Med.* 22: 469, 1957.
6. Glick, S. M., J. Roth, R. S. Yalow and S. A. Berson, Immunoassay of human growth hormone in plasma, *Nature* 199: 784, 1963.
7. Glick, S. M., R. S. Yalow and S. A. Berson, Hypoglycaemia: a potent stimulans to secretion of growth hormone, *Science* 140: 987, 1963.

8. Greenspan, F. S., C. H. Li, M. E. Simpson and H. M. Evans, Bioassay of hypophyseal growth hormone: the tibia test, *Endocrinology* 45: 455, 1949.
9. Kember, N. F., Cell division in endochondral ossification, *J. Bone Joint Surg.* 42B: 824, 1960.
10. Levie, L. H., *Skeletgroei en interne secretie*, Diss. Amsterdam, 1939.
11. Marks, V. and R. G. Bannister, Pituitary and adrenal function in undernutrition with mental illness, *Brit. J. Psychiat.* 109: 480, 1963.
12. Milch, R. A., D. P. Rall, and J. E. Tobie, Bone localisation of the tetracyclines, *J. Nat. Cancer Inst.* 19: 87, 1957.
13. Perloff, W. H., E. M. Lasché, J. H. Nodine, N. G. Schneeberg and C. B. Vieillard, The starvation state and functional hypopituitarism, *J. Am. Med. Ass.* 155: 1307, 1954.
14. Ray, R. D., C. W. Asling, D. G. Walker, M. E. Simpson, C. H. Li and H. M. Evans, Growth and differentiation of the skeleton in thyroidectomized-hypophysectomized rats treated with thyroxin, growth hormone, and the combination, *J. Bone Joint Surg.* 36a: 94, 1954.
15. Smeenk, D., J. van der Sluys Veer, J. C. Birkenhäger and R. O. van der Heul, Rate of calcification of the proximal tibial epiphyseal cartilage of rats studied with the aid of tetracycline labelling, *Proc. Second Europ. Symp. Calcified Tissues,* 1965 : 199, Ed. Univ. de Liège.
16. Walker, D. C., M. E. Simpson, C. W. Asling and H. E. Evans, Growth and differentiation in the rat following hypophysectomy at 6 days of age, *Anat. Rec.* 106: 539, 1960.

EFFECTS OF HORMONES ON THE MICROSTRUCTURE OF BONE, WITH SPECIAL EMPHASIS ON CORTISONE

ZVI LARON

Linear growth in man is directly related to the growth of bones, which consists of three basic phenomena: cell multiplication, increase in cell size and formation of bony tissue itself. In long bones, these processes take place in the epiphyseal cartilage plates. Bone growth is controlled and influenced by genetic and nutritional factors, and by hormones .

The hormones which exert the most apparent stimulating effects on skeletal growth are: growth hormone, thyroid hormone and androgenic hormone of gonadal or adrenal origin. Insulin seems to have a permissive action necessary for the effect of growth hormone. In the absence of these hormones skeletal growth is impaired. It is not known whether the adrenal glucocorticoids exert an important effect on the growth of bone under physiological conditions; excessive amounts, secreted or administered, exhibit an inhibitory effect.

Little is known concerning the exact mode of action of hormones on bone, and it is probable that not all hormones act through the same mechanism. Growth hormone probably affects the rate of multiplication of cells in the proliferative cell layer (4, 14). The presence of insulin seems necessary to enable growth hormones to exert its stimulating action (16), but insulin also plays a role in the early stages of the maturation of the cartilage cells, by influencing glycogen formation on the cells (6, 14). Glycogen is a precursor of phosphatases which play an important role in calcification (9, 11). Thyroxine plays an important role in the maturation of the cartilage cells until they reach the point at which they burst (10, 31). A schematic presentation of the locus of hormone action in the process of growth in the epiphyseal cartilage is given in fig. 1.

As it is very difficult to study processes in children, one is compelled to retreat to the laboratory and produce artificial states in animals with the aim to further our understanding of the physiologic and pathologic processes in man. This is very risky if we assume that the laboratory animal behaves in a similar fashion as the human being; also we

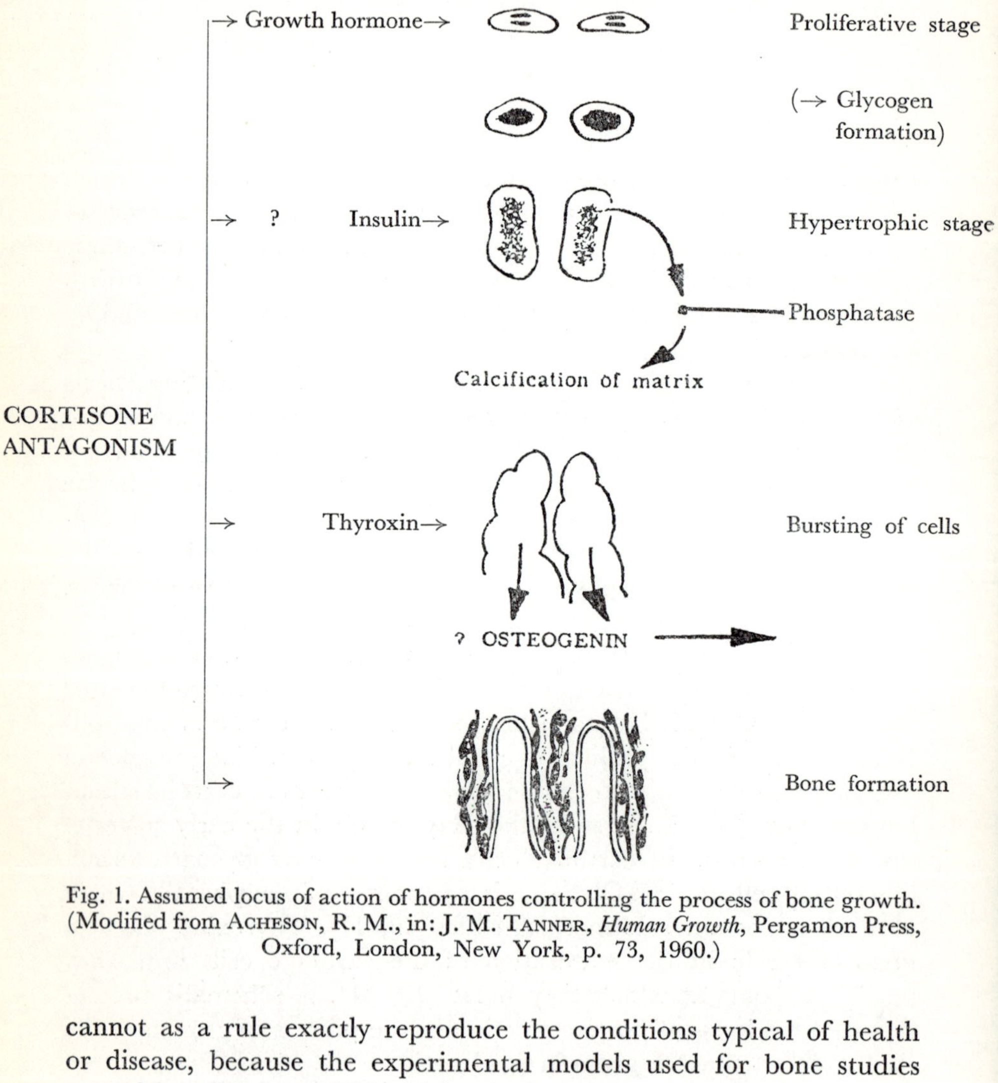

Fig. 1. Assumed locus of action of hormones controlling the process of bone growth. (Modified from ACHESON, R. M., in: J. M. TANNER, *Human Growth*, Pergamon Press, Oxford, London, New York, p. 73, 1960.)

cannot as a rule exactly reproduce the conditions typical of health or disease, because the experimental models used for bone studies necessitate the use of fairly high, pharmacological, doses of hormones. Calculated per unit of body weight, the doses used in laboratory

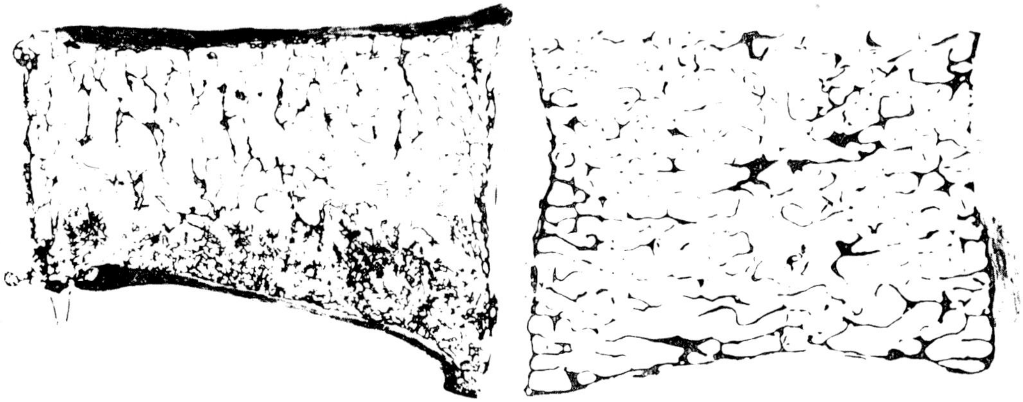

A B

Fig. 2. Structure of vertebral body in Cushing's disease (a) as compared to a normal vertebra (b), from SISSON, H. A., *J. Bone and Joint Surg.* 38B: 418, 1956

Fig. 4. Histological appearance of the proximal epiphysis and metaphysis of the rat tibia: A. control untreated and B. rat having received 10 mg cortisone intraperitoneally for 6 days (for explanation see text)

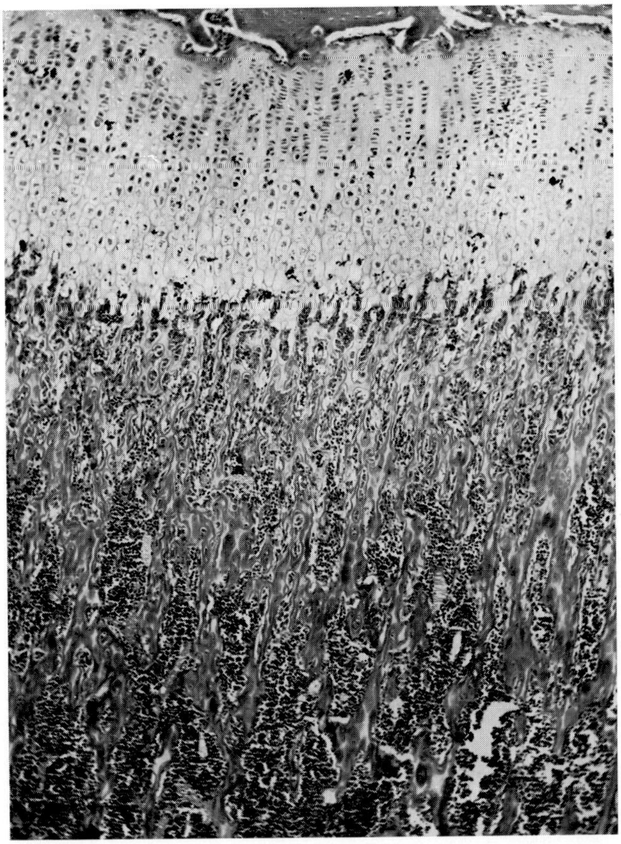

Fig. 4A

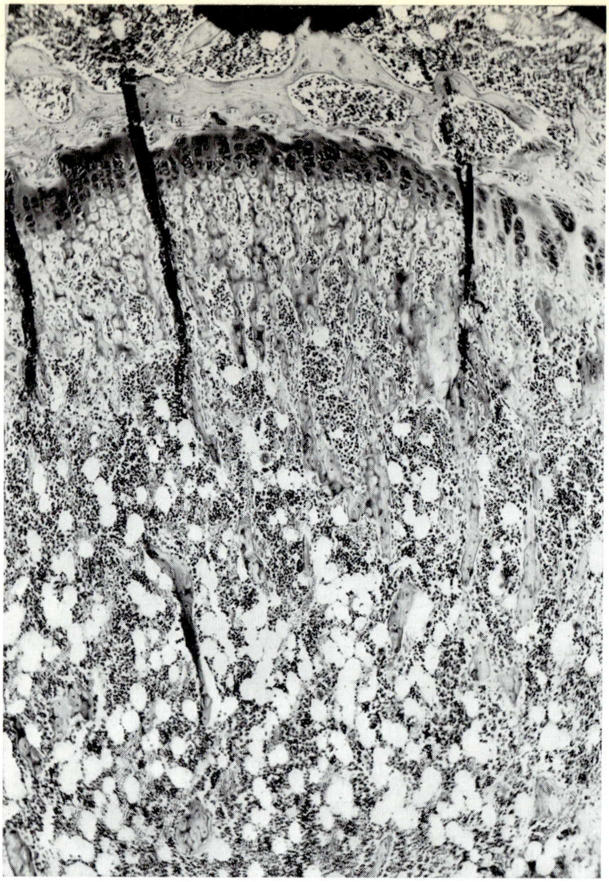

Fig. 4B

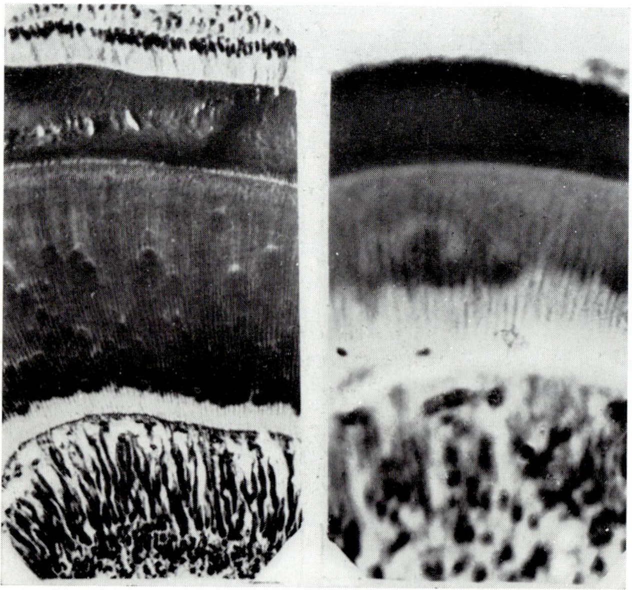

A B

Fig. 5. Action of cortisone on the calcification of the upper incisor of a rat treated with 10 mg cortisone (B) as compared to the tooth of an untreated rat (A)

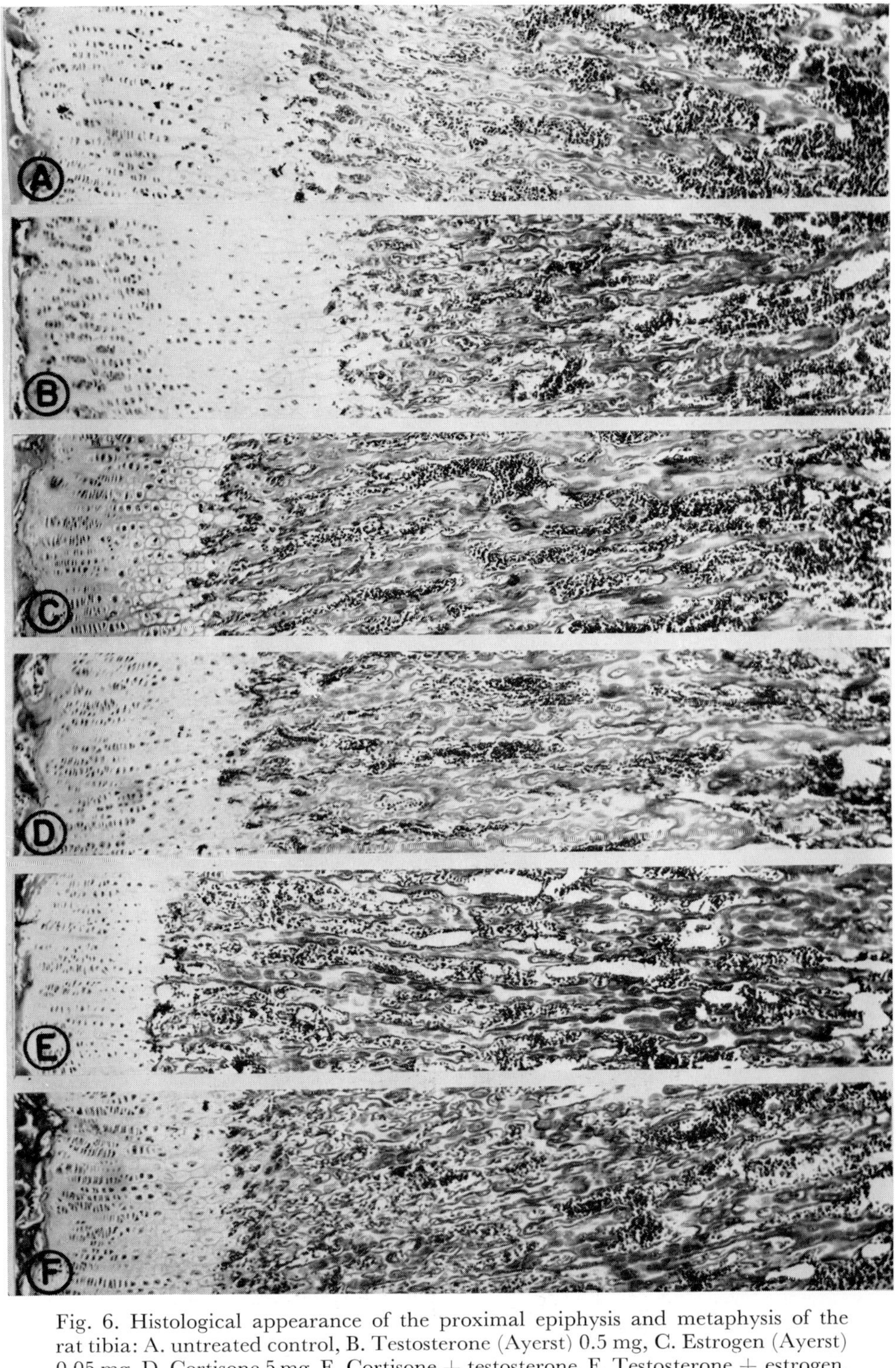

Fig. 6. Histological appearance of the proximal epiphysis and metaphysis of the rat tibia: A. untreated control, B. Testosterone (Ayerst) 0.5 mg, C. Estrogen (Ayerst) 0.05 mg, D. Cortisone 5 mg, E. Cortisone + testosterone, F. Testosterone + estrogen. All hormones were administered daily by the intraperitoneal route for three weeks

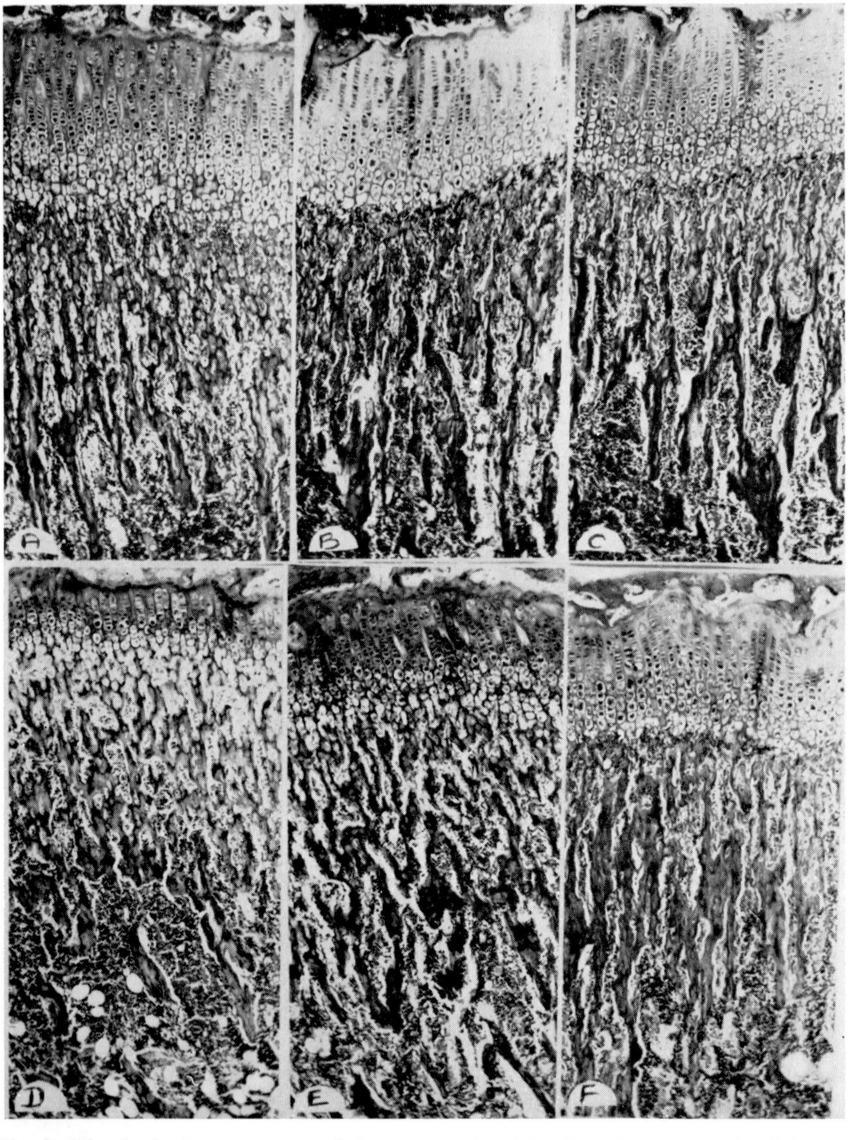

Fig. 7. Histological appearance of the proximal epiphysis and metaphysis of the rat tibia: A. untreated control, B. bovine growth hormone, 0.5 mg/day, C. sheep growth hormone 1 mg/day, D. Medrol 1 mg/day, E. Medrol 1 mg and bovine growth hormone 0.5 mg/day, F. Medrol 1 mg and sheep growth hormone 1 mg/day. Treatment was given for 2 weeks (from LARON et al, *Endocrinology* 72: 470, 1963)

experiments are sometimes of an astronomical order, in comparison with those given to the human.

I shall now review the effects of corticosteroid hormones, alone or in combination with other hormones, on the microscopical appearance of the growth area of long bones.

In 1932 Cushing (7) described the syndrome later to be called after him, and which was found to be caused by secondary adrenal hyperfunction. In 6 out of 8 of his young adult patients, osteoporosis — especially of the vertebrae — was found. Lescher and Robb-Smith (29) showed that primary hyperplasia of the adrenals also led to these bone changes (fig. 2). Albright (1) postulated the theory that increased amounts of glucocorticoids interfere with protein synthesis, including bone matrix formation, through their anti-anabolic action. This process, disturbance of new bone formation in the presence of a continued bone resorption, will lead to disturbed bone growth and osteoporosis. Albright's theory has been challenged (33) but a good alternative explanation for the corticosteroid action on bone is still lacking.

Among the first to study the effect of cortisone on the bone of growing rats was Follis (12); he was followed by Sissons and Hadfield (32), who also studied the rabbit, Duthie and Barker (8), Laron et al. (19, 24, 27) and Storey (33, 34, 35). The changes induced by cortisone administered subcutaneously or intraperitoneally for one to three weeks in doses ranging from 10 to 50 mg per kg body weight, can be summarized as follows: the animals that received cortisone either stopped growing or grew much slower than control animals (fig. 3). Sections through long bones — usually the tibia or femur — revealed: (fig. 4) a. narrowing of the epiphyseal cartilage due to a retardation in both the proliferative and the hypertrophic cell layer; b. an increase in the provisionally calcified cartilaginous matrix persisting within the trabeculae of the primary spongiosa; c. irregularity in shape of the trabeculae; d. decrease of the osteoid seams, and e. reduction of the penetrating connective tissue carrying the osteogenic cells. The underlying spongiosa is also rarefied. These changes indicate an arrest of the normal process of resorption and remodelling of the calcified cartilaginous matrix. Treatment with cortisone also led to an increase of the medullary fat.

Corticosterone, the predominant corticosteroid in the rat, produces the same histological alterations as those caused by cortisone (20) the most easily available corticosteroid.

The osteoporotic changes caused by cortisone become more evident if treatment is continued for months (15) or if cortisone is administered to an already diseased bone, such as in rickets (24). As already stated the exact mechanism by which cortisone suppresses the growth processes in the bone is not known. It is possible that it antagonizes the effect of growth hormone; that its anti-anabolic effect reduces the formation of protein substances necessary for the bone matrix. Cortisone is also known to influence glycogen metabolism which, as already stated, is a source of phosphatases. Small doses of cortisone stimulate alkaline phosphatase activity, whereas larger doses inhibit this enzyme (26). Cortisone or its derivatives also depress acid phosphatase activity (17, 21). It has also been found that cortisone interferes with the polymerization of the mucopolysaccharides in the ground substance (3) and this could explain the interference with the process of calcification of the cartilaginous core. The impairment of cartilage resorption has been recently demonstrated by the use of tritiated thymidine (36). Cortisone interferes also with the healing of bone fractures (5)

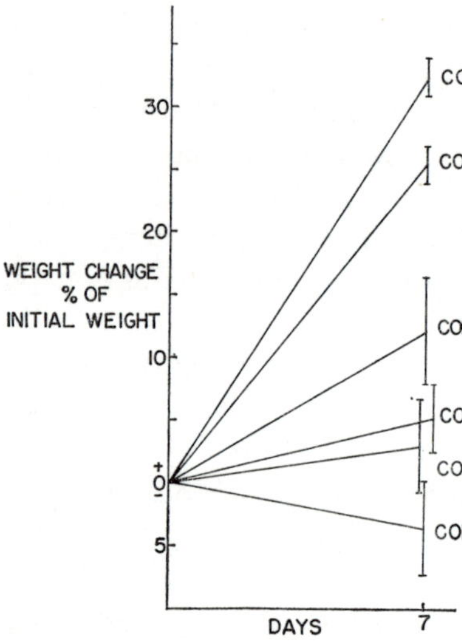

Fig. 3. Growth of rats: untreated and groups treated with different doses of corticosterone (from 19)

and prevents the formation of ectopic bone (20). The hypercalcaemia in cortisone-treated nephrectomized dogs (13) may be caused by interference with the process of calcification but could also reflect increased resorption of bone. All of these processes together could lead to the picture of osteoporosis that cortisone and its analogues may cause.

Cortisone also disturbs calcium deposition in the teeth as demonstrated by the widening of the predentin layer (23, 27) (fig. 5).

Having summarized the main ill effects of cortisone on the growing bone, the question arises whether there are means to counteract or prevent these changes. Much has been written about the protective value of androgenic and anabolic steroids against the deleterious effects of cortisone (18, 30) and beautiful drawings have been used to schematically dramatise this effect. To my regret we have not been able to confirm these results or expectations. Testosterone, which if administered alone causes no changes in the bone structure other than slight widening of the epiphyseal cartilage plate in the rat, failed to counteract the bone changes induced by cortisone (fig. 6) (25). Similar findings were obtained when 19-nor androstenolone phenylpropionate (Durabolin) was used (19). There was also no effect on body growth as a whole. Our sad experience has been confirmed by other investigators (2). Some protection of Durabolin against the deleterious effects of 6-methyl prednisolone (Medrol) has been observed in bones of rats made rachitic by a low calcium diet (28); similar results were obtained with vitamin D (24). In the latter two instances the improvement concerned bone that remained sick. Of utmost interest are the findings that growth hormone prevented the histological changes in the rat bone, although it dit not affect the weight changes induced by 6-methyl prednisolone (Medrol) (fig. 7).

Because of the lack of sufficient amounts of human growth hormone it is not yet possible to repeat this experiment in man, but at least some hope exists now that it will be possible to prevent the undesirable effects of cortisone and analogous substances.

ACKNOWLEDGEMENT

These studies were supported by grants from the Upjohn Company, Kalamazoo, Michigan, U.S.A.

REFERENCES

1. ALBRIGHT, F., *Harvey Lectures* 38: 123, 1943.
2. BAVETTA, L. A., I. BEKHOR, R. SHAH, P. O'DAY and M. E. NIMNI, *Endocrinology* 71: 221, 1962.
3. BERNICK, S. and B. H. ERSHOFF, *Endocrinology* 72: 231, 1963.
4. BLUMENTHAL, H. T., K. M. HSIEH and T. Y. WANG, *Amer. J. Path.* 30: 771, 1954.
5. BLUNT, J. W. JR., C. M. PLOTZ, R. LATTES, E. L. HOWES, K. MEYER and C. REGAN, *Proc. Soc. Exp. Biol. and Med.* 73: 678, 1950.
6. CHEN, M. J., *J. Physiol.* 125: 148, 1954.
7. CUSHING, H., *Bull. Johns Hopkins Hosp.* 50: 137, 1932.
8. DUTHIE, R. B. and A. N. BARKER, *J. Bone & Joint Surg.* 37B: 691, 1955.
9. EEG-LARSEN, N., *Acta Physiol. Scand.* 38: suppl. 128, 1956.
10. FELL, H. B. and E. MELLANBY, *J. Physiol.* 127: 427, 1955.
11. FOLLIS, R. H. JR., *Bull. Johns Hopkins Hosp.* 85: 360, 1949.
12. FOLLIS, R. H. JR., *Proc. Soc. Exp. Biol. and Med.* 76: 722, 1951.
13. GROLLMAN, A., *Proc. Soc. Exp. Biol. and Med.* 85: 582, 1954.
14. HAY, M. F., *J. Physiol.* 144: 490, 1958.
15. KAHN, D. S. and S. C. SKORYNA, *Lab. Investig.* 8: 763, 1959.
16. KORNER, A., in: F. GROSS, Ed., *Protein metabolism*, Springer Verlag, Berlin-Göttingen, Heidelberg, p. 8, 1962.
17. KOWADLO, A. and Z. LARON, *Metabolism* 12: 176, 1963.
18. KOWALEWSKI, K., in: F. GROSS, Ed., *Protein Metabolism*, Springer Verlag, Berlin, Göttingen, Heidelberg, p. 238, 1962.
19. LARON, Z. and J. H. BOSS, *Arch. Path.* 53: 274, 1962.
20. LARON, Z. and A. LAUFER, *Endocrinology* 70: 437, 1962.
21. LARON, Z. and A. KOWADLO, *Metabolism* 10: 1100, 1961.
22. LARON, Z., B. Z. ARIE and S. KENDE, *Endocrinology* 72: 470, 1963.
23. LARON, Z., B. D. CANLAS JR. and J. D. CRAWFORD, *A. M. A. Arch. Path.* 61: 177, 1956.
24. LARON, Z., B. D. CANLAS JR. and J. D. CRAWFORD, *A. M. A. Arch. Path.* 65: 403, 1958.
25. LARON, Z., H. R. DUDLEY and J. D. CRAWFORD — unpublished data.
26. LARON, Z., J. FORTUNATO and R. KLEIN, *Endocrinology* 61: 483, 1957.
27. LARON, Z., J. P. MUHLETHALER and R. KLEIN, *A. M. A. Arch. Path.* 65: 125, 1958.
28. LARON, Z., A. KOWADLO, B. Z. ARIE, I. KALISH and S. KENDE, *Israel J. Exp. Med.* 11: 41, 1963.
29. LESCHER, F. G. and A. H. T. ROBB-SMITH, *Quart. J. Med. N.S.* 4: 23, 1935.
30. REIFENSTEIN, E. C. JR., *Metabolism* 7: 78, 1958.
31. SIMPSON, M. E., C. W. ASLING and H. M. EVANS, *Yale J. Biol. Med.* 23: 1, 1950.
32. SISSONS, H. A. and G. J. HADFIELD, *J. Anat.* 89: 69, 1955.
33. STOREY, E., *Australasian Ann. Med.* 9: 318, 1960.
34. STOREY, E., *Australian and New Zealand J. Surg.* 30: 36, 1960.
35. STOREY, E., *Endocrinology* 68: 533, 1961.
36. YOUNG, M. H. and W. A. J. CRANE, *Ann. Rheum. Dis.* 23: 163, 1964.

DISCUSSION

Steendijk: In animal experiments, Storey (quoted by Dr. Laron) has been able to induce changes ranging from severe osteoporosis to severe osteosclerosis by dietary measures, particularly through altering the calcium: phosphate ratio in the diet, and by adding various amounts of cortisone.

Van der Sluys Veer: I just wanted to add to Dr. Laron's paper that we have studied the influence of cortisone on tetracycline labelling. The picture we obtained corresponds with Dr. Laron's findings; these animals were tube-fed with the same diet as the controls, so that there was no variation in diet. I know that this is an important factor, because when you give large doses of cortisone, they stop eating.

Sobel: I did not grasp the conditions of the experiment in which Dr. Laron found that androgen had no effect on the skeletal maturation of the rat. Could you mention the age and sex of the animals used?

Laron: They were male rats, and the initial weight was usually between 90 and 130 grams.

Sobel: We have found that testosterone can advance skeletal maturation of young female rats treated for 6 weeks beginning at age 28 days, when weight is approximately 65 to 75 gm (Joss, E. E., K. A. Zuppinger and E. H. Sobel , *Endocrinology* 72: 123, 1963). Perhaps the differences in our findings can be explained by the differences in the sex and age of the animals treated, and the duration of the experiments.

Van Wersch: We have studied the influence of Durabolin in rats. There is no doubt that this drug caused an increase in the alkaline phosphatase in the kidney by histochemical and biochemical parameters, but there was no increase in the serum alkaline phosphatase.

Laron: We did not study alkaline phosphatase activity during or after testosterone or any anabolic substance, so I would not be able to comment on your results. The alkaline phosphatase response to cortisone is dose-dependent. Small doses of cortisone stimulated alkaline phosphatase whereas higher doses depressed alkaline phosphatase activity. This may be important in the physiological homeostasis, where under stress conditions in the human we would also have weak stimulation of cortisol secretion. Possibly Dr. SOBEL would like to comment; when she was still at the Massachusets General Hospital, they were giving cortisone to children with growth retardation, thinking that the catch-up might afterwards overcome the growth lag.

Sobel: I was no longer at the Massachusets General Hospital when those studies were undertaken, and don't recall the details of the published findings.

Prader: I have just one remark to make. Dr. LARON has shown that testosterone does not correct the influence of cortisone on bone, but that growth hormone does correct it, in rats.

In the last issue of the *Lancet* there was a paper by the group of FRASER in London, (*Lancet* 2 : 376, 1964), showing that in the human large amounts of cortisone may suppress the secretion of growth hormone, because it was found that cortisone suppressed the insulin-induced rise in growth hormone. I think this fits in very well with what Dr. LARON found in rats.

Van der Linden: I should like to ask a practical question about the technique of tetracycline labelling. Is it possible to label two or three times?

Van der Sluys Veer: It is possible to label twice and we have done it on several occasions. A complication is that the labels become mixed, so that one has to use different substances. However, it is not necessary to do double labelling, because you can easily distinguish between the calcified non-labelled part and the un-calcified epiphyseal cartilage, because the latter does not show fluorescence. It is just as blue as the background light of the fluorescence microscope.

Croughs: Dr. VAN DER SLUYS VEER showed that there was a delay in the growth of the epiphyseal cartilage with malnutrition. I am astonished that there was not a real catch-up, with a growth rate above the normal.

Van der Sluys Veer: We might have seen catch-up growth if we had continued the experiments longer. There might be an increase in the epiphyseal cartilage width, and more obviously in the calcification rate, to a level above that of the controls. That is a significant difference which may compensate the retardation caused by fasting. That is a point still under study.

CHAPTER IV

GROWTH IN CHILDHOOD

THE GROWTH CURVE FOR HEIGHT, AND EFFECTS OF 'NORMAL' VARIABLES

J. J. VAN DER WERFF TEN BOSCH

The variations in stature among healthy children of a common racial stock who live in the same country, can be attributed to a number of factors (see 17). The most obvious factors are the age and the sex. Less obvious, perhaps, are the ill-defined rate of general physical maturation and the timing of the onset of sexual maturation. Superimposed upon or subordinate to these factors is the family background in terms of genetic constitution, early childhood care and family size.

At birth boys are slightly longer (and heavier) than girls and a smaller difference may persist for some time (11), but between 5 and 10 years there seems to be no or only a slight sex difference. From birth until the age of 10 years a child grows from about 50 cm to a size of nearly 140 cm. The gain of 90 cm is not spread evenly over the ten intervening years. At first the child gains far more than 9 cm in a year, in fact about 25 cm during the first year of life. The gain in length or height per unit of time (e.g. expressed as cm per year) is the rate of growth in height or the height velocity; the growth rate falls sharply after the first year and reaches values of 3—6 cm per year when the child is ten years old (fig. 1). During sexual maturation the sex hormones secreted by the ovaries or testes cause a great rise in the growth rate so that the child suddenly outgrows its age peers which have not yet started to come in puberty. This pubertal 'spurt' in growth is a self-limiting process, since the sex steroids secreted by the maturing gonads do not only stimulate the cartilaginous epiphyseal cells of the long bones to multiply more quickly (and thereby to cause the long bones to become longer), but the sex hormones also accelerate the final ossification of the discs which leads to complete cessation of growth in height. The pubertal spurt in height occurs earlier (because puberty begins earlier), and is of shorter duration and of lesser intensity in girls than in boys. These sex differences (fig. 1) in the pubertal spurt are the main causes of the sex difference in adult stature, which is about 13 cm in the Netherlands.

In children of the same sex, the stature and the age at which puberty occurs are interrelated. By and large the gain in height from

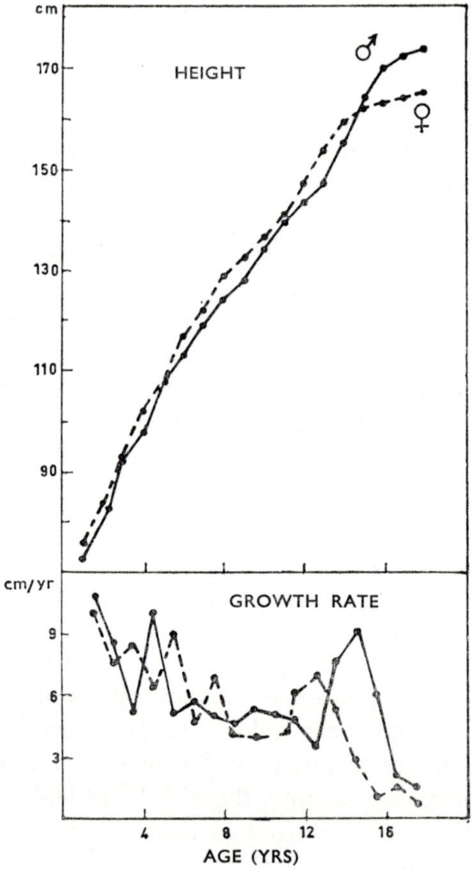

Fig. 1. Height and growth rate of a boy and one of his sisters (data from 7)

the beginning of the pubertal spurt until cessation of growth, is greater in children with early puberty and smaller in children with late puberty (table 1). This may be due to the fact that the skeleton is less mature in the first category, and more mature in the latter, when the spurt begins. The effect of this difference in height gained during

Table 1. *Difference in pre-pubertal and pubertal growth in height between early and late maturing girls (derived from 16).*

		Early girls	Late girls	Difference
Age at menarche (yrs.-months)		10-0 — 11-11	13-0 — 15-5	
Approximate average age at onset of pubertal spurt (yrs.)		9	11	+ 2
Increment in height (cm)	7 yrs. till onset of spurt	12.6	22.6	+ 10.0
Increment in height (cm)	onset of spurt till 17 yrs.	27.8	22.5	— 5.3
Increment in height (cm)	7 — 17 yrs.	40.4	45.1	+ 4.7

puberty upon adult stature is partly neutralized by the difference in height at the time of onset of the pubertal spurt (table 1). A child with late puberty will have had more years of growth at a pre-pubertal rate than the child with early puberty, and will have reached a greater stature by the time that puberty begins. Marked differences in adult height therefore occur only between individuals with excessively advanced or delayed puberty, in other words in abnormal children. When children who come in puberty within the normal time limits are considered, another fact can be noted. In such children height during infancy is related to the age at which puberty begins. Girls with relatively early puberty, are taller from a very early age (table 2) and have a more mature skeleton from the age of six years or earlier (see p. 41), than girls who have menarche relatively late. The early maturers of this type tend to become taller adults than the late maturers. It is clear that if age in terms of years elapsed since birth could be substituted by age in terms of physical maturity (developmental age), puberty might be found to set in at the same developmental age in all children. This may be illustrated by the use of skeletal age as a specimen of developmental age. Fig. 2 shows the skeletal or bone age of nine normal girls around the time of menarche. Plotted against the

Table 2. *The average heights at various ages, of groups of girls who showed no signs of puberty at all (A) one sign only (B) or two or three (C) at the age of 11 years. The signs of puberty were breast development, pigmented pubic hair and menarche (data from 5).*

Age when measured	Average height (cm)		
	A	B	C
2 years	84.8	84.6	85.8
$4^1/_2$ years	102.2	103.1	104.3
6 years	112.4	114.3	115.7
7 years	118.8	120.2	122.7
11 years	138.9	142.0	147.0

chronological age the bone ages vary tremendously, but when the same data are plotted against the distance in time from menarche the bone ages follow a uniform pattern. The same phenomenon can be observed when other changes are recorded, e.g. the changes in height or in sex hormone excretion which occur during puberty. Such

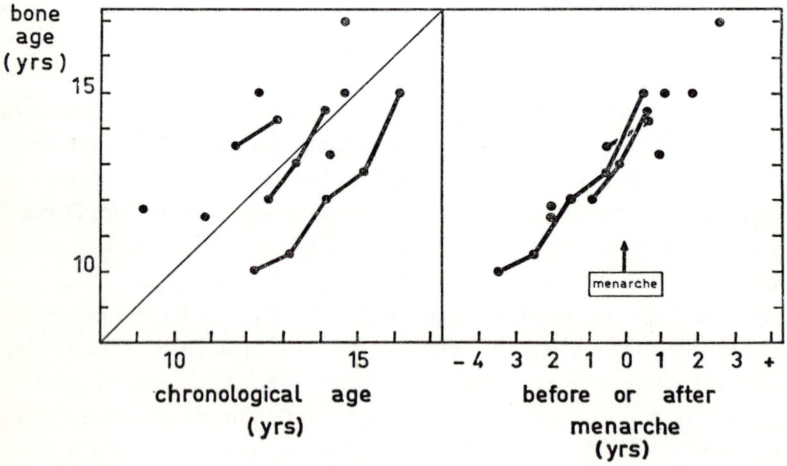

Fig. 2. To show that the bone age of (9 normal) girls near puberty is related more to the time of menarche than to the chronological age

data appear to be much better related to the degree of sexual maturity than to the chronological age.

There is no doubt that the chromosomes within the ovum and the sperm of the parents contain the genotypical potential of the size that the offspring may eventually reach. The magnitude of the paternal as

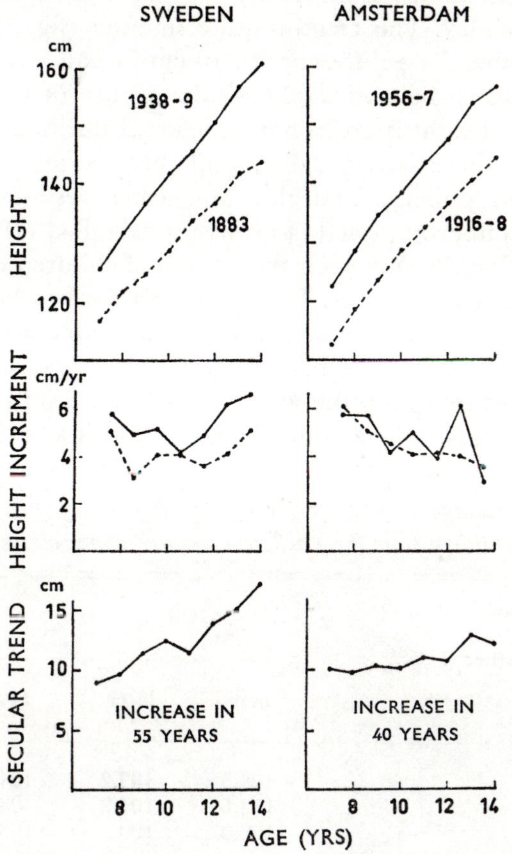

Fig. 3. The secular trend in height of schoolboys in Sweden (3) and in Holland (15)

compared to the maternal genetic contribution is not known. The mother's influence is complicated by the fact that pregnancy itself, through uterine blood supply, placental size and length of gestation, can modify the size of the newborn and the postnatal rate of growth (13, 14, 10, 6). It is perhaps not surprising, therefore, that the weight at birth correlates better with the height of the mother than with the father's height (4).

The influence of the early childhood environment on the growth rate of healthy young children has been demonstrated in a number of ways. The secular trend in height, the greater size of children in subsequent generations, is probably an effect of the environment during early infancy. This trend is quite marked (fig. 3) at the age of 7 years, when there is a difference of 10 cm in half a century, and its effect may already be noticeable within a year of birth (18). The secular trend in height is much more apparent during infancy than in adults because there is a parallel, probably related, trend towards earlier onset of puberty and thus to earlier cessation of growth, sothat the pre-pubertal period of growth is curtailed (12, 8).

The effect of family size upon the growth of children is perhaps also due to environmental factors. Later children tend to be shorter, and to come in puberty later, than first children. Table 3 shows that the difference in height may begin to appear at an early age.

It is of interest that both the secular trend and family size (table 3) are effective at all socio-economic levels, sothat it seems unlikely that

Table 3. *The average heights at the age of 4 years of first born and later born children from three different socio-economic classes (data from 5).*

Occupation of father	Girls		Boys	
	first	later	first	later
non-manual	104.5	103.2	104.3	103.9
skilled manual	102.6	101.2	103.4	102.3
other manual	102.0	100.4	103.4	101.9

the degree of prosperity plays a major role. Also in both instances the greater stature during infancy is associated with earlier onset of puberty, sothat it would seem that some general developmental factor is involved.

Curiously enough a secular trend is quite clear in Japanese data from the beginning of the twentieth century, notwithstanding the fact that the beginning of this century saw the industrial revolution in Japan, accompanied by poverty, increased infant mortality rate and tuberculosis (9). This argues against BACKMAN's view (1) that the secular trend represents a recovery from the set-backs which were originally caused by the industrial revolution. There are some indications, that in the most prosperous and well-cared for categories of children the secular trend may now be completed (2).

REFERENCES

1. BACKMAN, G., Die beschleunigte Entwicklung der Jugend. Verfrühte Menarche, verspätete Menopause, verlängerte Lebensdauer, *Acta anat.* 4: 421, 1948.
2. BAKWIN, H. and S. M. MCLAUGHLIN, Secular increase in height. Is the end in sight?, *Lancet* 2: 1195, 1964.
3. BROMAN, B., G. DAHLBERG and A. LICHTENSTEIN, Height and weight during growth, *Acta paed.* (*Upps.*) 30: 1, 1942.
4. CAWLEY, R. H., T. MCKEOWN and R. G. RECORD, Parental stature and birth weight, *Amer. J. hum. Genet.* 6: 448, 1954.
5. DOUGLAS, J. W. B., The height of boys and girls and their home environment, *Mod. Probl. Pediat.* 7: 178, 1962.
6. FALKNER, F., C. R. de la Réunion annuelle des équipes chargées des études sur la croissance et le développement de l'enfant normal, p. 33, Centre International de l'Enfance, Paris 1964.
7. FORD, E. H. R., Growth in height of ten siblings, *Hum. Biol.* 30: 107, 1958.
8. FROE, A. DE, On the increase of stature and the age of maximum height, *Proceed. Kon. Ned. Akad. Wetensch.* 53: 1276, 1950.
9. HAGEN, W., The secular acceleration of growth and the individual, *Mod. Probl. Pediat.* 7: 8, 1962.
10. HEALY, M. J. R., A. MCLAREN and D. MICHIE, Foetal growth in the mouse, *Proc. roy. Soc. B.* 153: 367, 1960.
11. HEIERLI, E., Longitudinale Wachstumsstudie. Resultate von Länge, Gewicht und Kopfumfang in den ersten vier Lebensjahren, *Helv. Paed. Acta* 15: 311, 1960.
12. KIIL, V., Stature and growth of Norwegian men during the past two hundred years, *Skr. norske Vidensk.-Akad., Oslo I, Mat.-naturv. Kl.* 2: 1, 1939.
13. MCKEOWN, T. and R. G. RECORD, Observations on foetal growth in multiple pregnancy in man, *J. Endocrin.* 8: 386, 1952.
14. MCKEOWN, T. and R. G. RECORD, The influence of placental size on foetal growth in man, with special reference to multiple pregnancy, *J. Endocrin.* 9: 418, 1953.
15. OPPERS, V. M., *Analyse van de acceleratie van de menselijke lengtegroei door bepaling van het tijdstip van de groeifasen*, M. D. Thesis, Amsterdam University, 1963.
16. SIMMONS, K. and W. W. GREULICH, Menarcheal age and the height, weight and skeletal age of girls age 7—17 years, *J. Pediat.* 22: 518, 1943.
17. TANNER, J. M., *Growth at Adolescence*, 2nd ed., Blackwell Sci. Publ., Oxford, 1962.
18. THOMSON, J., Birth weight and weight gain at six months, *Health Bull. Edinburgh* 12: 25, 1954.

SEASONAL CHANGES IN THE RATE OF GROWTH

J. F. DE WIJN and S. POSTMUS
with statistical assistance of CHR. DIRKS

Both health and growth are affected by a complexity of environmental factors, by past illnesses and nutrition. Although there is continual improvement in growth and physique with improvement of environmental conditions, indications are accumulating that the potential growth rates of the bulk of children are not being fulfilled. Many studies, also in prosperous countries such as the Netherlands, have indicated by comparison of groups of children of different social class or from regions in the same country different in hygienic conditions, family size or way of living, that the potential physique of a relatively large section of the schoolpopulation has not been achieved (7). Yet in the clinical assessment of the state of health or state of nutrition, the great majority of children in such surveys are generally classified as good, and so clinical assessment may easily lead to a more optimistic view about health conditions than is warranted from growth data.

The usual treatment of growth data of groups of individuals for the assessment of physique by the calculation of height and weight averages for various age groups, may be satisfactory for some purposes but has limitations for others. The growth rate (increment per unit of time) is a better index of the actual condition of a child than the attained physique, which is the end result of all health conditions which have prevailed over a number of years.

In this paper we shall try to evaluate weight and height increments as influenced by the occurrence of short-term fluctuations in growth rate. Short-term variations in growth rate will often add to the difficulties of assessing whether a child is growing properly or not. There are two types: 1. the variations in growth rate of individual children due to illness of short duration or to temporary lack of appetite; 2. the seasonal pattern of growth, with *regularly* occurring variations in the growth rate in groups of children, which occur every year on both the Northern and Southern hemisphere.

Seasonal variations in growth rate have often been considered to be natural and of little significance. It has been shown, however, that the magnitude of the seasonal variations in growth rate varies with the state of health, the variations being greatest in children of poor health. Observations made by BRANSBY (1) and others have shown that the irregularity in the seasonal weight increments became less as the annual increments in weight improved, so that sub-optimal health may be one of the causes of irregularities in the growth rate.

On the Northern hemisphere the *growth rate in weight* has been reported to be high during late summer and autumn and low in the spring and early summer, and this rule applied at all ages (4). However, the data on which this view is based were collected in the U.S.A. in 1933, and it seems possible that the children then studied were not of optimal health. This is indicated by the work of BRANSBY (2), who found no evidence that the average growth rate in *weight* of a *group of children* was less in spring than during the rest of the year. In *individual* 'healthy' children seasonal variations did occur, but in an irregular fashion. In the London group studied by BRANSBY $^2/_3$ out of 63 healthy boys failed to gain weight during at least one quarter, but seasonal patterns of the individual boys were not reflected in the average pattern of the group, which showed no seasonal fluctuation. Thus the fact remains that such short-term fluctuations in the growth rate in weight occur among children who have been medically examined and found to be healthy.

Unfortunately body weight alone is not a reliable index of growth and well-being of children; an increase in weight may result from deposition of fat, or retention of water. Taking *increments in height* as indices of growth, DREIZEN, MANN and SPIES (3) noticed that in *malnourished children* (1945—1946) a retardation occurred which could not be attributed to coinciding infectious diseases, and which was usually prevalent in the spring, summer and early autumn. The retardation in growth was associated with clinical manifestations of malnutrition, whereas a control group of the same genetic stock of North Alabama children grew at a normal rate, with the exception of a few individuals who showed retardation which was associated with acute infectious diseases. Observations made in post-war years in various

European countries agree with these findings that seasonal fluctuations with marked retardation of growth from early summer till autumn are most prevalent in undernourished children. Seasonal fluctuations in the growth rate in height occur also in clinically wellnourished children. The most frequently observed pattern is that with a period of greatest height gain in spring, which is associated with the smallest weight gain (5). These early observations made in countries of the Northern hemisphere, have recently been confirmed in the Southern hemisphere, in Tanganyika (6). Comparing growth patterns throughout the year for both healthy European children living in the highlands, and native boys of the hot and humid coastal areas with entirely different climatic conditions, there appeared to be seasonal patterns in the rate of weight increase and, in the opposite direction, in the rate of height increase, which were independent of climate, altitude and race.

OWN OBSERVATIONS

The following data are the result of calculating figures from routine examinations, which were not particularly planned to determine the seasonal pattern.

The first study was on 8-year-old middle class school children, in the Northern part of the Netherlands (Friesland). The children appeared to be of good health, and their average height and weight were at the 67 % level of the national averages. Wearing pants only, they were weighed and measured on 3 occasions, in February 1959, in July 1959 and in March 1960. As the intervals between the weighing sessions were of unequal length, mean changes were calculated per 26 weeks. In the period from late winter (February) to early summer (July), thus including spring, growth rates in height were significantly smaller than in the following period from midsummer into late winter (table 1). These findings contrast with the reverse trend which is usually observed; a possible explanation is that in Holland most of the school children of about 8 years receive codliver oil in autumn and winter. It is of interest that in cross-sectional data of various surveys in this country higher serum alkaline phosphatase levels have been found in autumn and winter, than in spring (fig. 1). This finding, in well-nourished children, cannot be interpreted in terms of ricktes, but

Table 1. *Seasonal variations in the rate of growth of boys and girls, age 7—9 years.*

	Mean growth rate (in cm and kg per 26 weeks)		
	February—July	July—March	
(no. of children)	late winter—early summer	summer-winter	difference
boys (46)	Ht 2.36 cm Wt 1.73 kg	2.95 cm 1.37 kg	0.59 cm —0.36 kg
girls (38)	Ht 2.43 cm Wt 1.74 kg	2.96 cm 1.04 kg	0.53 cm —0.70 kg
boys and girls (84)	Ht 2.39 cm s̄: 0.18	2.95 cm s̄: 0.09	0.56 cm* s.d.: 0.20
	Wt 1.73 kg s̄: 0.23	1.22 kg s̄: 0.10	—0.51 kg* s.d.: 0.25

* = significant at 5 % level

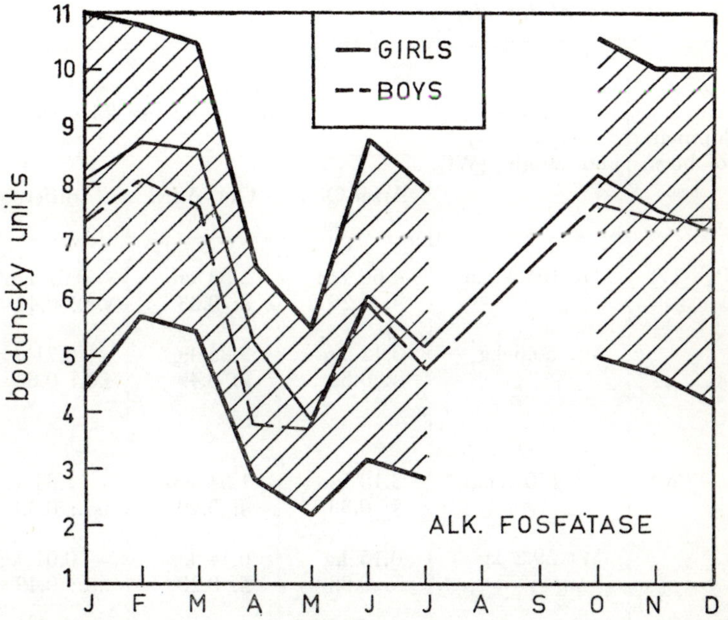

Fig. 1. Seasonal changes in alkaline phosphatase activity in the serum of 2082 school children in the Netherlands (age 8—9 years). Cross-sectional data per month during 1953—1958. In August and September no observations were made. The upper and lower lines represent the highest and lowest averages obtained in subgroups, differentiated for social class and family size (from 7)

possibly reflects increased activity of osteoblasts in the autumn and winter, which may be due to the use of codliver oil.

The second study was on adolescent boys, 14—16 years of age, pupils of a training school for mariners of the mercantile fleet. They were healthy and their averages for height and weight were slightly above the 50 % level of the national averages. The boys were arranged in a group of less advanced sexual maturity (P_2 and P_3) and a group of more advanced (P_4) sexual maturity. Measurements were taken on 3 occasions, in April 1963, in October 1963 and in April 1964. In this study the highest rate of growth in *height* was found to occur in both groups between April and October, and in one group the highest rate of growth in *weight* occurred between October and April (table 2); these findings are in agreement with many other reports.

Table 2. *Seasonal variations in the rate of growth of adolescent boys, age 14—16 years, grouped by the stage of sexual development at the beginning of the study.*

Stage of sexual development (no. of boys)	Initial height (Ht) and weight (Wt)	Mean growth rate (in cm and kg per 26 weeks)		
		April-Oct.	Oct.-April	difference
$P_2 + P_3$ (17)	Ht 161.4 cm	4.66 cm $\bar{s}$: 0.26	3.88 cm $\bar{s}$: 0.33	—0.67 cm* s.d.: 0.42
	Wt 50.6 kg	3.12 kg $\bar{s}$: 0.38	3.83 kg $\bar{s}$: 0.49	+ 0.71 kg* s.d.: 0.62
P_4 (20)	Ht 170.2 cm	3.18 cm $\bar{s}$: 0.33	1.54 cm $\bar{s}$: 0.20	— 1.64 cm** s.d.: 0.39
	Wt 59.2 kg	0.15 kg $\bar{s}$: 0.33	0.14 kg $\bar{s}$: 0.29	— 0.01 kg s.d.: 0.49

* = significant at 5 % level
** = significant at 1 % level

In summary it would seem that there occur short-term variations in the rate of growth which can be called seasonal variations. These occur in children of all ages on both hemispheres, even in the absence of ill health, and are independent of climate, altitude or race. Seasonal variations are more pronounced in undernourished than in healthy children. The most common pattern is characterized by maximal height gain and least weight gain in the spring.

From our own observations it appears that the pattern of seasonal variations in the rate of growth may not always be the same. Schoolchildren of 8 years, studied in 1960—61, grew slower in height and faster in weight during the late winter and spring (February—July), than during the rest of the year. Adolescents studied in 1962—63 appeared to grow faster in height in the spring and summer (April—October) than in the autumn and winter. These figures have a limited value because of the long and uneven intervals between measurements. The variations that were observed cannot be due to illnesses and their origin remains obscure.

It is recommended that when survey studies on the occurrence and magnitude of seasonal variations in growth rate are carried out, groups of children of similar growth pattern are selected (e.g. all children prepubertal), and that measurements are done frequently and with short intervals.

The setback in gain of height from February to July for schoolchildren (table 1) may be related to nutritional conditions in late winter and the more gain of weight in that period to lack of moving whereas abundant activity in the other part of the year might be responsible for less weight increment.

Of more interest is the question that arises, whether retardations of growth observed in certain seasons are of practical significance or not, because there are no medical signs of ill health; or whether signs of ill health are too slight to be detected by the clinician. So-called healthy children have enough reserves and elasticity of growth, which enables them to catch up short-term setbacks. Probably these setbacks are the result of a temporary unfavourable condition, and the only thing that matters in this case is whether they are made good or not. We agree with Bransby (2) when he points out that the setback may be the danger signal. The failure to make it good is the danger. We are of the opinion that subnormal health conditions which occur in spite of the absence of clinical manifestations of ill-health, often do not enable the individual child to catch up seasonal setbacks. Regular weighing and measuring are therefore valuable guides to a child's general condition, enabling the clinician or health officer to detect retardation of growth quickly and to find out what cause it may have. These conditions, improving in the course of time but still present, do contribute to subnormal growth and suboptimal health which for a part is illustrated for all groups of children up till now by the continuation of the secular trend of growth.

REFERENCES

1. Bransby, E. R., Seasonal growth of children, *The Medical Officer*, May 1945, Sept. 1945.
2. Bransby, E. R., The growth and health of children, *The Medical Officer*, March 1946.
3. Dreizen, S., A. W. Mann and T. D. Spies, Seasonal incidence of retarded growth in children with nutritive failure, *Lancet* I: 175, 1948.
4. Palmer, C. E., Seasonal variation of average growth in weight of elementary schoolchildren, *Publ. Hlth. Rep.* (Washington) 48: 211, 1933.
5. Reynolds, E. L. and L. W. Sontag, Seasonal variations in weight, height and appearance of ossification centres, *J. Pediat.* 24: 524, 1944.
6. Robson, J. R. K., Seasonal influence on height and weight increments of boys and girls in Tanganyika, *J. Trop. Med. and Hyg.* 67: 46, 1964.
7. Wijn, J. F. de, Kritische samenvatting van onderzoekingen naar de voedingstoestand van het schoolkind in Nederland (1953—1958), *Tijdschr. v. Soc. Geneesk.* 38: 141, 1960.

BODY COMPOSITION

A. HAAK

INTRODUCTION

The four principal chemical constituents of the human body are water, protein, fat and minerals. During the period of growth, and the attendant weight increase, these constituents do not all increase at the same rate.

The methods available for study of alterations in body composition can be arranged in three groups.

1. *Anatomical methods:* The thickness of the subcutaneous layer of fat can be measured on soft-tissue radiographs and with the aid of the skinfold caliper.

2. *Chemical methods:* Total body water and the extracellular water compartment can be measured by using suitable tracer substances in a test based on the dilution principle. Total fat content can be measured in comparable fashion when a fat-soluble gas is used. For minerals, such as potassium, the amount of exchangeable material can be estimated after the administration of a radioisotope.

3. *Physical methods:* The whole-body counter enables the estimation of the total amount of radioactive potassium, which occurs naturally, from which the total amount of potassium in the body can be calculated on the assumption that 0.012 % of the potassium is unstable. Other physical methods are used for the estimation of the specific gravity of the body, through measurement of the body volume; the specific gravity can, of course, be calculated when weight and body volume are known.

The volume can be measured in terms of the volume of water, air or helium displaced by the body, or by underwater weighing.

The helium-displacement method has the advantage that correction for the volume of the lungs is not necessary.

FAT AND LEAN BODY MASS

Methods for the estimation of the specific gravity of the body are essentially intended to yield information on a gross subdivision of the body into the fat compartment (F) and the fat-free compartment (FF). The two compartments have different specific gravities or densities (DF and DFF).

The specific gravity of the whole body (D) is calculated from body weight and body volume. The fat compartment, as a fraction of total body weight (f) can be calculated from the following equation.

$f = \left(\frac{DFF}{D} - 1\right) / \left(\frac{DFF}{DF} - 1\right)$, if density of fat and that of the fat-free mass is also known (14). The density of fat is 0.900, but the density of the fat-free mass is not known. Instead of this density, that of the leanest body ever reported, is often used: 1.097 from a study of BEHNKE (3). Taking into account the variable water content of the fat-free mass or lean body mass (L.B.M.), SIRI proposed a formula for the calculation of the fat content in which also the value of total water must be substituted (21).

The above subdivision of the human body into two compartments is valuable only if it makes sense from the physiological point of view. It has been shown that the fat-free compartment is a better yardstick than body surface for variables such as basal metabolic rate (4) and basal cardiac output (24). There are, nevertheless, some important criticisms that can be raised. The fat-free compartment is by no means homogeneous, but is composed of different tissues such as muscle, parenchymatous organs and bone, each of which have their individual physical and physiological characteristics.

The calculations are based on the wrong assumption that the fat-free compartment has a constant composition (25). The specific gravity of the L.B.M. cannot be estimated but only roughly approximated.

CLINICAL IMPORTANCE

Obesity is an important factor in diabetes mellitus, cardiovascular and other diseases. Thus quantitative estimation of obesity is of clinical importance. Usually standard tables of height and weight are employed to this end. The fact, however, such tables give an approximation of overweight. Overweight is not always due to obesity (increased fat content), whilst obesity may occur in individuals of normal weight for height. There is a place, therefore, for the estimation of the fat content of the body (plate 1).

Notwithstanding the shortcomings in the assumptions on which estimation of body fat and lean body mass are based, the methods seem acceptable for the purpose of longitudinal studies in single individuals so long as the lean body mass does not undergo marked changes in composition. When such changes may reasonably be expected to occur, due to illness or nutritional disorders, it is incorrect to use the assumption of the constant composition of the lean body mass.

The results obtained with different methods can be validated only by comparison with the results of other methods, because direct estimations cannot be carried out. Frequently the data from a few chemical carcass analyses are used for comparison. The validity of such a procedure is questionable. Their number is extremely small, and the physical state at the time of death may render the carcasses far from representative of individuals alive and healthy. Comparisons between different methods suffer from the lack of homogeneity of the entities measured. Anatomical methods measure fat tissue, which contains 60 % fat. Fat-soluble gasses yield data on chemically defined fat. The specific gravity methods require that a fixed value for fat is substituted in the equation.

Data obtained for adult males with the whole-body counter show significant correlations between total body fat and body weight (0.765), average skinfold thickness (0.721) of six sites (midbiceps, midtriceps, subcostal, abdominal, supra-iliacal, subscapular), and the circumference of the abdomen (0.860) and the nates (0.870). There was also a positive correlation of lean body mass with stature (0.624), but not with body weight, skinfold or circumferences. In adult women there was also a significant correlation between total body fat and body weight (0.762) and circumference of the nates (0.695), but much less with average skinfold thickness (0.434). Lean body mass was not correlated with stature (0.330) (2).

Young et al. (31) studied total fat content by underwater weighing, and subcutaneous fat by radiography, in adult women. The correlation coefficient between total body fat and the sum of 13 subcutaneous fat measurements was 0.742. The best correlation with an individual subcutaneous layer was with that over the iliac crest (0.709). The sites measured by the group of YOUNG, must be better indicators of fatness in females, than the sites studied by BARTER and FORBES (2).

CHANGES DURING GROWTH

Some of the work done with the methods indicated earlier, will be discussed here. More detailed accounts and discussions may be found in the papers of TANNER (22) and FORBES (5), and in a special issue of the *Annals of the New York Academy of Sciences* (27).

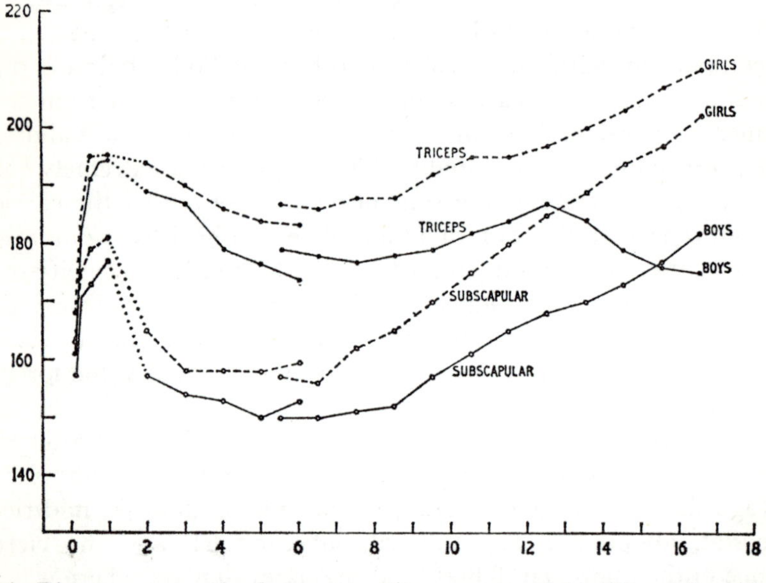

Fig. 1. Distance curve of subcutaneous tissue measured by Harpenden skinfold calipers over triceps and under scapula. Data 0-1 year, pure longitudinal core 4-6 and actual mean increments subtracted or added to get means at 2 and 3: 5-16 cross-sectional. (Skinfolds in log transformed units.) From 22

1. *Anatomical methods:* Fig. 1 shows the thickness of the subcutaneous fat layer in boys and girls from birth to 18 years. In both sexes the fat layers decrease between 1 and 7 years and then rise slowly. In girls, who have more fat than boys at all ages, the fat layer continues to increase in thickness during puberty. Boys show a different pattern; the subscapular skinfold continues to rise during puberty, as

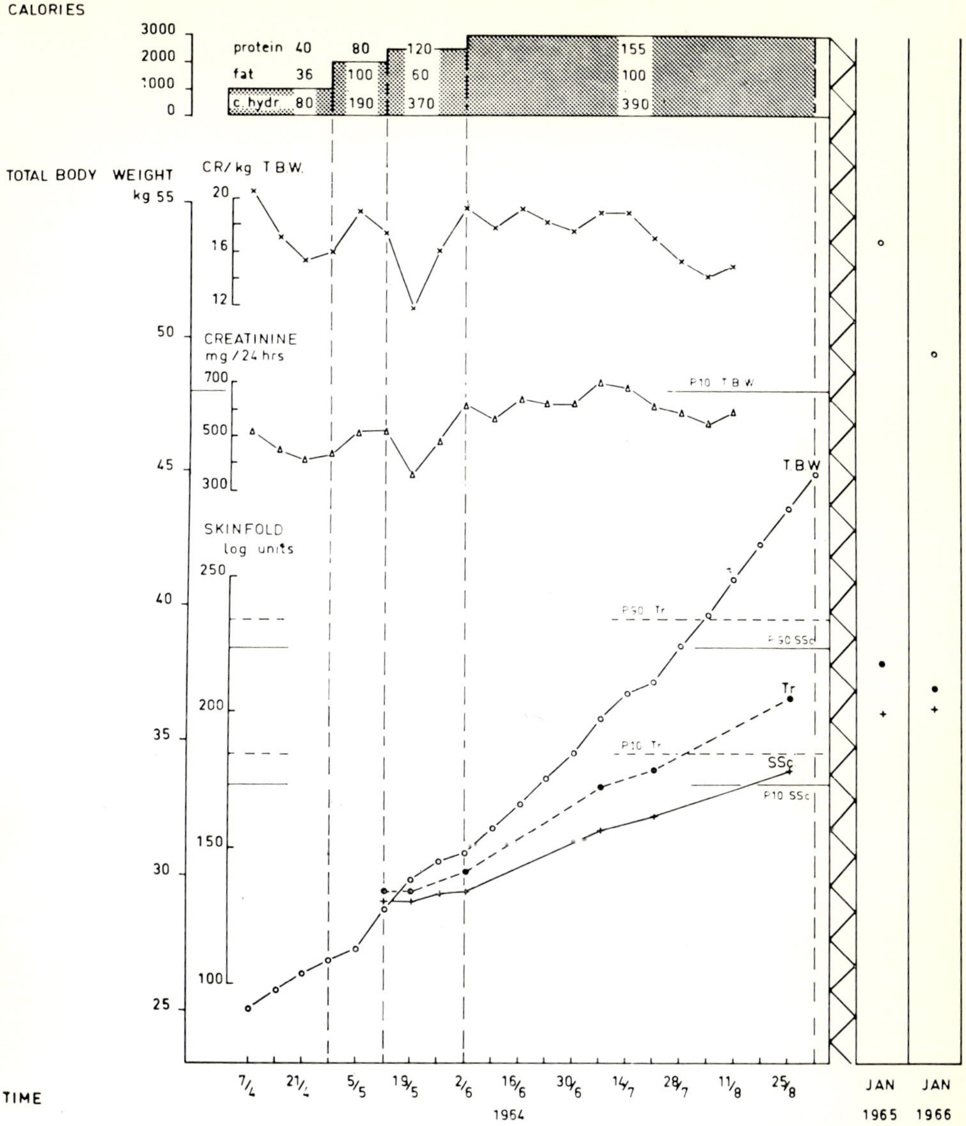

Plate 1. Example of a combination of underweight and high fat content.
Body weights, triceps and subscapular skinfold measurements and creatinine excretion of a girl with anorexia nervosa during refeeding. Height 161.3 cm. Chronological age 18 years, bone age 14 years. Percentiles for a girl of 16 years. Note that at a time when body weight is still below the 10th percentile, the triceps skinfold is in the normal range whilst the creatinine coefficient is subnormal (normal is about 21, see 18). Percentiles for weight: see 30; for skinfolds, see 23

in girls, but the fat layer over the triceps muscle of the arm falls sharply when puberty sets in.

A decrease in thickness of the fat layer may be due to fat loss or to growth of the limb which causes the same amount of fat to be spread over a greater surface. Considered in relation to such measurements as limb circumference, changes in skinfold thickness may indicate alterations in the relative amounts of the various components.

Experiments in animals have shown that testosterone may cause fat mobilization (20), along with nitrogen retention. There are large differences in the muscle response to androgens between different species and, within a species, between different muscles. The increase in trunk fat and the decrease in limb fat noted in boys during puberty, suggest that regional differences in testosterone sensitivity exist also for fat tissue.

An example of a clinical longitudinal study in which anatomical methods (skinfold caliper and soft tissue radiography), were used to a ascertain alterations in fat and muscle components, concerned a 13-year-old girl treated with a synthetic steroid. The girl was stunted in growth following tuberculous meningitis at 7 years; she had diabetes insipidus, her serum growth hormone level was too low to be demonstable by the radio-immune method, and she was prepuberal. Adrenal and thyroid function tests gave normal results. Treatment consisted of norandrostenolone-phenyl-proponiate, 25 mg intramuscularly every fortnight for 13 months. The growth rate in height was not affected, but an increase in muscle and a loss of fat were noted in the upper arm and calf (12, 26) (fig. 2). These changes are similar to those which occur in boys during puberty, with one exception: the trunk fat (subscapular skinfold) also decreased during treatment, while this is not seen in the cross-sectional data of boys during puberty.

2. *Chemical methods:* Friis-Hansen (10) has estimated the water content of children of different ages. After birth the total water content dropped from about 80 %, to a value of 60 % of the body weight at 2 years. Nearly all of this fall concerned the extra-cellular compartment. From 2 years the total water content remained constant, but a gradual shift took place from the extra-cellular into the intra-cellular compartment.

The body thus seemed to gain mainly cells with a relatively high water content, presumably muscle cells.

In Friis-Hansen's material there were no sex differences. Owen et al. (19) studied children at ages 131—270 days and found values for the total body water content of 59.9 % in 16 boys, and of 56.3%

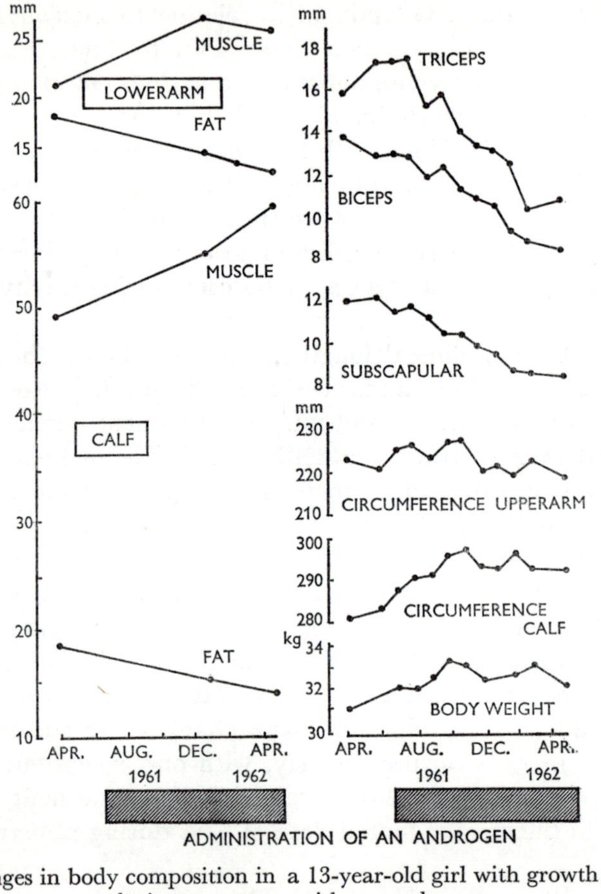

Fig. 2. Changes in body composition in a 13-year-old girl with growth retardation, during treatment with an androgen
On the left: measurements on soft tissue radiographs,
On the right: skinfold measurements, limb circumferences and body weight

in 10 girls. In adult males the water content is also higher than in adult females.

The method of Lesser (13) for the estimation of total body fat content by means of fat-soluble gasses (cyclopropane or Krypton), has not yet been applied to the study of children.

The method by which the fat compartment is calculated from data obtained by total body water estimations, is based upon the assumptions that fat tissue contains no water and that the fat-free compartment has a constant water content (of about 72 % for adults).

Table 1. *Total body water (T) extra-cellular (E) and water intra-cellular water (I) during growth, expressed as percent of total body weight (data from 10).*

Age	T	E	I
0— 1 day	79.0	43.9	34.7
1—10 days	74.0	39.7	31.8
1— 3 months	72.3	32.2	43.3
3— 6 months	70.1	30.1	42.1
6—12 months	60.4	27.4	35.2
1— 2 years	58.7	25.6	33.8
2— 3 years	63.5	26.7	38.3
3— 5 years	62.2	21.4	45.7
5—10 years	61.5	22.0	42.3
10—16 years	58.0	18.7	46.7

3. *Physical methods:* The body content of the natural radioisotope of potassium (K^{40}) can be measured with the whole-body counter. It is assumed that fat contains no potassium, so that the lean body mass can be calculated from the amount measured, the fact that 0.012 % of body potassium is radio active, and the assumption that the lean body mass has a constant potassium content. Forbes et al. (6, 7) found an average potassium content of four carcasses of adult men of 68.1 mEq K/kg. Anderson and Langham, taking into account the water content of fat tissue, used the value of .73m Eq K/kg (1). One of the technical problems involved is constituted by the facts that the body build varies from one individual to another, and that K is not uniformly distributed in the body (16).

Forbes and Hursh (6) studied males and females from the age of 7 years onwards. It appeared that the rise in body weight from that age is almost entirely attributable to a gain in lean body mass. The fat content is lower (in percent of body weight) in boys than in girls. At ages over 20 years body weight increments consist entirely of fat, while the lean body mass remains constant. Expressed as a percentage of total body weight, L.B.M. and fat remain constant, 75 % and 25 % respectively, from the age of 8 up to 40 in males, with the exception of a short period in puberty, in which L.B.M. increases and fat content decreases (15). This finding confirms the skinfold data described above. In females, fat content increases steadily from about 25 % at the age of 8 to 45 % up to the age of 70. Consequently

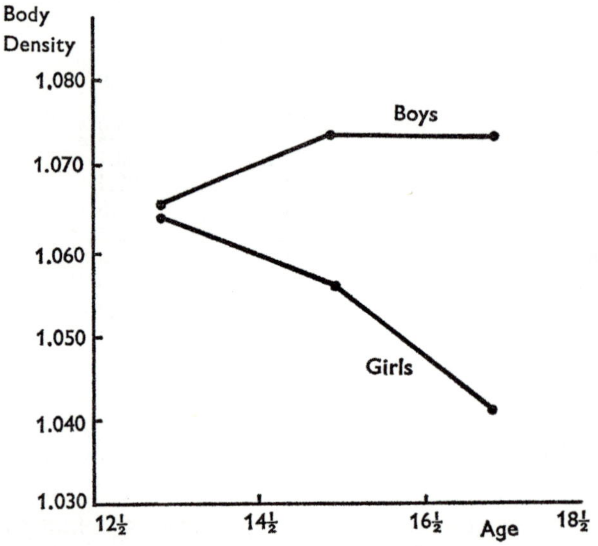

Fig. 3. Body density, measured by underwater weighing, in boys and girls according to age groups (data from 18)

L.B.M. decreases in the same period from about 75 % to 55 % (15).

Specific gravity determinations by measuring body volume are very well suited for physiological studies, and many such studies have been carried out. Novak (18) used the method of underwater weighing for a study of children aged 12—18 years (fig. 3). Over this age range the specific gravity of girls decreased while that of boys increased. A fall in specific gravity concomitant with a rise in body weight indicates a percentual increase in fat content.

CONCLUSIONS

The results of the studies discussed, show good agreement with the results of carcass analyses (table 2).

Table 2. *Results of carcass analyses of newborns and adults*

Subjects	Water	Fat	Nitrogen	References
	(in per cent of body weight)			
Six new-borns	69.1	16.1 (11—28)	1.9 (1.7—2.2)	27
Five adults	60 (55—70)	17.5 (4.3—28)	2.7 (2.3—3.1)	8, 9, 17, 29

The water content of the newborn is higher than that of the adult, its protein content is lower; the fat content is similar in the two categories.

Investigations in this particular field of human biology must be concentrated upon further 'dissection' of the lean body mass. The skeleton presents particular problems, which seem difficult to solve (11).

REFERENCES

1. ANDERSON, E. C. and W. H. LANGHAM, Estimation of total body fat from potassium-40 content, *Science* 133: 1917, 1961.
2. BARTER, J. and G. B. FORBES, Correlation of potassium-40 data with anthropometic measurements, *Ann. N.Y. Acad. Sci.* 110: 264, 1963.
3. BEHNKE, A. R., B. G. FEEN and W. C. WELHAM, The specific gravity of healthy men, *J.A.M.A.* 118: 495, 1942.
4. VON DÖBELN, W., Human standard and maximal metabolic rate in relation to fat-free body mass, *Acta Physiol. Scandinav.* (suppl. 126) 37: 1, 1956.
5. FORBES, G. B., Methods for determining composition of the human body, *Pediatrics* 29: 477, 1962.
6. FORBES, G. B. and J. B. HURSH, Age and sex trends in lean body mass calculated from K^{40} measurements, *Ann. N.Y. Acad. Sci.* 110: 255, 1963.
7. FORBES, G. B., J. GALLUP and J. B. HURSH, Estimation of total body fat from potassium-40 content, *Science* 133: 101, 1961.
8. FORBES, R. M., A. R. COOPER and H. H. MITCHELL, The composition of the adult human body as determined by chemical analysis, *J. Biol. Chem.* 203: 359, 1953.
9. FORBES, R. M., H. H. MITCHELL and A. R. COOPER, Further studies on the gross composition and mineral elements of the adult human body, *J. Biol. Chem.* 203: 969, 1956.

10. FRIIS-HANSEN, B., Changes in body water compartments during growth, *Acta Paediatrica* Suppl. 110: 1—67, 1956.
11. GARN, S. M., Human biology and research in body composition, *Ann. N.Y. Acad. Sci.* 110: 429, 1963.
12. HAAK, A., *Studies over de werking van humaan groeihormoon en testosteron op de eiwitstofwisseling van de mens*, J. J. Groen en Zoon N.V., Leiden, 1963.
13. LESSER, G. I., W. PERL and J. M. STEELE, Determination of total body fat by absorption of an inert gas; measurements and results in normal human subjects, *J. Clin. Invest.* 39: 1791, 1960.
14. LIM, T. P. K. and U. C. LUFT, Body density, fat and fat-free weight, *Am. J. of Med.* 30: 825, 1961.
15. MENEELY, G. R., R. M. HEYSSEL, C. O. T. BALL, R. L. WEILAND, A. ROSS-DORIMER and C. CONSTANTINIDES, Analysis of factors affecting body composition determined from potassium content in 915 normal subjects, *Ann. N.Y. Acad. Sci.* 110: 271, 1963.
16. MILLER, C. E. and A. P. REMENCHIK, Problems involved in accurately measuring the K content of the human body, *Ann. N.Y. Acad. Sci.* 110: 175, 1963.
17. MITCHELL, H. H., J. S. HAMILTON, F. R. STAPPERDEN and H. W. BEAN, The chemical composition of the adult human body and its bearing on the biochemistry of growth, *J. Biol. Chem.* 158: 625, 1945.
18. NOVAK, L. P., Age and sex differences in body density and creatinine excretion of high school children, *Ann. N.Y. Acad. Sci.* 110: 545, 1963.
19. OWEN, G. M., R. L. JENSEN, L. N. THOMAS and S. J. FOMON, Influence of age, sex and diet on total bodywater of four- to seven month old infants, *Ann. N.Y. Acad. Sci.* 110: 861, 1963.
20. SCOW, R. O., Effect of testosterone on muscle and other tissues and on carcass composition in hypophysectomized, thyroidectomized and gonadoectomized male rats, *Endocrinology* 51: 42, 1952.
21. SIRI, W. E., Gross composition of the body, *Advances in Biology and Medical Physics* 4: 239, 1956.
22. TANNER, J. M., *Growth at adolescence*, Blackwell Scientific Publication, Oxford, 2nd ed., 1962.
23. TANNER, J. M. and R. H. WHITEHOUSE, Standards for subcutaneous fat in British children, *Brit. Med. J.* 1: 446, 1962.
24. TAYLOR, H. L., J. BROZEK and A. KEYS, Basal cardiac function and body composition with special reference to obesity, *J. Clin. Invest.* 31: 976, 1952.
25. WERDEIN, E. J. and L. H. KYLE, Estimation of the constancy of density of the fat-free body, *J. Clin. Invest.* 39 I: 626, 1960.
26. WERFF TEN BOSCH, J. J. VAN DER, *Proteinmetabolism*, p. 401, Springer-Verlag, Heidelberg, 1962.
27. WHIPPLE, H. E., S. SILVERZWEIG and J. BROZEK (editors), Body composition, *Ann. N.Y. Acad. Sci.* 110, 1963.
28. WIDDOWSON, E. M., Chemical composition of newly born mammals, *Nature* 166: 626, 1950.
29. WIDDOWSON, E. M., R. A. MCCANCE and C. M. SPRAY, The chemical composition of the human body, *Clin. Sci.* 10: 113, 1951.
30. WIJN, J. F. DE and J. H. DE HAAS, Groeidiagrammen van 1—25 jarigen in Nederland, *Verhandelingen van het Ned. Inst. v. Praev. Geneesk.*, no. 49, Leiden 1960.
31. YOUNG, C. M., R. S. TENSUAN, R. S. SAULT and F. HOLMES, Estimating body fat of normal young women, *J. Am. Diet. A.* 42: 409, 1963.

CHANGING LEVELS OF BLOOD CONSTITUENTS DURING GROWTH

J. F. DE WIJN

In growth there is a fairly uniform pattern of changing levels for various blood constituents, which are often used for diagnosis of either somatic growth and development, or nutriture. Some of those reflect metabolic activity of the body as a whole, others are expression of the nutritional state. In either case, however, the constituents of the blood fail to reflect the dynamic action of metabolism in the cells but inform us about the concentration of nutrients on their way to the tissues and of metabolites in transport from one tissue to the other, on their way to depots or to the exit for excretion. Their concentrations in blood have been compared with people crowded in the streets of London on their way either to the coronation or to a royal funeral, but not attending the actual ceremonies.

One of the main characteristics of blood chemistry related to health is that findings in the blood are expressions of *individual biochemistry*, with a wide range of so-called normality. This wide variation no doubt includes also abnormal concentrations, both at the upper and lower limits of the range and in the middle of it. It is up to the clinician to decide which should be normal for the individual case which is under his care, using various diagnostic tools beside blood chemistry. In addition to individuality, the result of blood estimations depends on the techniques used in various laboratories and on the age and quality of the instruments as well as of the observer. Interlaboratory exchange of results and techniques is an indispensable means for the evaluation of data obtained, and will promote the standardization of techniques.

Nevertheless it is necessary to be informed about the usual pattern of growth and the 'range of normality' at each developmental age as found in healthy children, i.e. which are not obviously ill or undernourished. There is little information on chemical growth from longitudinal studies. We present the results of the estimation in the blood of some constituents from various cross-sectional or mixed longitudinal studies in the Netherlands, from school age through adolescence.

HAEMOGLOBIN

In infancy, at pre-school age and at school age, haemoglobin levels are not different for boys and girls. Tables 1 and 2 present averages from various surveys on toddlers, pre-school children and school children

Table 1. *Haemoglobin of infants and pre-school children in grams/100 ml (Unpublished data from the Netherlands Institute of Preventive Medicine, Leiden,* DONATH *and* LEEWIS, *1955). Siccameter method.*

Age	N	Boys s.d.	N	Girls s.d.
18 mth	34	12.3 1.1	29	12.7 1.0
24 mth	17	12.6 1.2	14	12.6 0.5
30 mth	23	12.6 1.0	25	12.7 0.8
36 mth	29	12.8 0.9	20	12.6 0.8
42 mth	15	12.6 0.9	15	13.1 0.7
48 mth	9	12.5 0.6	17	12.6 0.8
4—6 years	104	13.0 0.6	101	13.0 0.6

Table 2. *Haemoglobin at school age and during adolescence in grams/100 ml of healthy prosperous children (Eight-year-olds from the school children survey 1964, Nutrition Council of the Netherlands,* ADAM, *Siccameter method; others from the Central Institute for Nutrition and Food Research T.N.O., HiCN-method,* PIKAAR *and* DE WIJN).

Age (yrs)	N	Boys s.d.	N	Girls s.d.
8— 9	724	13.5 0.6	719	13.4 0.6
12—13	106	14.4 0.7	59	14.2 1.0
14—15	60	14.8 0.8	—	— —
16—19	109	15.5 0.8	—	— —
20—30	107	15.2 0.9	41	13.8 1.0

in the period 1955—1965. Haemoglobin levels go up from 12.5 to 13.5 g/100 ml. Standard deviations are higher for toddlers than at school age. In the latter a s.d. of 0.6—0.7 g is the usual finding. In a well-nourished population there is a tendency to lower averages in school children from a low social class and from large families, when compared with children from prosperous c.q. small families (5, 6, 16). From 10 years onwards, haemoglobin levels of boys and girls differ (fig. 1). At 13 years averages range from 13.5 to 14.5 g/100 ml for

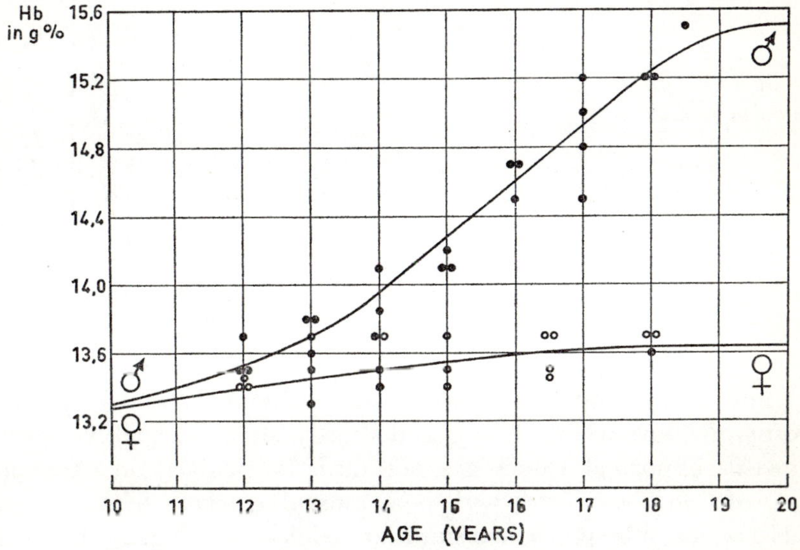

Fig. 1. Haemoglobin levels for boys and girls during adolescence in the Netherlands (1955—1960). From 16

boys and from 13.2—14.2 g/100 ml for girls, depending on the social class. In late adolescence (table 2) 15.5 g/100 ml for boys and 13.8 g/100 ml for girls, are normal averages in the Netherlands (12c, 4).

The increase in haemoglobin concentration in boys is due to an increase in red blood corpuscles which accompanies muscle growth. From 12 to 18 years a boy's Hb value therefore depends on his degree of maturity and on his physique or body build.

When maturity is the criterion of development, estimated by the appearance of pubic hair, the increase of Hb of boys from prosperous families appears to be sustained in the P_2 maturity-group, when the growth spurt commences. While in boys from non-prosperous families the overall level is low, the increase of Hb is sustained through P_3, when the growth spurt reaches its greatest velocity. Cross-sectional averages from each maturity group are presented in table 3. Standard deviations during adolescence are higher than at school

Table 3. *Haemoglobin during adolescent growth of boys at different maturity stages. Prosperous and non-prosperous families compared.*

	P_1	P_2	P_3	P_4	P_{5+6}
Prosperous families					
n	17	38	23	67	55
mean	14.4	14.2	14.7	15.2	15.9
s.d.	0.9	0.5	0.8	0.8	0.8
Non-prosperous families					
n	36	30	33	27	16
mean	13.8	14.3	14.3	14.7	15.2
s.d.	0.9	0.7	1.1	0.9	0.7

age and may be up to 1 g/100 ml and more in P_3 and P_4 for non-prosperous boys when, during and shortly after the peak velocity of growth, subnormal values are not rare. Particularly in ectomorph types of thin body build, with poor muscular development, the gain in Hb seems to be postponed until late adolescence (fig. 2). In a longitudinal follow-up of institutional boys from non-prosperous families (15) we estimated Hb every half-year; the actual increment per year for different maturity groups is shown in table 4. There is a significant rise in subsequent maturity groups except for the youngest still puerile boys among the P_1's, who after one year are still P_1. The older P_1-boys ($P_{1\frac{1}{2}}$) who proceed within one year to the P_2-stage, with first appearance of pubic hair, reached a higher level of Hb at the expense of serum iron (fig. 3). All the other maturity groups that proceeded to the next or second next P-stage within one year, showed an increase in Hb and serum iron content.

In girls, there is a small rise in Hb from 13.3 to nearly 13.7 g/100 ml with increasing age (fig. 1). Among adolescent girls from prosperous and non-prosperous families VAN 'T LAND and DE HAAS (13) and

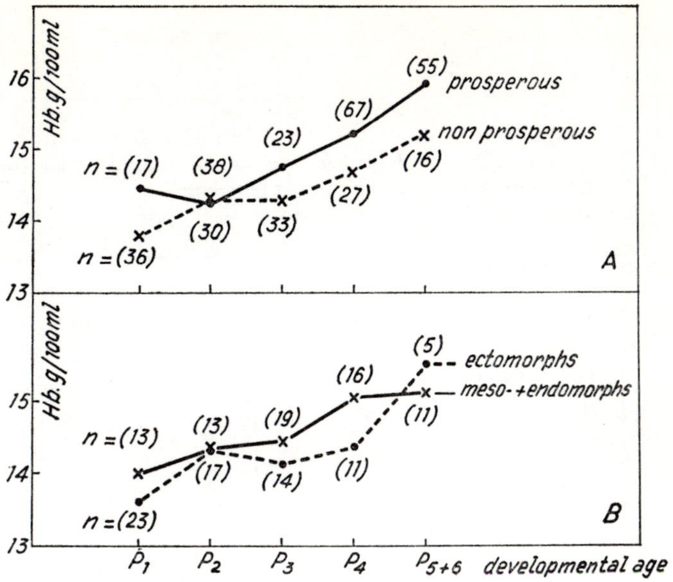

Fig. 2. Haemoglobin during adolescent growth for boys. Developmental age by maturity ratings from public hair appearance

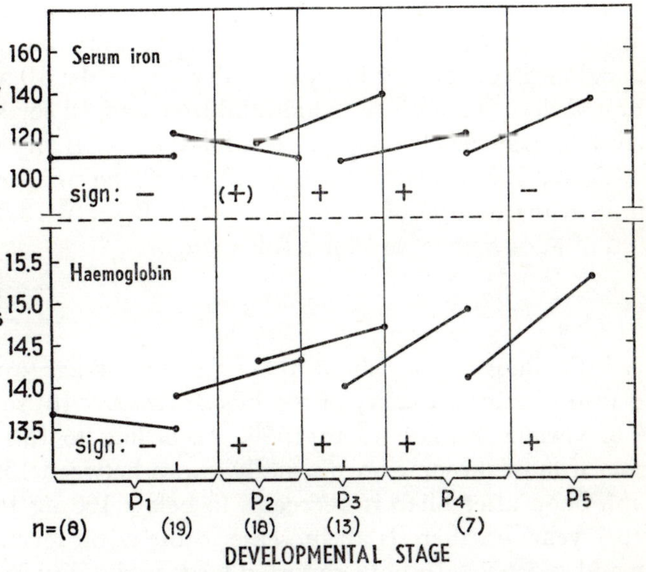

Fig. 3. Mean annual change in haemoglobin and serum iron in adolescent boys at different maturity stages

Table 4. *Mean increments of Hb per year in adolescent boys at different maturity stages.*

Central age (yrs)	Maturity group at 1st exam. and 1 year after	Number	Hb g/100 ml at 1st exam.	Increment after 1 year	s.d. of the mean
12.7	$P_1 \rightarrow P_1$	8	13.71	—0.2	0.46
13.5	$P_{1\frac{1}{2}} \rightarrow P_2$ or P_3	19	13.90	0.45*	0.21
13.7	$P_2 \rightarrow P_3$ or P_4	18	14.35	0.38	0.21
14.0	$P_3 \rightarrow P_4$ or P_5	13	13.98	0.92*	0.42
14.6	$P_4 \rightarrow P_5$	7	14.14	1.17*	0.54

* significant at 5 % level

SELTZER et al. (10) failed to find a difference in Hb-values between pre- and post-menarcheal girls in single age groups.

From these data on apparently healthy children and adolescents, as well as from other studies in the literature, it appears that the following haemoglobin concentrations are borderline levels: 10.5 g/100 ml blood for toddlers, 11 for pre-school children and 12 for school age and early adolescence (12 years). In adolescent girls the borderline level remains 12 g/100 ml and for boys 13 should be considered as the lower limit in the middle of adolescence (P_2—P_4) and 13.5 g/100 ml at the end of adolescence and for adult men.

SERUM IRON

There is little information about the influence of age upon serum iron and iron-binding capacity of the blood. RAMSAY (8) summarized findings of various studies up to 1956. According to this summary the plasma iron of the new-born usually varies between 150 and 200 μg/100 ml. Soon after birth it decreases to below 100 μg/100 ml and from 3 to 7 years on there is an increase to the adult level. SELTZER, WENZEL and MAYER (10) have reported large variability in the serum iron of adolescents, with sex differences as well as age variations. They found serum iron to be positively correlated with age in boys and negatively in girls. Obese boys and girls were found to have lower serum iron and greater iron-binding capacities than their non-obese counterparts. They summarized the findings obtained in various studies in adults, which varied from 105—145 μg/100 ml as group average for men, and from 95—125 μg/100 ml for women. Averages for unsaturated iron-binding capacities varied from 195—220 μg/100 ml in men and from 195—250 μg/100 ml in women.

In the Netherlands at 9 years serum iron (TRINDLER, colorimetric method) was found to average 93 ± 30 μg/100 ml in boys and 88 ± 29 μg/100 ml in girls in the Southern districts. In the Northern districts, where the general level of health is higher, averages were somewhat higher but not above 100 μg/100 ml (6). Unsaturated iron-binding capacities were 254 ± 47 μg/100 ml, and percentages of saturation 27.3 ± 8 for boys; in girls we found similar average levels, but higher standard deviations (table 5). Mean serum iron levels varied from 80 μg/100 ml in children from large families in non-prosperous socio-economic groups, to 105 μg/100 ml in prosperous groups and small families.

Table 5. *Serum iron and iron-binding capacity at school age and early adolescence (longitudinal).*

		Boys			Girls			
Central age (yrs)	Number	Serum iron μg/100 ml	Unsatur. iron-bind. cap. μg/100	Percent of saturation	Number	Serum iron μg/100 ml	Unsatur. iron-bind. cap. μg/100	Percent of saturation
9 1/4	55	93.4 ± 30.2	254 ± 47	27.3±8.1	62	88.3 ± 29.0	255 ± 58	26.1±9.9
13 1/4	55	96.1 ± 35.2	260 ± 54	27.4±10	62	93.8 ± 33.0	267 ± 57	26.5±9.7

When the same children were examined 4 years later, at the age of 13 years, approximately the same average levels were obtained in the same laboratory, though the standard deviations were higher. When we consider a combination of 50 μg/100 ml or less serum iron, and a percentage of saturation less than 15 % as diagnostic for iron deficiency in school children, 5—6 % of the 13-year-old children in this series had iron deficiency (9 cases out of 155 boys and girls together). Haemoglobin values in those iron deficient children ranged from 11.7 to 14.7 g %, and were less than 12 g % in two instances.

SELTZER, WENZEL, and MAYER (10) have published serum iron levels for boys and girls, that at 13½ years average 92 and 96 μg/100 ml, which is comparable to our figures. At an earlier age (before puberty or menarche, at 12½ years) a remarkable sex difference was found by these authors, with boys as low as 81 and girls 113 μg/100 ml. The small difference in our series between boys and girls at 13¼ years indicates an opposite trend, which was already noticeable at the age of 9 years.

In a mixed longitudinal study of growth in boys through puberty (12—17 years) (15) we found a steady rise of serum iron levels in subsequent maturity groups from 110 in the prepubertal P_1 stage up to 130 μg/100 ml in late adolescence (P_5) (table 6). The annual increment in different maturity groups was significant in the P_2 and P_3

Table 6. *Serum iron during adolescent growth of 12—17 years-old adolescent boys (mixed longitudinal).*

Developmental stage	P_1	P_2	P_3	P_4	P_5
Serum iron μg/100 ml	111	113	119	120	131
stand. dev.	31	45	38	34	38
number	36	30	33	27	16

stages. There was no increment, but rather a tendency to decrement, in P_1 maturity group (fig. 3). Also in this series, the thin boys (ectomorphs) had higher levels than the boys of medium and endomorph body build (fig. 4), which agrees with SELTZER's findings of low serum iron values in obese boys. Our starting level in early adolescence in this series is 15 μg higher than we found in the first series, at the age of 13 years (table 4). This difference may be due to the fact that estimations were done in a different laboratory. The trend however, of higher levels of serum iron through adolescence in boys, is evident, and the same was found in SELTZER's series, where serum iron varied with age from 81 to 131 μg/100 ml in boys. We do not know what

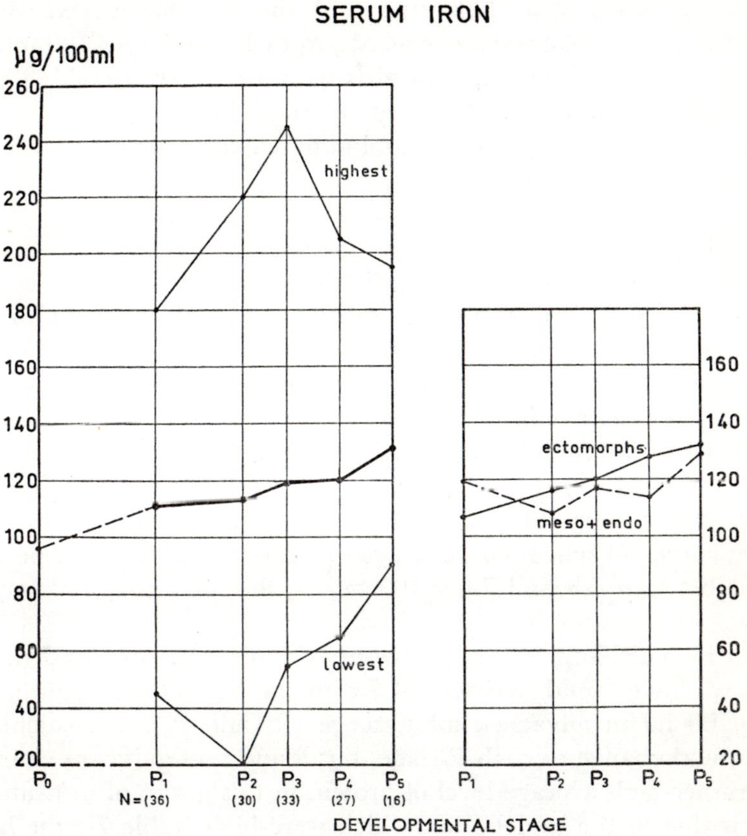

Fig. 4. Serum iron in adolescent boys. Developmental stage by maturity ratings from pubic hair appearance (mixed longitudinal) (From 15)

the lower limit of normality is for serum iron during adolescent growth. In adults, levels of 75 μg/100 ml and less, with unsaturated iron-binding capacity of 300 μg/100 ml or more, are considered subnormal by clinicians. Even if the borderline value for adolescent boys were 60 μg/100 ml, 7 out of 142 estimations in this group (5 %)

would be subnormal, and all of these occurred in maturity groups P_1 to P_3 (99 estimations), so that 7 % of the serum iron values in early adolescence were subnormal. In only two cases was the haemoglobin was less than 13 mg%, which we consider the lower limit of normality in adolescent boys.

In SELTZER's cross-sectional study (10) the trend for girls was downward from early adolescence onwards, from 113 to 86 μg/100 ml. We have only figures for adolescent girls with a central age of 13¼ years in our series (table 5). Contrary to SELTZER's findings, both the serum iron and unsaturated iron-binding capacity tend to be higher at 13 years than at 9 years, as in boys.

SERUM PROTEIN AND PROTEIN FRACTIONS

Results of the estimation of serum protein, and particularly of protein fractions, vary widely between laboratories. There is, however, general agreement that after 18 months of life the protein concentration does not alter with increasing age. From 1 to 14 years GEUDEKE en STAHLIE (2) found no variations in cross-sectional averages of serum protein (average of 7.04 g/100 ml, s.d. 0.59), in either healthy Dutch children or children with minor respiratory infections. In a Dutch survey of school children aged 9 years, mean levels of proteins varied between 7.3 and 7.6 g/100 ml (2) for both girls and boys of various socio-economic groups.

In a 1½ years' longitudinal follow-up of adolescent boys aged 12—15 years we have found averages of 7.6 in the P_1-maturity group, and 7.8 g/100 ml in advanced adolescence (P_4 and P_5). We calculated the annual change at each P-stage, but found no significant changes. The rather high average level of protein in this group of institutional boys is due to the γ-globulins, which were high (table 7); the latter finding may be due to the great number of minor infections which occur in children's homes. In these otherwise apparently healthy children, the serum protein level is probably related to physique or body-build. Ectomorphs tend to have higher levels, of up to an average of 8.0 g/100 ml in late adolescence (15).

More significance in terms of nutritional health, must be attached to the albumin fraction. In the Dutch school children survey (6), 60 % of total protein was derived from albumin, at 9 years, varying with socio-economic conditions; in intermediate social classes children from large families had 57 % albumin, against 62 % in children from small families (4.16 and 4.71 g/100 ml respectively). GEUDEKE and STAHLIE found an average value of 4.18 g/100 ml from 1 to 14 years, with no variations with age (2).

Table 7. *Total protein and protein fractions in g/100 ml serum during adolescent growth of 12—16-year-old boys (mixed longitudinal).*

	Developmental stage				
	P_1	P_2	P_3	P_4	P_5
total protein	7.64 ± 0.52	7.70 ± 0.57	7.68 ± 0.54	7.79 ± 0.54	7.79 ± 0.43
albumin	3.86	3.66	3.58	3.46	3.51
α_1-globulin	0.38	0.42	0.43	0.44	0.41
α_2-globulin	0.89	0.93	0.91	0.95	0.93
β-globulin	1.06	1.12	1.13	1.19	1.16
γ-globulin	1.48	1.57	1.63	1.75	1.78
number	28	27	30	24	16

In 12 to 16-year-old boys who were examined every half-year during 1½ years we found a trend of decreasing albumin levels as adolescence proceeded (table 7). These small differences will almost certainly be levelled out when chronological age is used instead of the developmental stage. In each maturity group up to P_3 the actual annual decrement of the albumin concentration is significant (table 8, fig. 5). The rather low level of albumin in this particular study may be artificial because of difficulties that have arisen with the standardisation of paper electrophoresis. Therefore the level may be higher but the trend towards lower levels throughout adolescence is suggestive for the influence of growth. After the administration of human growth hormone the first effect on protein metabolism is a lowering of amino acids and urea in plasma (9). There are also observations which indicate that androgens cause a decrease in serum albumin concentration (14). Also, with testosterone and other anabolic steroids, more sulphur is excreted with urine, which again indicates changes in protein substances in the body. Therefore, the change in albumin concentration noted during puberty is suggestive for an influence of either growth hormone or androgens on the metabolism of protein substances.

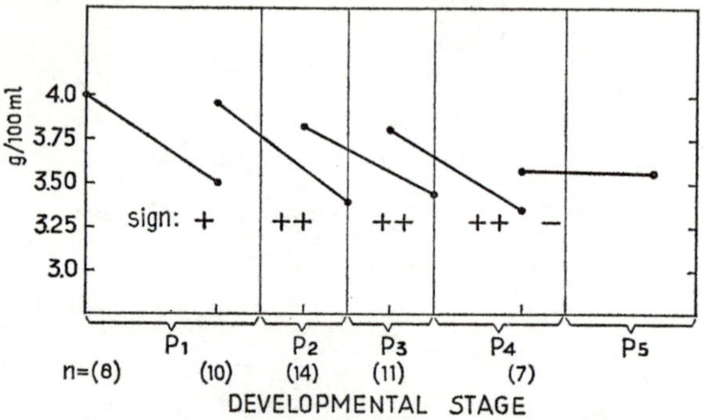

Fig. 5. Mean annual decrease of serum albumin in adolescent boys at different maturity stages

In the mixed longitudinal averages of table 7, most of the globulin fractions tend to rise, from P_1 up to P_4. An annual increment of the α_1- and β-fractions was noted (significant at either 5 % or 1 % level of significance) only at the P_1, P_2 and P_3 developmental stages, in a longitudinal study.

Table 8. *Mean annual decrease of albumin in serum of adolescent boys of different maturity groups.*

Central age (years)	Maturity group at 1st exam. and after 1 year	Number	Albumin g/100 ml at 1st exam.	Increment after 1 year	S.D. of the mean
12.7	$P_1 \rightarrow P_1$	8	4.07	—0.56*	0.22
13.5	$P_{1\frac{1}{2}} \rightarrow P_2$ or P_3	10	3.93	—0.55**	0.18
13.7	$P_2 \rightarrow P_3$ or P_4	14	3.83	—0.39**	0.14
14.0	$P_3 \rightarrow P_4$ or P_5	11	3.80	—0.45**	0.09
14.7	$P_4 \rightarrow P_5$	7	3.58	—0.03	0.10

* significant at 5 % level
** significant at 1 % level

ALKALINE PHOSPHATASE

Another blood constituent which may reflect hormone levels during growth, is the serum alkaline phosphatase. According to the earlier work by CLARK and BECK, alkaline phosphatase levels parallel the velocity curve for height during the growth period (1). The curve demonstrated a fall in the first 3 or 4 years of life, continuing at a fairly constant level till the age of 11 years, and followed in boys by a pubertal rise, with its peak at 13 years and a subsequent steep fall to the adult level. In girls there is no evidence for a pubertal rise in the figures of CLARK and BECK, but HARRISON et al. have found a small rise in girls too (3).

For alkaline phosphatase activity in serum of children (table 11), we have found that there was at each age a large variability, of 100 % and more below and above the average. Each child seems to have his own level, characteristic for the individual. At 9 years the alkaline phosphatase levels averaged 7.4 $\pm$ 2.1 (boys) and 7.9 $\pm$ 2.1 (girls) Bodansky units per 100 ml serum. There is some evidence in these cross-sectional data for a small rise at puberty in girls, with the highest level at 12 years. In boys a rise is evident, with its peak at 14 years (table 11, fig. 6). With the same technique 2.8 has been found in young adult males, and 3.6 B.U./100 ml in females.

In a group of 32 adolescent boys (age 12—16 years) who were examined at 6 months' intervals for 1½ years, we (5) found a cross-sectional average for the P_1 maturity group of 11.3 B.U./100 ml

Table 9. *Alkaline phosphatase in serum during adolescent growth of 12 to 16-year-old boys (mixed longitudinal).*

Developmental stage	P_0*	P_1	P_2	P_3	P_4	P_5
Height velocity (cm/yr)	5.3	4.9	7.1	8.2	6.4	3.4
Alkaline phosphatase (B.U./100 ml)	7.4	11.3	12.3	12.3	11.7	8.8
Stand. dev.	2.1	3.6	4.7	4.4	3.8	2.6
Number	141	36	30	33	27	16

* age 8—9, school children survey in the Netherlands (6)

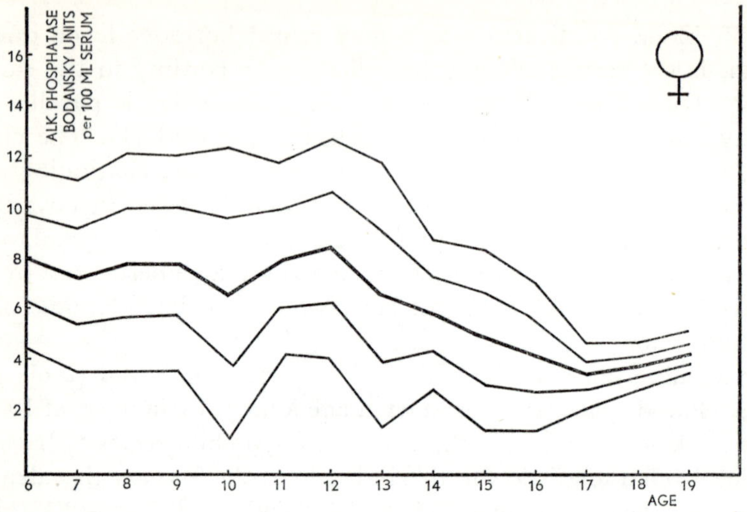

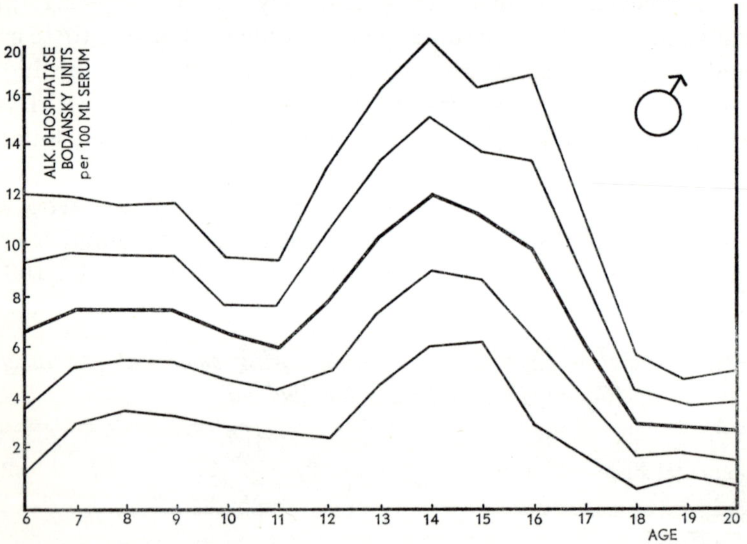

Fig. 6. Alkaline phosphatase in serum (Bodansky Units) by age, cross-sectional. The thinner lines indicate one and two standard deviationlevels above and below the mean (thick line). (Unpublished, Netherlands Institute of Preventive Medicine, Donath and De Wijn, 1952—1956)

(central age 12.7 years), and 12.3 B.U./100 ml in early adolescence, when pubic hair first appears (P_2, central age 13.6 years). This level was maintained through P_3, started to decrease in P_4 (central age 14.5 years), and had fallen markedly in P_5 (table 9). Ectomorphs had a higher average level than those with medium or endomorph types of body build (15).

For each developmental stage the actual change in alkaline phosphatase activity over the subsequent year was followed. In pre-

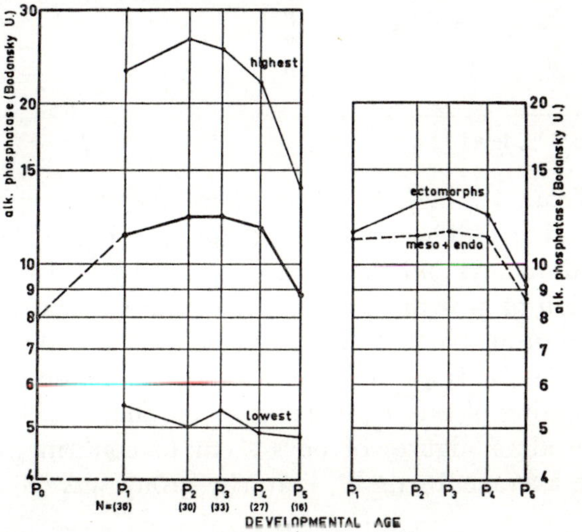

Fig. 7. Alkaline phosphatase activity of adolescent boys at different maturity-stages (mixed longitunidal)

pubertal P_1, when growth in height slowed down, there was a significant fall in phosphatase activity, when they did not reach P_2. For the older boys in P_1 ($P_{1\frac{1}{2}}$ in table 10), who proceeded to P_2, and for P_2's who reached P_3 or P_4 in the subsequent year, the large range of individual variations did not result in significant increments for these small groups. For P_3 there was a significant decrease during the year that followed (table 10).

INORGANIC PHOSPHATE

Serum inorganic phosphate is higher in children than in adults. Figures from the Netherlands are presented in table 11, (cross-

Table 10. *Mean annual changes in serum alkaline phosphatase activity at different maturity stages of adolescent boys between 12 and 15 years.*

Central age at 1st exam. (yrs)	Maturity 1st exam. — 1 year after	Number	Alk. phosph. at first examin. B.U. %	Increment per year	S.D. of the mean
12.7	$P_1 \rightarrow P_1$	8	11.2	—1.6*	0.6
13.5	$P_{1\frac{1}{2}} \rightarrow P_2$ or P_3	18	13.3	—0.2	0.7
13.7	$P_2 \rightarrow P_3$ or P_4	18	12.0	—0.8	0.6
14.0	$P_3 \rightarrow P_4$ or P_5	13	12.3	—1.9*	0.8
14.6	$P_4 \rightarrow P_5$	10	11.8	—3.3	1.9

* sginificant at 5 % level

sectional). From 4.7 mg/100 ml at school age there appears to be a fall before puberty. There is a trend towards higher levels from 12 years onwards in boys and girls, and again a fall from 16 years onwards. Administration of growth hormone raises the concentration of inorganic phosphate in blood (7). In adolescent boys, the physiological response to exercise is an increase of inorganic phosphate concentration in circulating blood (4), which may parallel muscle growth. Our mixed longitudinal figures of boys seem to confirm this view (15) (fig. 8). The average for the P_1 maturity group was 4.8 mg, which is

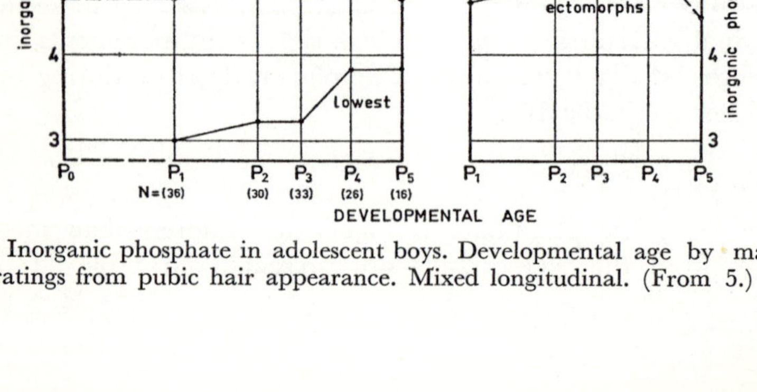

Fig. 8. Inorganic phosphate in adolescent boys. Developmental age by maturity ratings from pubic hair appearance. Mixed longitudinal. (From 5.)

the same as for the pre-adolescent boys from the cross-sectional data in table 11. It increases up to 5.3 mg in P_4.

When the ectomorphs are separated, the early rise in the curve for boys with medium and endomorph somatotype, and the constant level for the ectomorphs, support the idea of a relationship between muscle growth and inorganic phosphate levels. This may at the same time reflect the influence of either growth hormone or androgens.

In our study the actual annual increment at different maturity groups was not significant.

Table 11. *Alkaline phosphatase and inorganic phosphate in serum from 6—20 years (cross-sectional).**

Age (yrs)	Alkaline phosphatase Bod. Units/100 ml serum		Inorganic phosphate mg/100 ml serum	
	Boys (n)	Girls (n)	Boys (n)	Girls (n)
6	6.59 (22) ± 2.78	7.31 (31) ± 1.73	5.05 (22) ± 0.72	5.22 (30) ± 0.57
7	7.44 (118) ± 2.24	7.34 (108) ± 1.92	4.90 (119) ± 0.72	4.98 (108) ± 0.78
8	7.49 (141) ± 2.04	7.87 (124) ± 2.17	4.84 (141) ± 0.69	4.80 (106) ± 0.75
9	7.41 (136) ± 2.10	7.88 (119) ± 2.15	4.72 (136) ± 0.79	4.69 (118) ± 0.65
10	6.58 (46) ± 1.94	6.58 (34) ± 2.86	4.65 (46) ± 0.58	4.94 (26) ± 0.68
11	5.93 (35) ± 1.68	8.06 (5) ± 1.87	4.39 (35) ± 0.67	5.00 (5) ± 1.03
12	7.70 (19) ± 2.69	8.47 (14) ± 2.17	4.69 (19) ± 0.99	5.19 (14) ± 1.09
13	10.13 (21) ± 2.96	6.57 (8) ± 2.62	5.30 (26) ± 1.02	5.48 (8) ± 0.99
14	11.94 (28) ± 3.05	5.83 (13) ± 1.45	5.86 (30) ± 1.89	5.20 (15) ± 1.21
15	10.97 (14) ± 2.53	4.83 (16) ± 1.78	5.03 (19) ± 1.73	4.71 (16) ± 1.29
16	9.69 (10) ± 3.47	4.10 (18) ± 1.48	5.05 (14) ± 1.19	5.09 (19) ± 1.07
17—18	2.77 (23) ± 1.32	3.60 (20) ± 0.61	3.60 (23) ± 0.96	4.61 (28) ± 0.92
19—20	2.53 (23) ± 0.95	4.21 (16) ± 1.18	3.39 (38) ± 0.66	3.89 (7) ± 0.81

* The majority of these data are from blood samples taken in the autumn and winter, when alkaline phosphatase is higher and inorganic phosphate is lower than in the spring and summer (see table 12) data from 12a), ± indicates standard deviations of the individual observations

SEASONAL VARIATIONS

Apart from differences in blood constituents in relation to sex and age, important variations are found in relation to the seasons. Cross-sectional findings from healthy school children are summarized in table 12, dfferentiated for observations in the spring and in the autumn, for haemoglobin, alkaline phosphatase and inorganic phosphate. In all groups but one there is a lower haemoglobin level for girls in spring

Table 12. *Seasonal variations for haemoglobin, serum alkaline phosphatase and inorganic phosphate for 5 age groups of healthy school children (cross-sectional).*

Haemoglobin, g/100 ml blood

	Girls			
Age	Spring	(N)	Autumn	(N)
6	12.2	(4)	12.98	(24)
7	12.07	(21)	12.98	(42)
8	12.33	(26)	13.16	(70)
9	14.15	(14)	13.24	(66)
10	12.78	(30)	13.4	(3)

Inorganic phosphate, mg/100 ml serum

	Boys				Girls			
Age	Spring	(N)	Autumn	(N)	Spring	(N)	Autumn	(N)
6	5.10	(12)	4.76	(12)	5.40	(4)	5.19	(25)
7	5.42	(41)	4.98	(69)	5.61	(20)	4.93	(45)
8	5.42	(12)	4.92	(71)	5.18	(25)	4.72	(73)
9	5.33	(31)	4.77	(54)	5.33	(13)	4.68	(70)
10	4.64	(42)	4.52	(10)	5.39	(31)	4.49	(3)

Alkaline phosphatase, Bodansky Units/100 ml serum

	Boys				Girls			
Age	Spring	(N)	Autumn	(N)	Spring	(N)	Autumn	(N)
6	4.12	(12)	6.54	(12)	5.42	(4)	8.50	(25)
7	4.82	(41)	7.72	(69)	5.19	(20)	7.72	(45)
8	4.26	(12)	7.83	(71)	4.83	(25)	7.79	(73)
9	5.26	(31)	7.90	(54)	5.19	(13)	8.10	(70)
10	6.70	(42)	7.62	(10)	5.00	(31)	9.52	(3)

than in autumn. The lower spring values are possibly the result of winter diet and environmental conditions. Inorganic phosphate shows lower levels in autumn than in spring, while the winter has produced higher levels for alkaline phosphatase in all age groups from 6 to 10 years. Although active rickets was not observed, these figures suggest that the seasonal variations may be associated with a winter diet and decreased exposure to ultra violet rays.

The relationships of hormones or their metabolic products in blood and other blood constituents cannot be discovered until more longitudinal studies have been carried out. Also the truth about interrelationships between nutrients, metabolic enzymes and hormones requires further research under controlled conditions.

REFERENCES

1. Clark, L. C. and E. I. Beck, Plasma alkaline phosphatase activity. I. Normative data for growing children, *J. Pediat.* 36: 335, 1950.
2. Geudeke, M. and T. D. Stahlie, De invloed van lichte luchtweginfecties op de serumeiwitfracties bij kinderen, *Maandschr. Kindergeneesk.* 32: 530, 1964.
3. Harrison, A. P., C. Roderinck, M. Lesher, M. Kaucher, E. Z. Mayer, W. Lameck and E. F. Beach, Nutritional status of children VIII. *J. Amer. Diet. Ass.* 24: 503, 1948.
4. Morse, M., F. W. Schulz and D. E. Cassel, Relation of age to physiological responses of the older boy (10—17 years) to exercise, *J. Appl. Physiol.* 1: 683, 1949.
5. Nutrition Council of the Netherlands, Onderzoek naar de Voeding en Voedingstoestand van schoolkinderen in tien grote steden in 1951 en 1952, *Voeding* 19: 484, 1958.
6. Postmus, S., in: Th. F. S. M. van Schaik, De betekenis van gezinsgrootte en geboortenummer voor de voedingstoestand van schoolkinderen. Hoofdstuk III. *Voeding* 23: 104, 1962.
7. Raben, M. S., Treatment of a pituitary dwarf with human growth hormone, *J. Clin. Endocrin.* 18: 901, 1958.
8. Ramsay, W. N. M., Plasma iron. In: *Advances in clinical chemistry.* Vol. I. Acad. Press, New York, 1958.
9. Riggs, T. R. and L. M. Walker, *J. Biol. Chem.* 235: 3603, 1960.
10. Seltzer, C. C., B. J. Wenzel and Jean Mayer, Serum iron and iron binding capacity in adolescents, *Am. J. Clin. Nutr.* 13: 343, 1964.
11. Trindler, P., The improved determination of iron in serum, *J. Clin. Pathol.* 9: 170, 1956.

12. Unpublished figures from surveys:
(12a) from the Neth. Inst. of Prev. Med., Leyden, for age ½—6 year (1956, DONATH, W. F. and M. LEEWIS);
(12b) from the Nutrition Council of the Netherlands for age 8 (1964, Adam);
(12c) from the Centr. Inst. for Nutr. and Food Res. T.N.O. for age 12—19 year (1965, PIKAAR and DE WIJN).
13. VAN 'T LAND, G. M. and J. H. DE HAAS, Menarche leeftijd in Nederland, *Ned. Tijdschr. Geneesk.* 101: 1425, 1957.
14. WERNER, M., Stoffwechsel Untersuchungen am Menschen mit einem anabolen Steroid (Methandrostenolon), *Klin. Wochenschrift* 39: 998, 1961.
15. WIJN, J. F. DE, Somatische bevindingen bij jongens adolescenten van 12—16 jaar in een voogdij-inrichting. II. Groei en chemische groei, *Maandschr. Kindergeneesk.* 33: 49, 1965.
Also: Growth and chemical growth of adolescent boys, *Helv. Paed. Acta* 20: 497, 1965.
16. WIJN, J. F. DE and H. W. RUSBACH, Het hemoglobinegehalte van Nederlandse schoolkinderen en adolescenten, *Ned. Tijdschr. Geneesk.* 105: 1028, 1961.

DISCUSSION

Thomson: I would like to ask a question about the secular trend in adult stature. In the older data presumably a lot of the so-called adults measured may not in fact have been fully grown. Growth, perhaps 50 years ago, was not finished until one was in one's twenties, whereas now most people seem to be fully grown by about 18. This must have an effect on secular comparisons in groups aged about 20. I don't know of any longitudinal study from early adolescence right through until growth has obviously ceased. I was very interested in the Japanese data that were shown, I had not met them before. I wonder if Dr. VAN DER WERFF TEN BOSCH likes to say anything more about secular trend in adult stature.

Van der Werff ten Bosch: There are two main sources of data, KIIL and OPPERS.

The latter studied 19th century records of men who were examined twice, at about 20 years (for military service) and at about 25 years (for the municipal militia). Not only growth is hastened in our days, but also the onset of puberty; these two seem to be linked.

The secular difference in height before puberty is quite impressive, but since puberty now begins earlier, the adult difference in height is considerably smaller than the prepuberal difference.

Schwarz: When reading books, for instance SAMUEL PEPYS's diary, one is struck by the fact that girls used to marry at ages as early as 14 years.

Such girls must have been immature. The boys of 18 years seem to have had 15 tot 20 mistresses already. I wonder how this corresponds with the late onset of puberty in those days.

Van der Werff ten Bosch: Formal marriage may, of course, take place long before an individual is sexually mature. Your question really is: did people before the 19th century come in puberty as late as they did in the 19th century? This is a problem that has been much discussed. There are some indications that puberty occurred at the same age as at present. In India, 150 years ago, children came in puberty and had menarche at the same age as they do now, that is at about 13 or 14 years (see: KUSSMAUL, A., *Würzb. med. Z.* 3 : 321, 1862; ISRAEL, S., *J. Obstet. Gynaec. Brit. Emp.* 66 : 311, 1959). Then, probably, started the legend that in tropical climates children mature at an earlier age than in northern climates, because in Western Europe in those days menarche occurred later, at the age of 15—17 years.

Presumably something had changed in our part of the world, from which we have been recovering for the last hundred years or so. We don't know the cause of the set-back; it would seem that in India the set-back may not have occurred. Now puberty in tropical regions is later than in northern countries because of the differences in social and economic development, but exact data are scant.

Marshall: There is no doubt that this secular trend must have started at some time: if it has gone on back into history there would have been very little possibility for reproduction at all. There must have been some set-back. Whether this was purely related to the Industral Revolution, it is difficult to say. It very probably happened at about this time, but the fact that it seems to affect all social classes would tend in my view to eliminate the Industrial Revolution as being at least the only factor, because there were some people who did very well in the Industrial Revolution and the people in those classes are also undergoing a secular trend, although it is not quite so great as in the lower classes. Also this trend is apparent in some countries, notably the Scandinavian ones, who were not affected by an Industrial Revolution to the same extent as the countries like Great Britain. There has been a set-back, probably from around the Industrial Revolution time, but what part the revolution itself played in this, I think, is open to doubt.

Visser: Adult height is height at the moment the pubertal growth spurt starts, plus this growth spurt in centimeters. What, if any, is the difference in this growth spurt between girls and boys?

Van der Werff ten Bosch: I don't know whether there is a difference. There are two aspects. First: is the effect of sex hormones on skeletal maturation during the pubertal spurt greater in girls than in boys; in other words, is the spurt stopped sooner in the girl than in the boy.

I think this is an idea that most people would favour.

Another reason why growth could stop sooner in girls is that at all ages they are more mature than boys, if skeletal maturity is expressed in a neutral score.

Subsequent stages in the development of the bones are reached earlier by girls than by boys. Whether that is related to the fact that they come in puberty sooner, and what factors are involved in the co-ordination, if any, of two such widely different processes as sexual maturation and skeletal maturation, I cannot say. The conspicuous sex differences in the pubertal growth spurt are that this starts earlier and becomes less high in girls than in boys. The latter difference may be related to the fact (if this is a fact!) that girls have a more mature skeleton by the time that their pubertal spurt in height begins.

Van Gemund: I think that the secular trend starts before birth. It starts with taller mothers. It might be worthwhile to make a serial study of placental weights over a number of years.

I do not know of data in this context.

Van der Werff ten Bosch: Well, there are some data. Dr. FALKNER in Louisville, has been studying placentas of twins over the past 5 years or so. Identical twins who come at puberty at very nearly the same age, may have quite a marked difference in height (see TANNER, J. M., *Growth and adolescence*, 2nd ed. Blackwell, Oxford, 1962).

This difference seems to depend on the size of the portions of the placenta, that supply each of the two foetusses. FALKNER has found a correlation between the relative sizes of the placental portions and the sizes at birth of the identical twins nourished through them. A considerable difference in size at birth could persist during infancy, although the patterns of growth were remarkably similar.

Thomson: Perhaps I could just add to that question. I don't think there is any evidence in the literature about a secular increase in birth weight. I think the evidence is against such an increase.

Laron: I would like to ask Dr. VAN DER WERFF TEN BOSCH if he would agree with several assumptions. It has been assumed that the secular trend, if it exists, is due very much to improved nutrition. However, some data are available to-day to enable us to say that not only nutrition is involved but some higher regulation, possibly in the hypothalamus. This latter statement is based also on the data from the African and the Asian population, in general terms from countries that are underdeveloped and are in a stage that supposedly Europe was in 100 years ago. In Israel we have less industrialization, the food is poorer, nevertheless we see that maturation, menarche or puberty in general, may be slightly earlier. We also found that boys of oriental Jewish origin reach puberty earlier compared to Jews from Europe.

Van der Werff ten Bosch: What is the answer or assumption?

Laron: The assumption is that if there is a secular trend, there is more to it than just improved social conditions and improved nutrition; that there must be also something which regulates the start of puberty. What it is we don't know, but it would be nice to know what influences such a pace-maker.

Van der Werff ten Bosch: A priori one would expect a tendency for people of subsequent generations to become shorter, now that many people grow adult who would have been dead long ago in earlier days, because of peri-natal or post-natal diseases. It may be that potentially tall people are more apt to die in early infancy, and that with improved medical care in the neonatal and postnatal period a greater proportion of potentially tall people are enabled to reach adult age.

Stoelinga: Have the data of Dr. DE WIJN on seasonal variations in growth been collected during one year? Is it possible that in hot summers and cold winters the variations are greater or smaller?

De Wijn: Our own observations were made during one year, which was an average Dutch rainy and cloudy year. In tropical areas where seasonal fluctuations are observed too, these are probably not due to the high temperature, but to the undernourished condition of the population.

Querido: I think we have to realize and try to define for ourselves, what a skin fold measurement actually is. We measure two things, I think, the content of fat cells, and the number of layers of fat cells between the skin and the underlying muscles. I think there are data which indicate that the size of the fat-cells is related to the degree of overweight. A real question as to the final development of the body, I think, is whether the number of cells is pre-set at birth, or whether this may change in the course of life.

If overfeeding in the first years of life stimulates the formation of fat cells, then at a later age an identical fat content could result in a much thicker skin-fold than in individuals with a thin layer of fat cells. I could imagine that the subscapular measurements are an indication of changes in the number of cells, while the limb measurements could be indicative of changes in the fat content of a constant number of fat cells. This is a problem that has always puzzled me and I should like to hear whether Dr. HAAK or Dr. MARSHALL or anybody else can comment on this.

Marshall: I have no good answer. It is a definite weakness, I think, of the skin-fold technique that, although those who invent the instruments have gone to great lengths to compress the fat of the skin-fold by a constant amount, there is no way of saying, that the fat itself is always compressible by the same amount.

Prof. QUERIDO has said that there may be differences in the number of cells as well as differences in content of cells. These differences might well lead to fats of different compressibility, so that the same basic thickness of skinfold would give a different measurement on a caliper with exactly the same pressure. I don't think there are any data on this. It would be very useful to have some, because this might lead to re-interpretation of some of the skin-fold results that have been published.

Laron: Sometimes a nice scheme is not so simple as it looks, and the idea that the difference in fatlayer and muscle layer in males and females is androgen-determined, became confused when we found that oestrogens are better fat mobilizers, at least in rats, than androgens are.

Haak: It is possible that the disappearance rate of fat is influenced by oestrogens, why it does not work in girls I don't know. Can you give us some further data on fat mobilization?

Laron: I don't know if a factor of tissue sensitivity is involved. As I said I am now really confused. The nice explanation after finding that testosterone is a fat mobilizer is not so simple as it looks. We are now investigating what happens in vitro.

Querido: I should like to say something after the words of Dr. LARON on the oestrogen effect. In man observations of EDWARDS and his collaborators indicate that there is a parallelism between body weight and skin-fold measurements. That implies that the skin-fold thickness somehow reflects the fat content of the fat cells. During puberty two factors operate: re-shuffling within the body, and a change in caloric intake. Caloric intake will govern the overall excess which the individual must store. To demonstrate what actually happens in boys and girls during puberty is extremely difficult, and would involve the estimation of daily oxygen consumption, creatinine excretion etc., to see whether there is an excess of caloric intake.

Sobel: I would like to ask Dr. HAAK whether he thinks that it is possible for a clinician to estimate the relative amount of fat and muscle in a person by feeling in appropriate places for the thickness of the skin-fold and then feeling selected contracted muscles? Can you get an impression of the nutritional status, muscular development and muscle tone of the child?

Haak: You can get an impression of fat content by lifting the skin and subcutaneous tissue between thumb and index finger, without using mechanical devices.

CHAPTER V

GROWTH AROUND BIRTH

PRENATAL GROWTH

A. M. THOMSON

GENERAL FEATURES

Our knowledge of foetal growth depends almost entirely upon measurements made after the product of conception has been expelled or removed from the uterus. Except for those expelled normally at term, the great majority of the pregnancies concerned are unavoidably abnormal in some respect, and therefore the picture of foetal growth which emerges may not be physiological. Again, the data are cross-sectional, and a longitudinal picture derived from them does not necessarily show the pattern of growth of the individual foetus. Nevertheless, clinical experience suggests that the pattern of foetal growth so derived is not seriously misleading.

Fig. 1 shows the average weights and ranges of the foetus and placenta in a series of over 8000 births and therapeutic abortions of all parities in Aberdeen. Multiple births, stillbirths and spontaneous abortions have been excluded, as have all cases in which the date of the last menstrual period was uncertain, or the clinical progress of pregnancy apparently inconsistent with the date recorded.

The average curve shows the familiar sigmoid shape. Attention is drawn to the following characteristics.

1. During the first trimester, the placenta is larger than the foetus. Their combined weight at the end of the trimester is less than 100 g.

2. During the second trimester, foetal weight increases about 25 times, the acceleration of growth reaching a maximum about the 24th week. Average foetal weight at the end of the second trimester is about 1000 g. During the same period, placental weight increases about six times, to approximately 300 g. It should be noted that despite rapid growth during the second trimester, the combined weight of the foetus

and placenta at the end of this period is still quite small, so that the daily nutrient requirements imposed by their growth is small. Maternal weight gain is usually most rapid during this period, but relatively little of it is accounted for by the product of conception. The dramatic changes in the composition of maternal blood and other tissues which occur during the first six months of pregnancy can scarcely be explained as responses to nutritional 'stress' imposed by the requirements of the foetus.

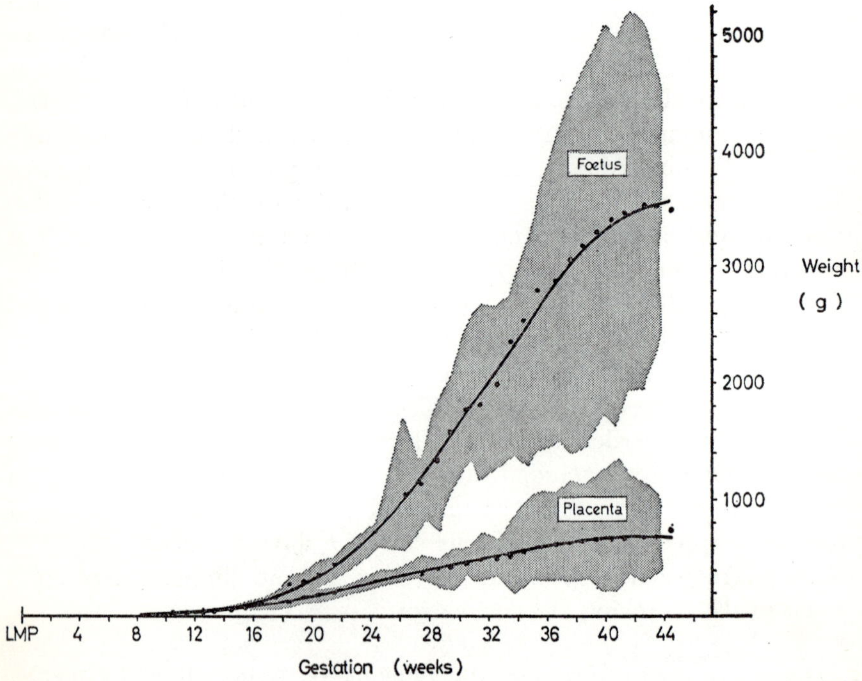

Fig. 1. Average weights of foetus and placenta by stage of gestation. The range of weights at each stage is indicated by hatching

3. The amount of new foetal tissue added per unit time appears to reach a maximum about the 32nd week, after which it seems to decrease. During this final stage, there is relatively little increase in the weight of the placenta. The capacity for transfer of nutrients through the placenta may fail to keep pace with foetal needs; but there is

little proof that this is so. The functional capacity of the placenta is not necessarily indicated by its weight.

4. Whether the marked slowing of growth at and after term (40 weeks) is 'real', or is due to selection of 'high risk' cases for termination of pregnancies that persist after term is difficult to say. Many clinicians believe that placental insufficiency often becomes clinically important after term. 'Postmature' pregnancy is certainly associated with a rise in foetal mortality (3, 11, 16).

5. At all stages of gestation, the range of foetal and placental weights is wide, increasing towards term. In the present series, the weights of babies born apparently at term ranged from 1757 to 5046 g. At any given stage of gestation, the distribution of weights round the mean is approximately symmetrical.

The problem is to find out what this wide range signifies.

FACTORS INFLUENCING FOETAL GROWTH

Male babies tend to be slightly heavier than female, at least during the final weeks of gestation, and multiparae have larger babies than primiparae. Singleton babies are larger than those from multiple pregnancies. But such factors do little to explain the very wide variation of birth weights at any given gestation period.

As would be expected, birth weight is appreciably influenced by maternal size. Cross-breeding experiments with animals of grossly different paternal and maternal size indicate that the size of the father has little or no influence upon the rate of growth *in utero* (9, 17). Extensive studies of birth weights by McKeown and Record (10) and by Morton (12) suggest that in man also, it is maternal rather than paternal size that is of importance.

Table 1, from Hytten and Leitch (8) shows that the babies of tall mothers were, on average, about 8 % heavier than those of short women; and the babies of overweight mothers were similarly heavier than those of underweight mothers. Babies of tall *and* heavy mothers were about 16 % heavier than those of short *and* light mothers. Such findings are of great importance in interpreting differences in birth weight (and in incidence of 'premature' babies, that is, babies of low birth weight) in different ethnic groups. It is often claimed that low average birth weights and high incidences of babies of low birth weight are due to differences in the nutrition of pregnant women. They are, however, more likely to be due to differences in maternal size. I shall be discussing the significance of differences of maternal size in a later paper (pag. 197).

Table 1. *Effect of maternal height and weight-for-height on mean birth weight (singletons) in primigravidae. (From 8).*

	Maternal height Under 155 cm	155—163 cm	Over 163 cm	Total
Maternal Weight-for-height	Mean birth weight (kg)			
Underweight	2.99	3.11	3.22	3.11
Average	3.11	3.23	3.40	3.25
Overweight	3.20	3.35	3.48	3.35
Total	3.10	3.23	3.37	3.24

Meanwhile, it has to be stated that birth weight appears *not* to be readily influenced by differences of maternal diet during pregnancy itself. During the famine in the Netherlands in 1945, average birth weights appeared to fall by about 240 g only during the height of the famine (13). The fall in birth weights recorded during the siege of Leningrad also appears to have been relatively small (1). While there are difficulties in the interpretation of such evidence, it can at least be said that within very wide limits of food intake during pregnancy foetal growth will proceed quite normally, if necessary at the expense of the maternal tissues. In this connection, it is interesting and significant that the average mother appears to lay down energy reserves, as fat, in her own tissues during a relatively early stage of pregnancy, while the needs of the foetus are still small (8).

Pathological interference with the adaptive processes of pregnancy may interfere with foetal growth. Fig. 2 from Baird, Thomson and Billewicz (2) shows that severe pre-eclampsia (hypertension with proteinuria) which occurs before term in first pregnancies appears

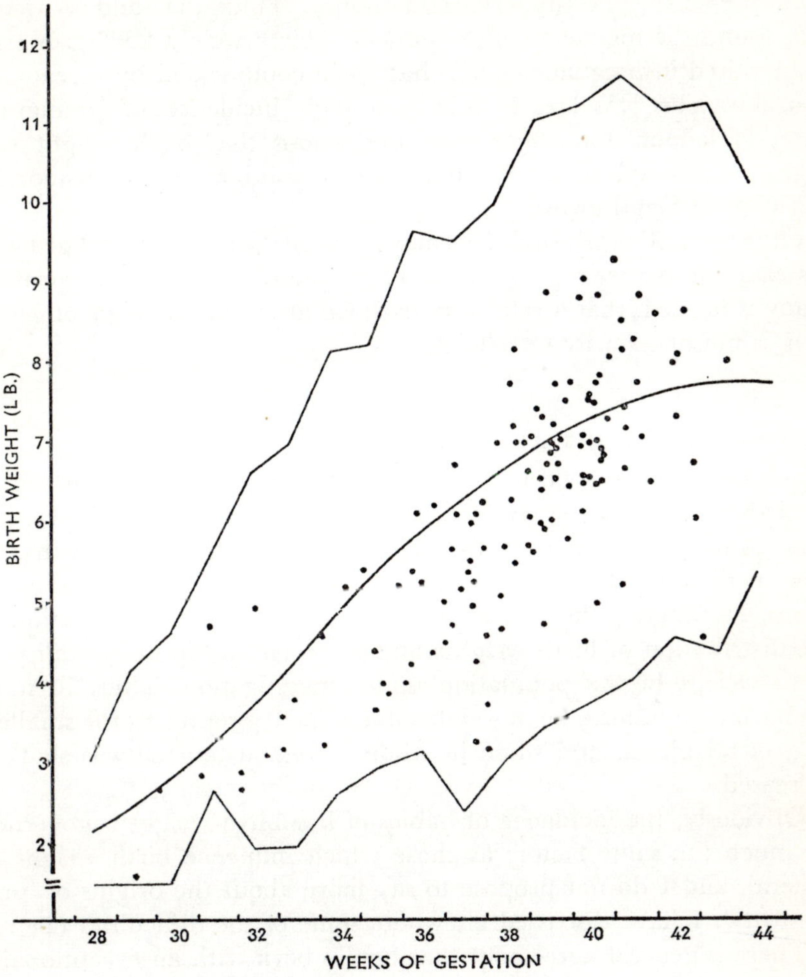

Fig. 2. Distribution of birth weights in cases of severe pre-eclampsia. (From 2.)

to result in depression of foetal growth. The same authors found little or no interference with the normal distribution of birth weights in mild pre-eclampsia (hypertension alone). TURNBULL and WALKER (15) found the incidence of prematurity (birth weight 2500 g or less) to be raised in pregnancies that had been complicated by threatened abortion. This was largely due to a high incidence of premature onset of labour, but there were indications that birth weight was slightly depressed at any given stage of gestation. Cigarette smoking can depress foetal growth (7).

Other pathological conditions may increase the rate of foetal growth, for example diabetic pregnancy. This example serves as a warning, if any is needed, that a relatively high foetal weight for stage of gestation, is not necessarily beneficial.

LOW BIRTH WEIGHT AND ITS CONSEQUENCES

Much confusion has been caused by defining 'prematurity' in terms of birth weight, and WHO (18) has recently recommended that the concept of 'prematurity' in the definition should give way to that of 'low birth weight'. The implication is not entirely clear in practical terms. Presumably 'low birth weight' should be defined in relation to the distribution of birth weights and the relationship of mortality to birth weight in the population under investigation. Thus, in most Western populations, birth weights under 2500 g represent the smallest 7 % of all births, and those in whom neonatal mortality is sharply increased.

Obviously, the incidence of babies of low birth weight is governed by much the same factors as those which influence birth weight in general, and I do not propose to say more about the origins of 'prematurity'. I have discussed elsewhere some of the difficulties (14).

There is general agreement that babies born with an exceptionally low birth weight are under both an immediate and a long-term disability. Certainly height and weight during childhood usually remain somewhat low and there is evidence that intellectual functions are impaired. But whether such disabilities are inherent in the prematurely born, or are due to defective conditions of upbringing, remains obscure. Mothers who live in poor social circumstances are themselves frequently undersized, and there is a high incidence of 'low birth weight' among their babies, who in later life are exposed to the effects of a poor physical and social environment. Under such circumstances, it is difficult or impossible to obtain a control series whose birth weights are not low, but who resemble the low birth weight series in all other relevant respects. Some of the difficulties have been discussed by DRILLIEN (5), DOUGLAS (4) and by FAIRWEATHER and ILLSLEY (6).

It is scarcely possible at present to decide whether the continued impairment of growth and function shown by the average premature child is congenital i.e. due to pre-natal causes, or is due to the effects of an adverse postnatal environment. Probably both kinds of aetiology are at work.

REFERENCES

1. ANTONOV, A., *J. Pediat.* 30: 250, 1947.
2. BAIRD, D., A. M. THOMSON and W. Z. BILLEWICZ, *J. Obstet. Gyn. Brit. Emp.* 64: 370, 1957.
3. BUTLER, N. R. and D. G. BONHAM, *Perinatal mortality*, Edinburgh and London, E. and S. Livingstone, 1963.
4. DOUGLAS, J. W. B., *Brit. med. J.* 1: 1008, 1960.
5. DRILLIEN, C. M., *The growth and development of the prematurely born child*, Edinburgh and London, E. and S. Livingstone, 1964.
6. FAIRWEATHER, D. V. I. and R. ILLSLEY, *Brit. J. soc. prev. Med.* 14: 149, 1960.
7. HERRIOT, A., W. BILLEWICZ and F. E. HYTTEN, *Lancet* 1: 771, 1962.
8. HYTTEN, F. E. and I. LEITCH, *The physiology of human pregnancy*, Oxford, Blackwell Scientific Publications, 1964.
9. JOUBERT, D. M. and J. HAMMOND, *Nature* Lond. 174: 647, 1954.
10. MCKEOWN, T. and R. G. RECORD, *Amer. J. hum. genet.* 6: 457, 1954.
11. MCKIDDIE, J. M., *J. Obstet. Gyn. Brit. Emp.* 56: 386, 1949.
12. MORTON, N. E., *Ann. hum. Genet.* 20: 125, 1955.
13. SMITH, C. A., *J. Pediat.* 30: 229, 1947.
14. THOMSON, A. M., *Mod. Probl. Pediat.* 8: 197, 1963.
15. TURNBULL, E. P. N. and J. WALKER, *J. Obstet. Gyn. Brit. Emp.* 63: 553, 1956.
16. WALKER, J., *J. Obstet. Gyn. Brit. Emp.* 61: 162, 1954.
17. WALTON, A. and J. HAMMOND, *Proc. roy. Soc.* B 125: 311, 1938.
18. WHO, *Tech. Rep. Series*, No. 217, 1961.

GROWTH IN EARLY INFANCY*

H. K. A. VISSER

INTRODUCTION

During the first year of postnatal life the infant grows rapidly in height. However, the velocity of growth, which is highest at birth, falls off rapidly. In fact growth velocity in height is at its maximum before birth, between the fourth and sixth month of intrauterine life, while maximal gain in weight occurs during the last months before birth.

There is evidence that the first two or three years after birth and particularly the first year, determine the subsequent pattern of growth.

LONGITUDINAL GROWTH STUDIES IN INFANCY

There are now data from several longitudinal growth studies in infancy and childhood (30, 48, 50, 54, 61). In Western countries the mean length at birth is about 50 cm and the increments are approximately 8 cm during the first three months, 6 cm during the second three months, 9 cm during the subsequent six months and approximately 12 cm during the second year of life. Mean birth weight for full-term infants is between 3 and 3.5 kg. During the first six months of life the infant gains about 4.5 kg, during the second six months about 2.5 kg.

Falkner (21) has reported longitudinal data for the first three years of life. Figures 1 and 2 show distance (attained size) and velocity (increment per unit of time) for recumbent length and weight in this study. Boys were taller than girls, but the growth velocity was very similar in both sexes. There was little relationship between recumbent

* Supported in part by a PHS retuining fellow grant (RF-41) from the Public Health Service, National Institutes of Health, Bethesda, Md., U.S.A., and a grant from the Netherlands Organization for the Advancement of Pure Research (Z.W.O.)

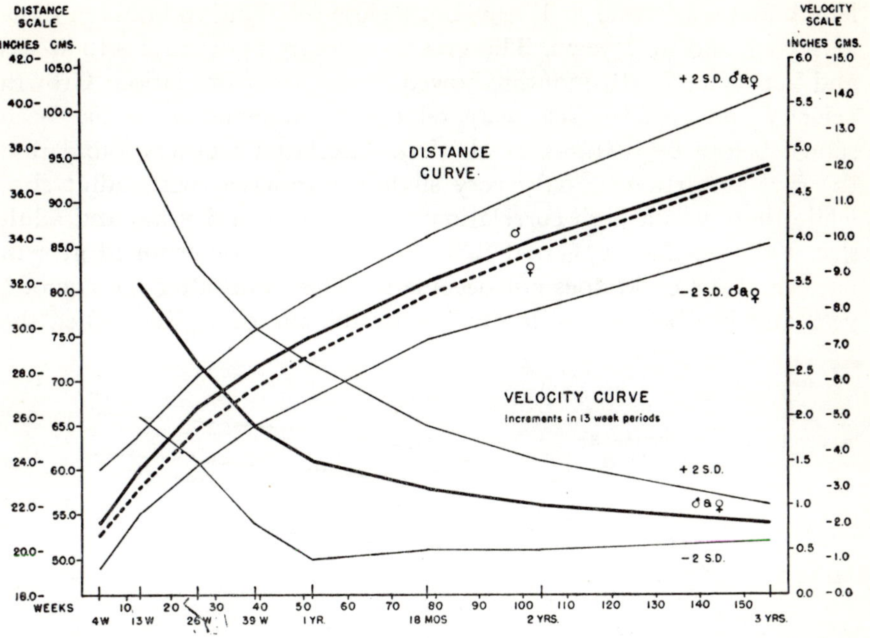

Fig. 1. Distance and velocity curves for recumbent length of boys and girls in Great-Britain between 4 weeks and 3 years of age (from 21)

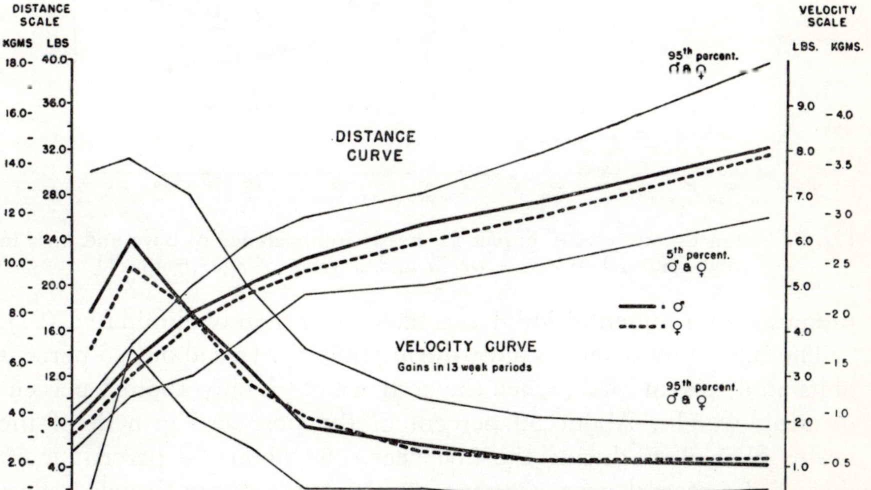

Fig. 2. Distance and velocity curves for weight of boys and girls in Great-Britain between 4 weeks and 3 years of age (from 21)

length at 4 weeks and at 1 year, but a close relationship between those at 1 year and at 2 years. The growth velocity between 4—13 weeks and between 12—18 months showed a very low correlation. Growth velocity and attained size were relatively independent, as has been shown before by TANNER et al. (58). The latter workers found that the size at birth was only very slightly correlated with adult size, while there was a high correlation between size at 3 years and adult size. FALKNER has suggested that the genetically determined growth pattern of the child does not become manifest until after the age of 1 year and has become quite obvious by the age of 2 years, when the

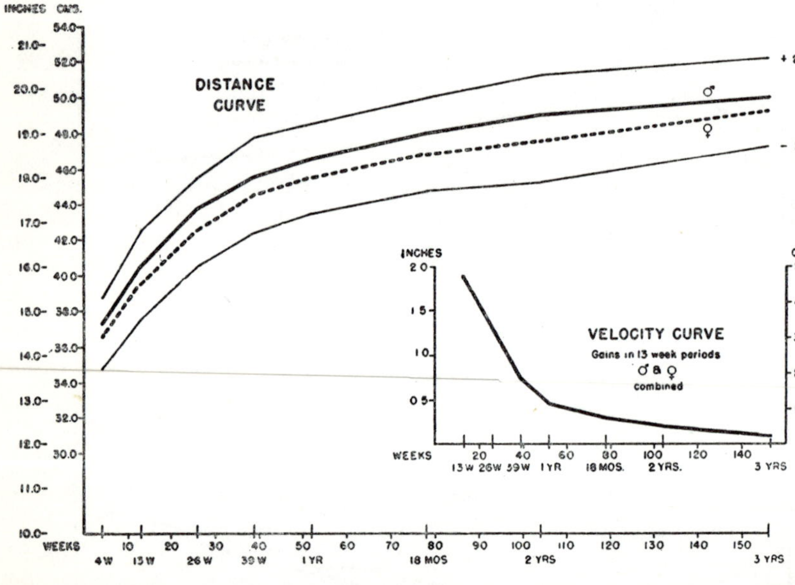

Fig. 3. Distance and velocity curves for head circumference of boys and girls in Great-Britain between 4 weeks and 3 years of age (from 21)

prenatal environmental influences have been mainly eliminated (21).

The brain grows very rapidly during infancy. It is about 25 percent of its adult size at birth, when the body weight is only about 5 percent of adult weight. About 50 percent of the postnatal growth of the brain takes place during the first year, and about 20 percent more during the second year. Changes in the head circumference reflect the general growth of the central nervous system (19, 30, 48, 50, 54, 61).

While growth of the body as a whole decelerates, the thickness of the subcutaneous tissue follows a unique pattern in that it increases rapidly during the first nine months after birth. Thereafter it diminishes in thickness and by 5 years it is approximately half as thick as at nine months (55).

Fig. 3 shows distance and velocity curves for head circumference in FALKNER's study. Mean head circumferences in boys were consistently larger than in girls, but curves for increments in boys and girls were about identical.

FACTORS WHICH INFLUENCE GROWTH

Birth weight and gestation period

'An immature infant is a liveborn infant with a birth weight of 2500 g or less, or specified as immature. In some countries, however, this criterion will not be applicable, if weight is not specified. A liveborn infant with a period of gestation less than 37 weeks or specified as 'premature' may be considered as the equivalent of an immature infant.' This definition of prematurity was proposed by the World Health Organization in 1948. Two years later, in 1950, the WHO Expert Group on Prematurity endorsed this definition, and since then it has been internationally accepted. Subsequent experience has shown, however, that in many cases of low birth weight this definition is not applicable. The definition of prematurity takes no account of gestation time unless birth weight is unknown. Several factors influence birth weight, e.g. racial and geographical factors, multiple pregnancy, social class, age of mother and, important in Western countries, complications of pregnancy as toxaemia. It has become quite clear that many babies by definition called 'premature', are in fact babies with low birth weight for gestational age, and many of these are born at or near term. As a result most of the studies on the relationship between low birth weight and subsequent growth are difficult to interpret, since gestational age is usually not known. Also, because of technical problems, only a few studies have, reported data on length, at birth and during infancy.

LUBCHENKO and collaborators (39) have recently published percentile curves on intrauterine growth, constructed from the birth weight of liveborn infants at gestational ages ranging from 24 to 42 weeks. These data, obtained at a high altitude, have certain limitations for use in other parts of the world. In an area of high altitude an excess of premature births (defined by weight at birth) and a lower mean birth weight have been found (37). Over 30 percent of infants in this area were less than 2500 g, compared with a State average of 10 percent. The percentile curves of LUBCHENKO et al. are the only intrauterine growth curves available at this time, and in spite of the limitations they can be very useful to differentiate the infant with low birth weight for gestational age from the prematurely born infant with a birth weight normal for gestation age. It is unfortunate that there are no intrauterine percentile curves for length. Measurements of length at birth and during infancy are technically difficult, but have to be employed in future studies on 'dysmaturity' or 'low birth weight for gestational age' or 'intrauterine growth retardation'.

DRILLIEN has carried out longitudinal studies on 600 children, including 100 pairs of twins. Approximately one-third of the total had a birth weight of 2000 g or less, one-third between 2000 and 2500 g and one-third 2500 g or more. Prematurity was defined as a birth weight of less than 2500 g (16). Throughout a five year period, weight and height were followed in the three groups of children. Figures 4 and 5 represent the results for male and female singletons and twins respectively. It can be seen that the growth rates in weight and height are not much different for the three groups. Infants with the lowest birth weights failed to overcome their initial birth weight handicap. Means for height show that at 5 years the prematurely born were still shorter than their mature controls. There is thus no correlation between birth weight and subsequent growth rates. In 55 percent of the infants with birth weight between 2000 and 2500 g, the estimated gestation time was 38 weeks or more. At 4 years these small full-term babies were 1100 g lighter and 1.9 cm shorter than babies of the same birth weight group whose estimated gestation time was less than 38 weeks. KUNNAS (35) has found that premature infants with a longer gestation period grew more rapidly in the first two to three months, but lagged behind at 39 weeks and at 1—1½ years.

LUBCHENKO et al. (39) also studied the relationship of fetal size to later physical growth of prematurely born children (see also 16). Fifty children with birth weight 1500 g or less were measured at the age of 10 years. At birth 80 percent were below the 50th weight percentile for gestational age, 22 percent below the 10th percentile. At the age of 10 years again 80 percent was below the 50th weight

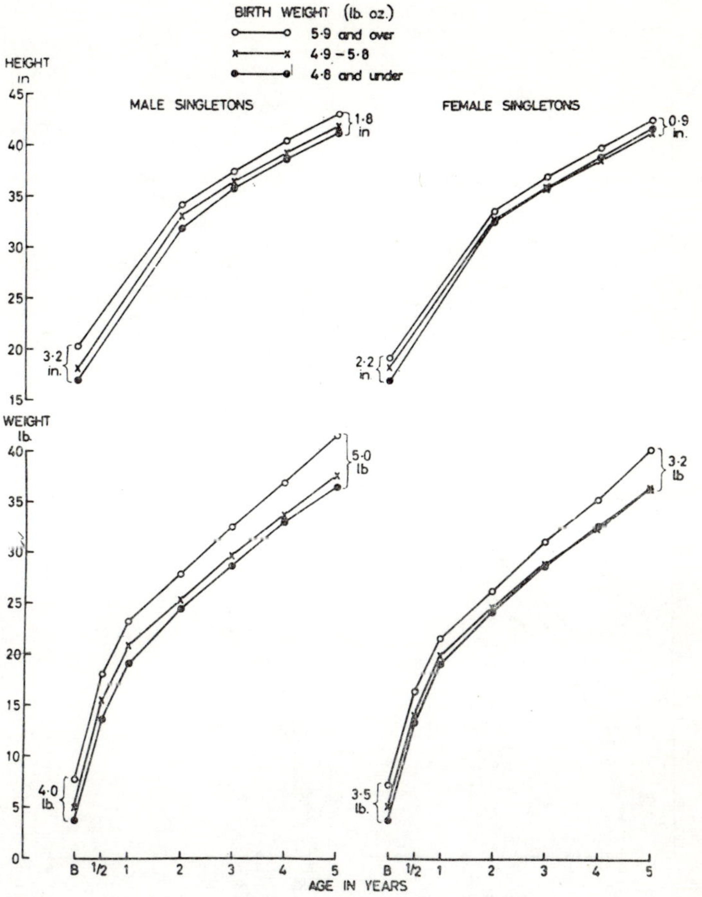

Fig. 4. Mean weights and heights at ages from birth to 6 years for male and female singletons in three birth weight groups (from 11)

percentile, but 42 percent were below the 10th percentile. Thus premature infants who at birth were small for their gestation age were also small at the age of 10 years. BABSON et al. (4) have recently reported a study on growth and development of twins of dissimilar size at birth. Sixteen pairs of twins (nine pairs were homozygotic) were examined at the age of 8½ years. The smaller twin at birth weighed less than 2000 g and this was at least 25 % less than the weight of the

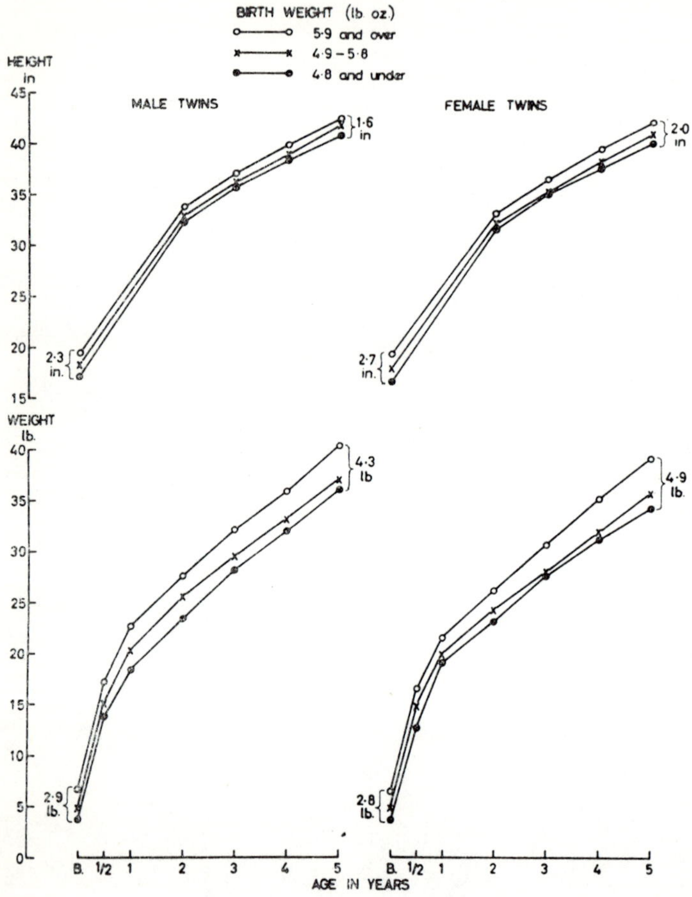

Fig. 5. Mean weights and heights at ages from birth to 5 years for male and female twins in three birth weight groups (from 16)

larger twin. At 8½ years a highly significant difference was present in height, weight and head circumference. There were also significant differences in intelligence and in levels of language comprehension and expression. FALKNER (22) is studying twins from birth on, and he is particularly interested in the relationship between differences in height and weight and differences in placental circulation during intrauterine life. Details of these studies are not yet available but will be most important for our knowledge on the permanent effects of intrauterine malnutrition on ultimate height and weight.

Maternal height

Environmental and genetic factors influence prenatal and postnatal growth. At birth male infants are generally taller and heavier than girls and there is good evidence that birth weight correlates more with the height of the mother than that of the father (13). Although heights of the parents are mainly genetically determined, it is clear that environmental factors as social class, maternal efficiency, illness and nutrition have also affected the growth of the parents. DRILLIEN (15) has shown that mothers of premature babies were significantly shorter than mothers of mature controls, and that average maternal height was related to women's childhood environment. BAIRD and ILLSLEY (6) found maternal height to be correlated with premarital environment and BAIRD (5) has also demonstrated an association between small stature and lower-than-average intelligence in mothers. This brings us to the problems of the influence of maternal care on postnatal growth (see below). DRILLIEN has stated that 'if height of the mother had no independent association with size of child, one would still expect children of short mothers to be smaller than average because they are likely to have received less adequate care from less intelligent mothers in poorer homes' (16). In DRILLIEN's studies mean weight and height increments at the age of 4 years were compared for children born to short, medium and tall mothers in three maternal efficiency groups. Rate of growth increased with height of mother for all grades of care and decreased with declining maternal standards for all heights of mother.

Maternal care

DRILLIEN (16) has studied the influence of maternal care on height and weight in the three groups of children with different birth weight (less than 2000 g, between 2000—2500 g, and more than 2500 g). Maternal efficiency was graded as very good, fair and poor by considering several points as cleanliness of the house, the child and its clothes; feeding habits and diet; advantage taken of wellfare facilities as immunization and infant clinics; management of training problems; and the relationship of mother and child, other children in the family and the father. Fig. 6 shows mean weights and heights at ages up to 5 years for singletons and twins, of birth weight 2000 g or less and 2500 g or more, receiving the best and the worst care. Mean weight and height of children receiving inadequate care was less than those from a better environment. This effect of environment was more obvious in the prematurely born (lowest birth weight group). Mean weight and height increments at 2 and 4 years were also related to maternal care for both singletons and twins. The average standard of care was lower for twins in all birth weight groups as compared with singletons and maternal care decreased with increasing size of the family.

Patton and Gardner have made fascinating observations on six children with severe growth retardation, delayed skeletal maturation and retarded psychomotor development. These authors found a close association with a 'specific disturbance of maternal behaviour and family organization: maternal deprivation' (44). There was a rapid and impressive early physical and behavioural response when environmental circumstances improved. Patton and Gardner state that 'the children failed to regain age norms completely in physical development' and they observed 'a tendency to residual defects in intellect and personality structure'. The authors suggest that 'the existence of critical periods in the early phases of post-natal somatic growth and neural organization during which unfavorable environmental factors may lead to an irreversible reduction in growth and developmental potential'. The follow-up periods of the patients studied are however too short to conclude that permanent effects of maternal deprivation have been demonstrated. It is very difficult to see how nutritional, hormonal and other factors in this deprivation syndrome can be separated from psychological factors, which Patton and Gardner suggest as most important in this growth-failure syndrome. However, whether the intrinsic mechanism for this growth-failure syndrome is regulated by nutritional, hormonal or other factors, it all seems to be secondary to the emotional disorder. In this way delay in growth and development may at times be a psychosomatic disease. The studies of Patton and Gardner present many challenges for the future and

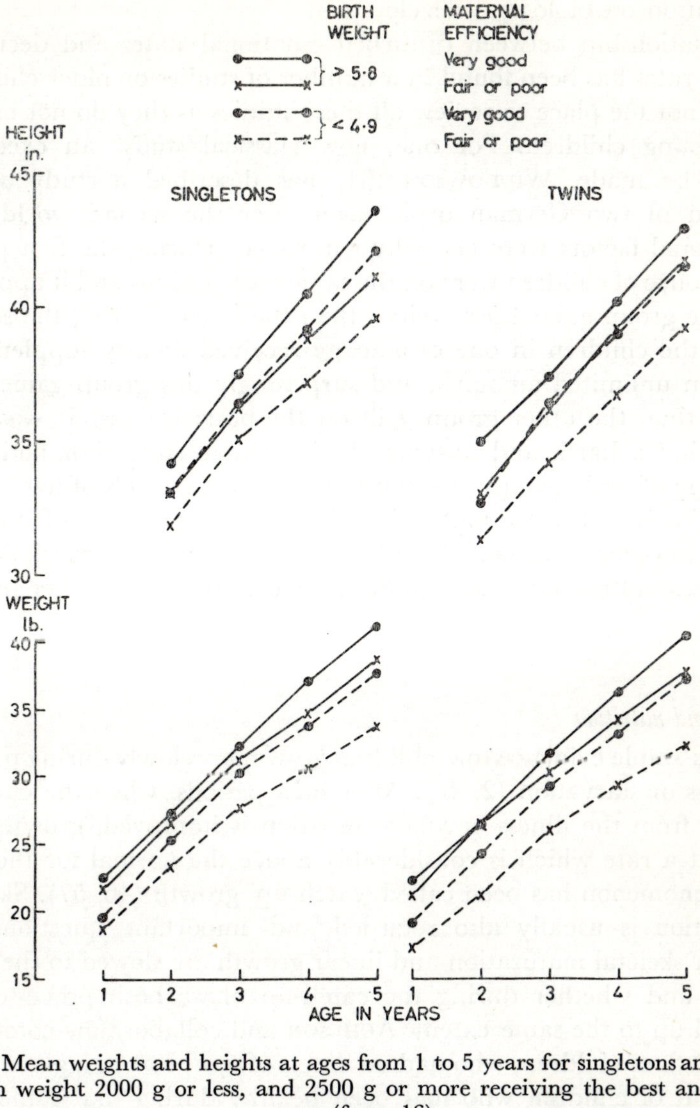

Fig. 6. Mean weights and heights at ages from 1 to 5 years for singletons and twins, of birth weight 2000 g or less, and 2500 g or more receiving the best and worst care (from 16)

are most important for our knowledge on the influence of early sensory deprivation on biological development.

A relationship between disturbed emotional states and decreased growth rates has been found in a number of studies on older children. This is not the place to review all these studies as they do not involve very young children. For one, now classical study, an exception should be made. WIDDOWSON (64) has described a study among children in two German orphanages after the second world war. Nutritional factors were carefully controlled. During the first period both groups of children were on the same basic rations and it appeared that one group gained less weight than the other. During the second period the children in one orphanage received dietary supplements, bread in unlimited amounts, and surprisingly this group gained less weight than the other group, still on the basic rations. It was then found that a harsh and unsympathetic woman supervisor had been in charge of both groups of children during the periods of less weight gain. This is a clear example of the influence of emotional factors on growth in older children. There is no reason why these psychological factors should not play an important role during the earlier periods of life.

Illness and nutrition

There is ample evidence that children grow more slowly during periods of illness or starvation (2, 46). After such periods, when the children recover from the illness or when nutrition is improved, growth may occur at a rate which is considerably above the normal for the age; this phenomenon has been called 'catch-up' growth (46, 57). Skeletal maturation is usually also retarded and important questions are whether skeletal maturation and linear growth are slowed to the same extent, and whether during the catch-up phase both processes are speeded up to the same extent. ACHESON and collaborators compared the growth of children, who had an illness of some sort in a given year, with that of children who had been healthy during that same year (2, 31). No child was ill for more than a few weeks. There was a significant effect on linear growth, whereas the effect on skeletal maturation was negligible; it was postulated that these differential effects would cause a loss in subsequent adult stature. PRADER, TANNER and VON HARNACK (46) have questioned this view. In some of their patients with catch-up growth, the acceleration of growth in height surpassed the acceleration of skeletal maturation. In such cases the final relation of height to bone age may become normal again, when skeletal maturation was initially less retarded than linear growth.

It can be expected that during infancy, a period with the highest growth rate after birth, periods of illness or undernourishment will have a considerable effect on linear growth and skeletal maturation. DRILLIEN (16) has studied the effect of illness on growth in length and weight in the three groups of infants (singletons and twins) with different birth weight. The effect of frequent illnesses during the first two years of life on height and weight at 2 years was most evident in singletons who were less than 2000 g at birth and in twins who were 2500 g or less. No data are given for skeletal maturation, however, and the long-term effects are not yet known.

Growth and nutrition studies of the first year of life have generally been short-term studies of groups of infants, and only a few longitudinal studies are available (54, 61, 48, 7, 33). RUEDA-WILLIAMSON and ROSE (48) have recently presented the results of a longitudinal study in Boston of 67 full-term infants from 2 to 15 months. Correlation coefficients were calculated for the increments of length and weight from 2 to 10 months, and the average daily calorie and protein intakes during those 8 months. There was a significant correlation between weight increment and calorie intake, but not between length increment and calorie or protein intake. The studies suggested that 'infants have genetically or physiologically predetermined maximums of statural growth which they cannot exceed no matter how much they increase calorie or protein intake'. Consumption of calories in excess of what was required for this 'maximum' stature resulted in weight gain, without further increase of length. Individual case studies indicated that the most important variables in the energy balance, beside food intake and growth, were illness and physical activity.

In animal experiments permanent effects of malnutrition in early postnatal life have been observed. WIDDOWSON and MCCANCE (11, 65) studied the effects of ad libitum feeding in rats who had suffered undernutrition for some time after birth. Rats undernourished during the first three weeks of life, continued to grow slowly on an unlimited supply of food and they became small adults. Rats allowed to grow normally during the first three weeks of life and then undernourished for three weeks, displayed catch-up growth when fed ad libitum. However, the ultimate weight of the undernourished animals did not reach the control level. If the period of undernutrition was longer, catch-up growth was also observed, but the difference in adult weight between undernourished and control rats was greater. When rats were undernourished at a later age, from the 9th to the 12th week, a complete catch-up growth followed and their mean weight even surpassed that of control animals. Experiments with cockerels (47) gave similar results. The long bones grew very slowly during undernutrition, and very fast when the birds got extra food. However, the bones stopped growing before they reached the length of bones of cockerels well-nourished throughout.

It seems then, that the younger the animal, the more serious the effects of undernutrition. Animals which are relatively mature at birth may, perhaps, be influenced at the same stage of development by malnutrition in utero (12, 65). Earlier in this paper we have reviewed studies which indicate that premature infants, small for their gestational age (at birth), are likely to remain relatively small (16, 35, 39).

It is possible that periods of malnutrition in infancy or early childhood may leave permanent marks, particularly on brain development. GRAHAM (28) studied children recovering from severe infantile marasmus in Peru, and found incomplete catch-up for head circumference and length. The deficit in length of these children was inversely proportional to the duration of breast feeding. STOCH and SMYTHE (53) have followed for two to seven years a group of children who at the age of one year were half their expected weight. Brain growth of the undernourished group, as reflected by head circumference and I.Q., and height were significantly lower than in a control group. DOBBING (17) studied the influence of undernutrition during the first week after birth on the development and myelination of the rat brain; he found large differences in the rate of cholesterol deposition in the brain between undernourished rats and their normal controls.

These recent observations, particularly in animal experiments, have indicated the great significance of nutrition in early life and have given a new stimulus for the research in infant nutrition.

HORMONES

Thyroid hormone is essential for the development of the central nervous system and for normal growth during infancy and childhood. Although in the first few months of life the infant with athyroidism may not be much shorter than the normal infant of the same age, the retardation of growth usually becomes apparent at a very early age (24, 66). This 'normal' somatic development at birth demonstrates that maternal thyroid hormones can protect the athyrotic foetus from the intrauterine thyroid deficiency. However, in newborn infants with athyroidism, skeletal maturation is usually retarded and there is evidence that at least in some of these infants the development of the central nervous system is retarded irreversibly during intrauterine life (41, 4). This points to an important role of thyroid hormone on intrauterine growth and development. There is good evidence that the foetal thyroid gland in the human is functionally active from the 12th week of gestation on (3).

The role of pituitary growth hormone during foetal and neonatal life is not clear. All available evidence suggests that absence of the foetal hypophysis does not influence, to any degree, embryonic and foetal growth. Hypophysectomy of mother and foetus has been reported to have no effect, or only a slight one, upon foetal growth in the chick, rat, rabbit, or mouse (34, 49). Apituitary and anencephalic human foetuses were of normal length (8, 9, 45, 59). An infant born of a mother, hypophysectomized during the 25th week of pregnancy for carcinoma of the breast, was of normal size (38). There is no direct evidence that growth hormone is transferred across the placenta. Administration of growth hormone to the pregnant rat gave different results (20, 60) and infants born of mothers with active acromegaly were of normal size (1, 32). It is not at all sure that the large size of babies born to prediabetic or diabetic mothers is due to an excess of maternal growth hormone (23, 27).

Idiopathic hypopituitary dwarfs are usually normal in size at birth and slowing of growth may not be apparent until they are 2 to 4 years of age (40). At least growth during early infancy seems to be normal. However, in familial hypopituitarism infants may have a birth weight less than 2000 g and they grow slowly from birth on (36).

Rats hypophysectomized at 6 days of age grew at about half the rate of the unoperated control group, until about 30 days after birth when growth stopped completely. Hypophysectomy at the age of 28 days resulted in an abrupt cessation of growth (51, 62). A strain of mice with hereditary anterior pituitary dwarfism shows normal size at birth and normal rate of growth during the first week of life, but degenerative changes in the eosinophilic cells of the anterior hypophysis are detectable microscopically before birth (25).

Ducharme and Grumbach (18) administered human growth hormone to premature infants and concluded that these infants were relatively unresponsive. However, human growth hormone was given in low doses for very short periods and several metabolic changes, typical after administration of this hormone, were observed. In the light of recent findings of high serum levels of growth hormone in premature infants, as will be discussed below, another explanation is that the infants were already stimulated by endogenous growth hormone. In this respect it is interesting that one of these infants, on a high dose of 10 mg human growth hormone per day for three days, showed an increase of the growth rate of the fibula.

Recently direct measurements of pituitary growth hormone in serum have become available. High serum levels were found in the neonatal period, in premature infants higher than in full-term infants (14, 29). The newborn infant is able to secrete growth hormone in response to acute hypoglycaemia (14). In a number of children with documented evidence of growth failure as early as 3, 6 and 9 months of age, no demonstrable growth hormone levels before or after insuline-induced hypoglycaemia were found (52). Administration of human growth hormone to these children increased the growth rate significantly. These findings are of utmost importance and suggest that pituitary growth hormone has an important role in early infancy. The role of growth hormone in intrauterine growth remains uncertain. There is still a possibility that the human placenta produces growth hormone (26) and until growth hormone levels have been determined in the serum of anencephalic human foetuses we cannot definitely accept that foetal growth in the human is independent of growth hormone.

The influence of androgenic hormones on intrauterine and neonatal growth is not understood. Newborn infants with congenital adrenal hyperplasia are of normal size and generally skeletal maturation is not advanced. After birth these children grow much faster than normal children, but accurate data on growth rate of untreated infants are not available.

The urinary excretion of 17-ketosteroids in the newborn period is higher than during the whole period of childhood before puberty starts. We do not know whether these urinary ketosteroids represent the secretion of biologically active androgenic steroids; highly elevated plasma levels of dehydroepiandrosterone and androsterone have been found in newborn infants and during the first weeks of life (41).

REFERENCES

1. Abelove, W. A., J. J. Rupp and K. E. Paschkis, Acromegaly and pregnancy, *J. Clin. Endocrin.* 14: 32, 1954.
2. Acheson, R. M., Effects of nutrition and disease on human growth, in: *Human Growth*, Symp. Soc. Human Biology, J. M. Tanner, ed., vol. III, p. 73, Pergamon Press, Oxford, 1960.
3. Andersen, H. J., *Studies of hypothyroidism in children*, thesis Copenhagen, Aarhuus Stiftsbogtrijkkerie, 1960.
4. Babson, S. G., J. Kangas, N. Young and J. L. Bramhall, Growth and development of twins of dissimilar size at birth, *Pediatrics* 33: 327, 1964.
5. Baird, D., The contribution of obstetrical factors to serious physical and mental handicap in children, *J. Obstet. Gynaec. Brit. Emp.* 66: 743, 1959.
6. Baird, D. and R. Illsley, Environment and child bearing, *Proc. R. Soc. Med.* 46: 53, 1953.
7. Beal, V. A., Nutritional intake of children: I. Calories, carbohydrates, fat and protein, *J. Nutr.* 50: 233, 1953. II. Calcium, phosphorus and iron, *J. Nutr.* 53: 499, 1954.
8. Blizzard, R. M. and M. Alberts, Hypopituitarism, hypoadrenalism and hypogonadism in the newborn infant, *J. Pediat.* 48: 782, 1956.
9. Brewer, D. B., Congenital absence of the pituitary gland and its consequences, *J. Path. Bact.* 73: 59, 1957.
10. Broman, B., G. Dahlberg and A. Lichtenstein, Height and weight during growth, *Acta Pediat.* 30: 1, 1942.
11. McCance, R. A., Food, growth and time, *Lancet* II: 621, 671, 1962.
12. McCance, R. A., The bearing of the plane of nutrition on growth and endocrine development, in: *Protein Metabolism*, Ciba symp., F. Gross, ed., p. 109, Springer-Verlag, Berlin, 1962.
13. Cawley, R. H., T. McKeown and R. G. Record, Parental stature and birth weight, *Amer. J. Hum. Gen.* 6: 448, 1954.
14. Cornblath, M., S. H. Reisner, M. L. Parker and W. H. Daughaday, Growth hormone levels in premature and full term infants, *Abstract Soc. Ped. Res.*, 34th Ann. Meeting, p. 14, 1964.
15. Drillien, C. M., The social and economic factors affecting the incidence of premature birth, *J. Obstet. Gynaec. Brit. Emp.* 64: 161, 1957.
16. Drillien, C. M., *The growth and development of the prematurely born infant*, E. S. Livingstone, Ltd., Edinburgh, 1964.
17. Dobbing, J., The influence of early nutrition on the development and myelination of the brain, *Proc. Roy. Soc. B.* 159: 503, 1964.

18. Ducharme, J. R. and M. M. Grumbach, Studies of the effects of human growth hormone in premature infants, *J. Clin. Invest.* 40: 243, 1961.
19. Ellis, R. W. B., in: *Child Health and Development*, p. 151, J. A. Churchill Ltd., London, 1962.
20. Engfeldt, B. and G. T. Hultquist, Administration of crystalline growth hormone to pregnant rats, *Acta Endocrinol.* 14: 181, 1953.
21. Falkner, F., Some physical measurements in the first three years of life, *Arch. Dis. Childh.* 31: 1, 1958.
22. Falkner, F., Personal communication.
23. Farquhar, J. W., The child of the diabetic woman, *Arch. Dis. Childh.* 34: 76, 1959.
24. Fisher, D. A. and D. E. Pickering, Infantile hypothyroidism, diagnosis and treatment, *Ped. Clin. North Am.* p. 863, 1957.
25. Francis, T., *Investigations into the development of the pituitary at hereditary anterior pituitary dwarfism in mice, with reference to the pathogenesis of the anterior pituitary dwarfism*, E. Munksgaard, Copenhagen, Denmark, 1944.
26. Gemzell, C. A., Das Wachstumshormon in retroplazentärer Blut und in Nabelschnurblut, in: *Probleme der fötalen Endocrinologie*, 3. Symp. Deutsche Gesellsch. f. Endocrin., Springer-Verlag, Heidelberg, 1956.
27. Gilbert, J. A. L., The association of maternal obesity, large babies and diabetes, *Brit. Med. J.* 1: 702, 1949.
28. Graham, G., in: *Diet and bodily constitution*, discussion, p. 14, G. E. W. Wolstenholme and M. O'Connor, eds., J. A. Churchill Ltd., London, 1964.
29. Greenwood, F. C., W. M. Hunter and A. I. Klopper, Assay of human growth hormone in pregnancy at parturition and in lactation, *Brit. Med. J.* 1: 22, 1964.
30. Heierli, E., Longitudinale Wachstumsstudie, Resultate von Länge, Gewicht und Kopfumfang in den ersten vier Lebensjahren, *Helv. Ped. Acta* 5: 311, 1960.
31. Hewitt, D., C. K. Westropp and R. M. Acheson, The Oxford Child Health Survey. Effect of childish ailments on skeletal development, *Brit. J. Prev. Soc. Med.* 9: 179, 1955.
32. Jackson, W. P. U., The prediabetic syndrome. Large babies and the (pre) diabetic father, *J. Clin. Endocrin.* 14: 177, 1954.
33. Jeliffe, D. B., *Infant nutrition in the subtropics and tropics*, WHO monograph 29, Geneva, 1955.
34. Jost, A. and L. Picon, Hormonal factors in the growth of the foetus, in: *The biological actions of growth substances*, Symp. Soc. Exp. Biol. 11: 228.
35. Kunnas, M., Gestation age and growth of premature infant, *Ann. Paed. Fenn.* 6, fasc. 2, 1960.
36. Laron, Z., Personal communication.
37. Lichty, J. A., R. Y. Ting, P. D. Burns and E. Dyar, Studies of babies born at high altitudes, 1. Relation of altitude to birth weight, *Am. J. Dis. Child.* 93: 666, 1957.
38. Little, B., O. W. Smith, A. G. Jessiman, H. A. Selenkow, W. van 't Hof, J. M. Eglin and F. D. Moore, Hypophysectomy during pregnancy in a patient with cancer of the breast: case report with hormone studies, *J. Clin. Endocrin.* 18: 425, 1958.
39. Lubchenko, L. D., C. Hansman, M. Dressler and E. Boyd, Intrauterine growth as estimated from liveborn birth-weight data at 24 to 42 weeks of gestation, *Pediatrics* 32: 793, 1963.

40. Martin, M. M. and L. Wilkins, Pituitary dwarfism, diagnosis and treatment, *J. Clin. Endocrin.* 18: 679, 1958.
41. Migeon, C. J., The endocrine function of the newborn, in: *The somatic stability of the newly born*, Ciba symp., G. E. W. Wolstenholme and M. O'Connor, eds., p. 215, J. A. Churchill Ltd., London, 1961.
42. Myers, B., cited by F. Falkner, reference 8. *Brit. J. Child. Dis.* 23: 87, 1926.
43. Oppers, V. M., *Analyse van de acceleratie van de menselijke lengtegroei door bepaling van het tijdstip van de groeifasen*, Thesis, Amsterdam, 1963.
44. Patton, R. G. and L. I. Gardner, *Growth failure and maternal deprivation*, Charles C. Thomas Publ., Springfield, Ill., 1963.
45. Pennell, M. T. and A. J. Kukral, An unusual case of holo-acephalus, *Amer. J. Obstet, Gynaec.* 52: 669, 1946.
46. Prader, A., J. M. Tanner and G. A. von Harnack, Catch-up growth following illness or starvation, *J. Pediat.* 62: 646, 1963.
47. Pratt, C. W. M. and R. A. McCance, Severe undernutrition in growing and adult animals: 6. Changes in the long bones during the rehabilitation of cockerels, *Brit. J. Nutr.* 15: 121, 1961.
48. Rueda-Williamson, R. and H. E. Rose, Growth and nutrition of infants, the influence of diet and other factors in growth, *Pediatrics* 30: 639, 1962.
49. Seckel, H. P. G. Concepts relating the pituitary growth hormone to somatic growth of the normal child, *Amer. J. Dis. Childh.* 99: 349, 1960.
50. Sempe, M., C. Tutia et N. P. Masse, La croissance de l'enfant de 0 à 7 ans, *Extr. Arch. Franç. Péd.* 21: 111, 1964.
51. Simpson, M. E., C. W. Asling and H. M. Evans, Some endocrine influences on skeletal growth and differentiation, *Yale J. Biol. Med.* 23: 1, 1950.
52. Spector, S., O. H. Pearson, S. Stratman and B. Likly, Pituitary somatotropic hormone and growth, *Abstract Amer. Ped. Soc.* 74th Ann Meeting, p. 133, 1964.
53. Stoch, M. B. and R. M. Smythe, Does undernutrition during infancy inhibit brain growth and subsequent intellectual development?, *Arch. Dis. Childh.* 38: 546, 1963.
54. Stuart, H. C., et al., Longitudinal studies on child health and development — series II — reports based on completed case studies, *Pediatrics* 24: 875, 1959.
55. Stuart, H. C. and E. H. Sobel, The thickness of the skin and subcutaneous tissue by age and sex in childhood, *J. Pediat.* 28: 637, 1946.
56. Tanner, J. M., *Growth at adolescence*, 2nd ed., Blackwell Scient. Publ., Oxford, 1962.
57. Tanner, J. M., The regulation of human growth, *Child Developm.* 4: 817, 1963.
58. Tanner, J. M., M. J. R. Healey, R. D. Lockhart, J. D. Mackenzie and R. H. Whitehouse, Aberdeen growth study, I. The prediction of adult measurements from measurements taken each year from birth to 5 years, *Arch. Dis. Childh.* 31: 372, 1956.
59. Thomas, A., F. Lepage et Mme. Sorel-Dejerine, Examen anatomo-clinique de deux anencéphales protubérantiels, *Rev. neurol.* 76: 173, 1944.
60. Tuchmann-Duplessis, H. et L. Mercier-Parot, Hypophyse et développement prénatal. L'hormone somatotrope est-elle responsable du gigantisme foetal? *Presse Méd.* 86: 1831, 1955.
61. Vickers, V. S. and H. C. Stuart, Anthropometry in the pediatrician's office. Norms for selected body measurements based on studies of children of North European stock, *J. Pediat.* 22: 155, 1943.

62. WALKER, D. G., C. W. ASLING, M. E. SIMPSON, C. H. LI and H. M. EVANS, Structural alterations in rats, hypophysectomized at six days of age and their correction with growth hormone, *Anat. Rec.* 114: 19, 1952.
63. WERFF TEN BOSCH, J. J. VAN DER and R. ENTHOVEN, De normale lengtegroei, *Ned. Tijdschr. v. Geneesk.* 108: 1174, 1964.
64. WIDDOWSON, E. M., Mental contentment and physical growth, *Lancet* 1: 1316, 1951.
65. WIDDOWSON, E. M., Early nutrition and later development, in: *Diet and bodily constitution*, p. 3, G. E. W. WOLSTENHOLME and M. O'CONNOR, eds., J. A. Churchill Ltd., London, 1964.
66. WILKINS, L., *The diagnosis and treatment of endocrine disorders in childhood and adolescence*, 2nd ed., Blackwell Scientific Publ., Oxford, 1957.

DISCUSSION

Schwarz: I don't want to sound anti-feministic, but I would like to know whether the stature of the father is somewhere reflected in the birth weight of the child.

Thomson: The answer is no. This has been shown in animals by cross-breeding experiments (Walton and Hammond, 1938). The off-spring at birth is proportional to maternal size and it is only after birth that the father's size begins to come out. There have been at least two studies in man (Morton in Japan and McKeown in England); both indicate that paternal size has little or no influence upon birth weight.

Tiddens: Dr. Visser, one of the reasons why you expect an influence of illness in early infancy on final stature is the result of experiments in rats. Isn't the postnatal rate of growth far higher in the rat than in the human, relatively speaking, so that data obtained on rats may be more comparable to the intrauterine phase of human life.

Visser: I think for the human there are no accurate data available today, which give definite proof that malnutrition or illness during early infancy, and also before birth, may leave permanent marks, but evidence is accumulating. The studies of Drillien on the effect of illness in early infancy suggest that those children never catch up, at least not by the age of 5 years, and one could expect the catch-up before that. The experience with marasmic infants in Africa and South-America, who do not catch up, particularly not in brain development, support this view. The effects of illness are particularly difficult to study, because so far there are no data on skeletal maturation during illness and during catch-up growth in infants. And these data are needed to evaluate the effect on ultimate height.

CHAPTER VI

HORMONES, FOOD AND ACUTE NON-ENDOCRINE DISEASES

VARIATIONS IN ACTIVITY OF SOME ENDOCRINE ORGANS

J. J. VAN DER WERFF TEN BOSCH

Nearly all endocrine disorders become associated with gross abnormalities in the growth rate and stature, when they occur in childhood and remain untreated for a sufficiently long time. This is one of the reasons why the endocrine organs are supposed to be responsible for the normal variations in the growth rate. Until recently there have been few data to substantiate this view (38). The notable exception is the pubertal growth spurt, which has long been recognized to be due to sex steroids, that are secreted in increased amounts at this time. The lack of evidence for fluctuations in hormone secretion by other endocrine organs has been interpreted to indicate that their significance for growth is limited to a permissive action. There is now a clear indication that growth hormone may be secreted at different rates, with peaks which coincide with peaks in the growth rate.

The thyroid gland. The blood thyroid hormone level and the rate of thyroidal uptake of labelled iodine seem constant throughout childhood, except for the first week or weeks of life, when higher values are found (see 38). However, in groups of normal individuals the range of data for these measurements is so wide, that it seems possible that individual variations may not be discernable; it may be that more refined techniques employed in longitudinal studies would reveal significant differences. The possible regulatory function of thyroid hormone-binding serum proteins must also be considered. If the free thyroid hormone, less than 10 % of the value obtained in a PBI determination, is the biologically active component, then even major variations in the blood level of this fraction may go undetected. Large differences in serum PBI have been noted between different species (26, 31) and in sheep of different ages (11), which are possibly due to differences in the level of thyroid hormone-binding capacity of the serum. The high PBI values in newborn infants have been attributed to a similar mechanism (8), although the validity of this explanation has since been questioned (30).

The adrenal steroids. From the first week after birth the glucocorticoid level in the blood, determined as 17-hydroxycorticosteroids, remains constant and similar to that found in adults. Urinary excretion values rise slowly but are probably also constant, per unit of body surface area, if one takes into account the fact that conjugation by glucuronidation is impaired in the newborn (32).

During pregnancy, the maternal plasma 17-hydroxycorticosteroids rise, with a peak during parturition (2). The cord plasma level at birth equals about half of the maternal plasma level (15, 33), but during the first week after birth the newborn level falls from an average of 20 μg per 100 ml to less than 10 μg (3). The high levels at birth are partly due to the stress of birth, since they are much lower after birth by caesarean section (15, 33), and for the remainder they may be attributed to adrenal stimulation by maternal or placental ACTH or chorionic gonadotrophin, or to a high demand for corticoids during pre-natal life which is met through foetal pituitary ACTH (28). The production rate of hydrocortisone is constant throughout life, when calculated per unit of body surface area (27).

Plasma levels of 17-ketosteroids (14), particularly the androgenic fractions dehydroepiandrosterone and androsterone, are relatively high in newborn children, but after a few weeks only undetectable amounts are present (34). Dehydroepiandrosterone has been detected in the urine of premature babies, but not in the urine of children born at term (4).

Recently attention has been drawn to hitherto unidentified steroids, which can be found in the urine of newborn infants (5), in the urine of children 8—12 years old (21), and in the urine of adults during stimulation with ACTH (21). By one group of workers the steroid has been provisionally identified as a 3β,21-dihydroxypregn-5-ene-20-one (5); the other workers, who may be dealing with the same steroid, have suggested the provisional name 'childhood steroid' (21). It is of interest that the greatest amount of the childhood steroid has been found in children with lipodystrophy and progeria (21).

The sex hormones. Indirect evidence for secretion of sex steroids long before puberty, has been available for quite a long time, and consists of the alterations which occur in the sex organs and in the morphological appearance and gonadotrophin content of the pituitary gland and in the urinary gonadotrophin level, after removal of the gonads from immature members of a variety of species, and in children who lack functioning testes and ovaries (7). With customary methods it is difficult to estimate sex hormone levels in blood and urine of children

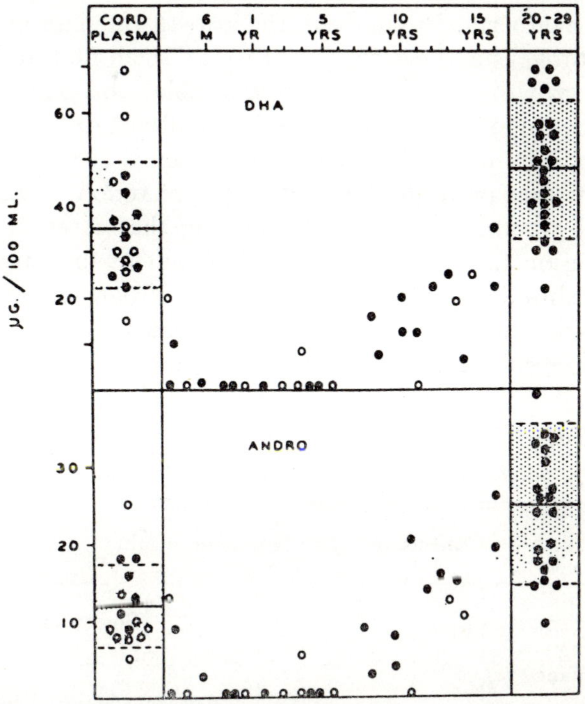

Fig. 1. Plasma levels of dehydroepiandrosterone (DHA) and androsterone (ANDRO) at birth, during infancy and adolescence, and in adulthood. ∘ = females, • = males. Shaded areas delimit one standard deviation below and above the mean levels (from 34)

before puberty. Except for the immediate post-natal period (see above) androgens are not demonstrable in plasma until the age of about 8 years, from which time both androsterone and dehydroepiandrosterone rise steadily (fig. 1). The shape of the curves is rather similar to those of the urinary androgenic activity published 25 years ago (35, 20). It is certain that a longitudinal study would yield considerably steeper curves. From a longitudinal study it might be learnt whether a slow rise precedes a steep increase, and at what level of androgen the secondary sex characters, the onset of the pubertal spurt in height, and the pubertal changes in body composition begin to appear. Similar considerations apply, of course, to data on oestrogen levels.

There is no doubt that sex hormones are *sine qua non* for most if not all of the somatic alterations that may be observed in the normal child during puberty. In children, the growth rate can be stimulated both by androgens and oestrogens. It would seem that androgens can act only if growth hormone is also available, and one possibility is that the secretion of growth hormone is stimulated under the influence of androgen. The mode of action of oestrogen is even less clear. One hypothesis is that oestrogens stimulate the secretion of androgens by the adrenal glands, possibly by promoting the secretion of ACTH. Much confusion has arisen from the fact that in the rat the growth rate is not stimulated, but depressed by oestrogens. The difference in the growth response to oestrogens between the child and the rat could be the result of a difference in adrenal response, with a greater

Tabel 1. *Some differences between rat and man, in their growth response to gonadectomy and sex hormone administration.*

Effects on body length or height			
Treatment during early infancy	Rat	Boys and girls	
		first decade	third decade
Gonadectomy	♂ shorter ♀ longer	?	taller
Intact, with testosterone			
'high dose'	♂ shorter	taller	shorter
'low dose'	♂ longer ?	?	?
Intact, with oestrogen	♀ shorter	taller	shorter

rise in androgens in the child and a greater rise in corticosteroids in the rat. The species difference is not confined to the effect of oestrogens (table 1), but also exists for the effect of exogenous androgen; in the young rat, both a single dose (36) and continued treatment with androgens (12, 13) cause depression of growth of male rats, while they stimulate the growth of females. These effects of androgens are comparable to those obtained after early gonadectomy (10).

Pituitary growth hormone. The foetal pituitary gland contains an appreciable amount of growth hormone, in one study in fact as much, per gland, as those of a 12-year-old boy and an adult (17). Yet the rate of intrauterine growth is believed to be independent of the foetal pituitary gland (24,25) and of growth hormone secreted by the maternal pituitary gland (1, 23, 29, 25). There is clinical (16) and experimental (6) evidence that the placenta may produce a growth promoting substance. It should not be overlooked that growth hormone simply happens to bear its present name, and that it has many other actions besides the stimulation of growth, so that there remains plenty of scope for a foetal growth hormone if it should indeed be found that pituitary growth hormone cannot promote foetal growth. The latter conclusion has been reached from a study in which prematurely born children, in contrast to older children, failed to show an increase in the growth rate during growth hormone administration (9).

The estimation of plasma levels of growth hormone by the radio-immuno-electrophoretic method has confirmed the finding that the foetal pituitary secretes growth hormone. Umbilical arteries and veins were found to contain identical and high (about 50 μmg per ml) plasma levels of growth hormone. In maternal blood the level was also considerably higher than in non-pregnant women, but less than half that of cord blood (18).

The role of growth hormone in the regulation of post-natal growth is uncertain. There have not yet been published longitudinal studies of children in whom the variations in the growth rate of single individuals could be related to variations in their plasma level of growth hormone. In cross-sectional studies, the results of growth hormone assays in children have been inconclusive. In one study (37) the range and the mean value for 12 normal children (7—17 years old) were identical with those obtained for 16 normal adults (20—92 years old).

In another study it has been reported that in 68 children and adolescents, plasma taken 2—3 hours after a meal had a growth hormone concentration about 20 times that found in adults, but that the values in children did not seem to correlate with age (19). In a table from the same laboratory, however, the mean values at various ages of a group of 84 children show marked fluctuations which seem to follow the fluctuations in growth rate: 18.6 μmg/ml under 1 year, 8.5 between 1 and 8 years, 2.8 between 9 and 10 years and 14.0 between 11 and 17 years (22). For adults these workers obtained an average value of 0.55 μmg/ml. These findings show that children have higher blood levels of growth hormone than adults, and that there may be a relationship between the growth rate and the growth hormone level.

It will be of extreme interest to see results of growth hormone assays in longitudinal studies of normal children (particularly before, during and immediately after puberty), in studies of children of short stature during treatment with growth stimulating substances, and in studies of children with growth retardation in consequence of specific non-endocrine diseases during specific treatment, e.g. coeliac disease and gluten-free diet. It may be, that effects of diseases and of effective therapy on the rate of growth are always mediated by changes in the plasma level of growth hormone. There is also the fascinating question through which channels the normal variations in the growth hormone level are brought about, and how adverse conditions or restorative measures exert their influence.

REFERENCES

1. Abelove, W. A., J. J. Rupp and K. E. Paschkis, Acromegaly and pregnancy, *J. Clin. Endocrinol.* 14: 32, 1954.
2. Bayliss, R. I. S., J. C. McC. Browne, B. P. Round and A. W. Steinbeck, Plasma-17-hydroxycorticosteroids in pregnancy, *Lancet* i: 62, 1955.
3. Bertrand, J., R. Gilly and B. Loras, L'étude des variations de la concentration plasmatique des formes libres et conjuguées des 17-hydroxycorticostéroides avant et après ACTH chex le nouveau-né et lors des huit premiers jours de la vie, *Arch. franç. Pédiat.* 17: 1257, 1960.
4. Birchall, K., D. M. Cathro, C. C. Forsyth and F. L. Mitchell, Separation and estimation of adrenal steroids in the urine of newborn infants, *Lancet* i: 26, 1961.
5. Cathro, D. M., K. Birchall, F. L. Mitchell and C. C. Forsyth, The excretion of neutral steroids in the urine of newborn infants, *J. Endocrinol.* 27: 53, 1963.

6. CONTOPOULOS, A. N. and M. E. SIMPSON, Growth-promoting activity of pregnant rat plasma after hypophysectomy and after thyroidectomy, *Endocrinology* 64: 1023, 1959.
7. DONOVAN, B. T. and J. J. VAN DER WERFF TEN BOSCH, *Physiology of Puberty*, London, 1965.
8. DOWLING, J. T., N. FREINKEL and S. H. INGBAR, Thyroxine-binding by sera of pregnant women, newborn infants, and women with spontaneous abortion, *J. clin. Invest.* 35: 1263, 1956.
9. DUCHARME, J. R. and M. M. GRUMBACH, Studies on the effects of human growth hormone in premature infants, *J. clin. Invest.* 40: 243, 1961.
10. ENTHOVEN, R., H. E. SWANSON and J. J. VAN DER WERFF TEN BOSCH, in preparation.
11. FALCONER, I. R. and H. A. ROBERTSON, Changes in thyroid activity during growth in the sheep, *J. Endocrinol.* 22: 23, 1961.
12. FUJII, T. and R. KOYAMA, Sex difference of rat growth after administration of testosterone propionate, *Endocrin. Japon* 9: 161, 1962.
13. FUJII, T., Y. MORITA and R. KOYAMA, Effects of some anabolic steroids on the growth in male and female rats, *Endocrin. Japon* 9: 93, 1962.
14. GARDNER, L. I. and R. L. WALTON, Plasma 17-ketosteroids of full-term and premature infants, *J. clin. Invest.* 33: 1642, 1954.
15. GEMZELL, C. A., Variations in plasma levels of 17-hydroxycorticosteroids in mother and infant following parturition, *Acta endocr. Copenhagen* 17: 100, 1954.
16. GEMZELL, C. A., Das Wachstumshormon im retroplacentären Blut und im Nabelschnurblut, *III Symp. Dtsch. Gesellsch. Endokrin.* 179, 1956.
17. GERSHBERG, H., Growth hormone content and metabolic actions of human pituitary glands, *Endocrinology* 61: 160, 1957.
18. GREENWOOD, F. C., W. M. HUNTER and A. KLOPPER, Assay of human growth hormone in pregnancy, at parturition and in lactation. Detection of a growth-hormone-like substance from the plasma, *Brit. med. J.* i: 22, 1964.
19. GREENWOOD, F. C., W. M. HUNTER and V. J. MARRIAN, Growth-hormone levels in children and adolescents, *Brit. med. J.* i: 25, 1964.
20. GREULICH, W. W., R. I. DORFMAN, H. R. CATCHPOLE, C. I. SOLOMON and C. S. CULOTTA, Somatic and endocrine studies of puberal and adolescent boys, *Monographs Soc. Res. Child Developm.* 7: no. 3, 1, 1942.
21. GUPTA, D. and J. M. TANNER, A new steroid found in the urine of children but not of adults, *Nature* 203: 187, 1964.
22. HUNTER, W. M. and F. C. GREENWOOD, A radio-immunoelectrophoretic assay for human growth hormone, *Biochem. J.* 91: 43, 1964.
23. JACKSON, W. P. U., The prediabetic syndrome. Large babies and the (pre) diabetic father, *J. clin. Endocrinol.* 14: 177, 1954.
24. JOST, A., Hormonal factors in the development of the fetus, *Cold Spr. Harb. Symp. quant. Biol.* 19: 167, 1954.
25. JOST, A. and L. PICON, Hormonal factors in the growth of the foetus, *Biological action of Growth Substances, Symp. Soc. exp. Biol.* 11: 228, 1957.
26. KELSEY, F. O., A. GULLOCK and H. J. CLAUSEN, Plasma protein-bound iodine in the beaver and other animals, *Acta endocr. Copenhagen* 35: 495, 1960.
27. KENNY, F. M., P. MALVAUX and C. J. MIGEON, Cortisol production rate in newborn babies, older infants and children, *Pediatrics* 31: 360, 1963.
28. LANMAN, J. T., The adrenal gland in the human fetus. An interpretation of its physiology and unusual developmental pattern, *Pediatrics* 27: 140, 1961.

29. LITTLE, B., O. W. SMITH, A. G. JESSIMAN, H. A. SELENKOW, W. VAN 'T HOFF, J. M. EGLIN and F. D. MOORE, Hypophysectomy during pregnancy in a patient with cancer of the breast: case report with hormone studies, *J. clin. Endocrinol.* 18: 425, 1958.
30. MARKS, J., J. WOLFSON and R. KLEIN, Neonatal thyroid function: erythrocyte T_3 uptake in early infancy, *J. Pediat.* 58: 32, 1961.
31. MATTY, A. J., Thyroid protein-bound iodine of a teleost fish (Scarus guacamaia), *J. Endocrinol.* 19: 353, 1960.
32. MIGEON, C. J., The endocrine function of the newborn, in: *Ciba Found. Symp. on Somatic stability in the newly born*, Ed. G. E. W. WOLSTENHOLME and M. O'CONNOR, London, 215, 1961.
33. MIGEON, C. J., A. R. KELLER and E. G. HOLMSTROM, Dehydroepiandrosterone, androsterone and 17- hydroxycorticosteroid levels in maternal and cord plasma in cases of vaginal delivery, *Johns Hopk. Hosp. Bull.* 97: 415, 1955.
34. MIGEON, C. J., A. R. KELLER, B. LAWRENCE and T. H. SHEPARD, Dehydroepiandrosterone and androsterone levels in human plasma. Effect of age and sex; day-to-day and diurnal variations, *J. clin. Endocrinol.* 17: 1051, 1957.
35. NATHANSON, I. T., L. E. TOWNE and J. C. AUB, Normal excretion of sex hormone in childhood, *Endocrinology* 28: 851, 1941.
36. SWANSON, H. E. and J. J. VAN DER WERFF TEN BOSCH, Sex differences in growth of rats, and their modification by a single injection of testosterone propionate shortly after birth, *J. Endocrinol.* 26: 197, 1963.
37. UTIGER, R. D., Extraction and radioimmunoassay of growth hormone in human serum, *J. clin. Endocrinol.* 24: 60, 1964.
38. WERFF TEN BOSCH, J. J. VAN DER, Anterior pituitary function in infancy and puberty, in: *The Pituitary Gland*, Eds. B. T. DONOVAN and G. W. HARRIS, London, 2: 324, 1966.

GROWTH OF CHILDREN IN WEST AFRICA: EFFECTS OF NUTRITION AND DISEASE

A. M. THOMSON, W. Z. BILLEWICZ and BARBARA THOMPSON*
and
I. A. MCGREGOR and A. K. RAHMAN**

There is remarkable unanimity in the literature that even where undernutrition and malnutrition are widespread and where breast feeding is customary, babies grow very well during the first few months of life. Growth in weight is usually as good as, and may even surpass standards that are regarded as 'optimum' in Western countries. Thus, for example GOPALAN and BELAVADY (1) found that the monthly weight increments of babies in a poor South Indian community were comparable with those of American infants. Similarly, OOMEN and MALCOLM (3) say that in Papua: 'The rate of weight increase during the first three months is usually not less than that observed in more propitious surroundings'.

Such high growth rates imply that breast feeding is as a rule extremely satisfactory. If the maternal diet is insufficient in quantity or of poor nutritive value, this apparently has little effect on lactation.

But the baby soon becomes too large to grow satisfactorily on a diet of breast milk alone. Other foods are introduced after a few weeks or months, though breast feeding may continue for a year or more. It is generally found that growth falters about the same time, and when the babies are one year of age or more they are usually much lighter than their Western counterparts. Mortality and morbidity begin to increase during the second half of the first year, and forms of protein-calorie malnutrition are described as being most common in many communities during the second year.

This kind of pattern has been described in many parts of Africa and the present report deals with some recent data from The Gambia,

* Obstetric Medicine Research Unit (Medical Research Countil), University of Aberdeen.

** Medical Research Council Laboratories, The Gambia, West Africa.

West Africa. It should be understood that the material is still being analyzed, and that this is no more than a preliminary report.

Keneba is a small village near the tidal creeks of the Gambia river. Its 800 inhabitants are Mohammedans, practising polygamy and living according to a traditional subsistence economy: the village is in a rather remote situation, and has not been greatly affected by Western ideas or technology. The women grow most of the food, the main cereals being rice, millet, findo and maize, while the men cultivate groundnuts as a cash crop. Small quantities of fish, meat and milk are available from time to time, and the diet is filled out with cultivated or wild fruits and vegetables. Young children are breast fed for up to two years, cereal paps being introduced during the first few months of life. By the time a child is weaned, it receives meals of the adult pattern. Care of children is somewhat haphazard, as the mothers must work extremely hard in the fields as well as in the village in order to subsist. Malaria is hyperendemic and stimulates a distinct pattern of immunity. During the first few months of life, children are protected by immunity inherited from their mothers, and seldom develop clinical malaria. In older children and in adults, a strong acquired immunity usually prevents parasitaemia developing to a level at which there are obvious clinical manifestations. The highest levels of parasitaemia, and the severest degrees of associated illness, are seen during the transitional stage between the passive and active phases of immunity, i.e. between about 6 months and 4 years of age. In children of this age, we have found remarkable seasonal fluctuations in blood haemoglobin concentrations, which are probably due to malaria.

Nearly all young children suffer more or less chronically from respiratory infections, skin sepsis and intestinal infections and infestations. Nearly half the children die before the age of five.

Children in the village have been weighed and measured each April since 1950. Fig. 1 shows the average growth in weight of children up to age 7 years. It is obvious that growth between about 6 months and 2 years of age is much less than in Britain; subsequently annual increments are much the same, but the African children do not 'catch-up'. Fig. 1 also shows that children who failed to survive until 7 years of age, or who died before the next annual examination had average weights very close to those of survivors. Fig. 2 indicates the pattern during the first year of life in more detail. A rapid survey of babies in

Keneba and three adjacent villages showed that during the first 6 months weights were evenly distributed around the British standard; during the next six months, most weights were below the standard.

Mortality was relatively low during the first 6 months of life, rose to a peak at about one year, and remained high until about the end

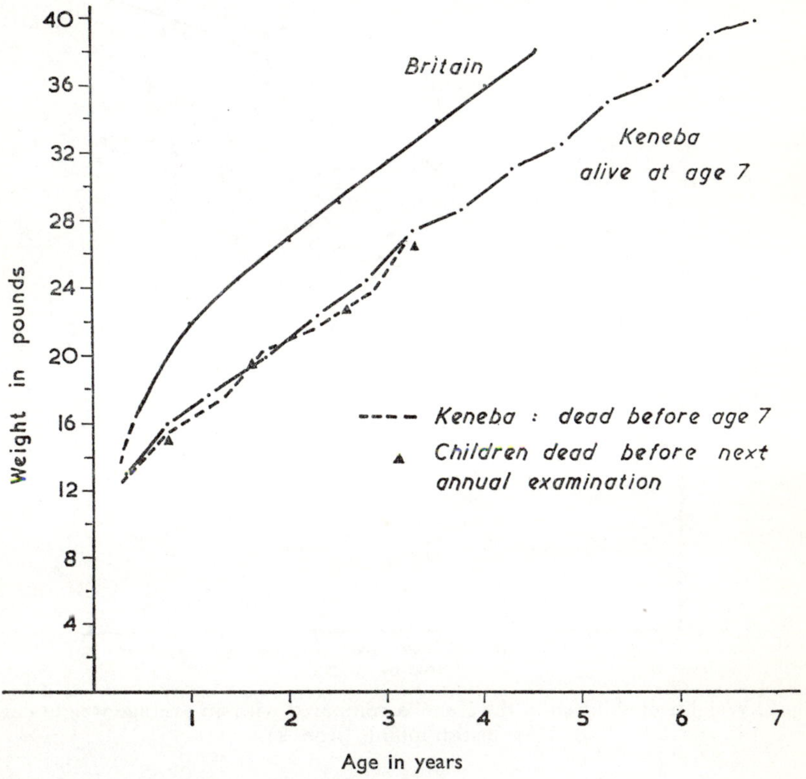

Fig. 1. Average weight curves of Keneba children alive at 7 years of age, and of those who died before 7 years, compared with British averages (from 2)

of the fourth year. Deaths occurred most frequently during the rainy season — roughly, mid-May until mid-November — when malaria and other insect-borne diseases reach their maximum incidence.

We described and discussed these phenomena three years ago and suggested that they were more likely to be explained by the impact of disease and changing patterns of immunity, than by primary malnutrition (2).

We have since studied the patterns of growth in more detail, by measuring all children aged under five years at intervals of two weeks or one month, and at the same time collecting as much information

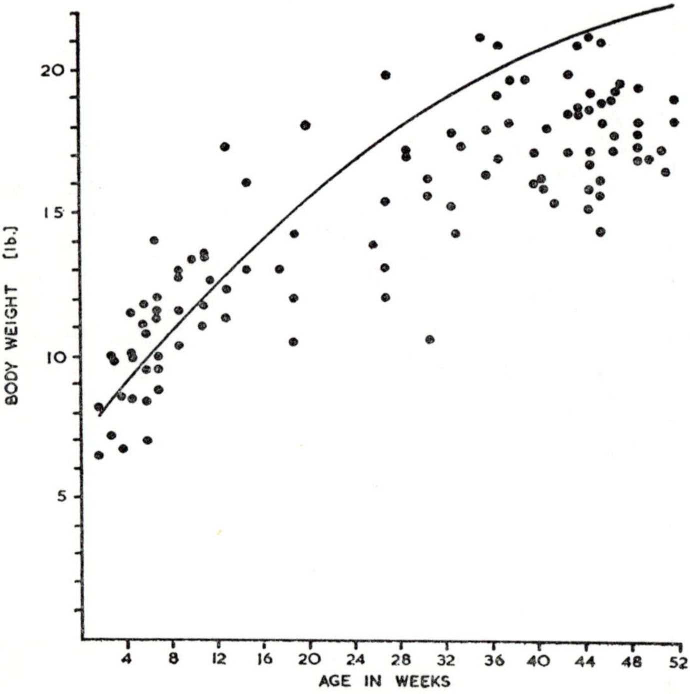

Fig. 2. Weights of children in the Keneba compared with an average weight curve for British infants (from 2)

about their health and conditions of living as was possible with very limited resources.

It soon became evident that the smooth average growth pattern already demonstrated does not tell the whole story. The annual measurements previously available naturally failed to show a remarkable seasonal cycle of growth. Fig. 3 differentiates four cohorts of children born at different times of year. In all, average growth during the first few months of life is very satisfactory, regardless of season.

Subsequently, the pattern of growth depends on season: for all practical purposes it ceases entirely during the rainy season, with recovery during the dry season. Thus, a child born just before the rains is likely to grow fairly well until it is almost a year old, whereas the growth of one that is about six months old in May is halted. Nevertheless, children born at different seasons appear to be of much the same average weight by two or more years of age, and even at one year the differences are small. The seasonal cycles of growth are

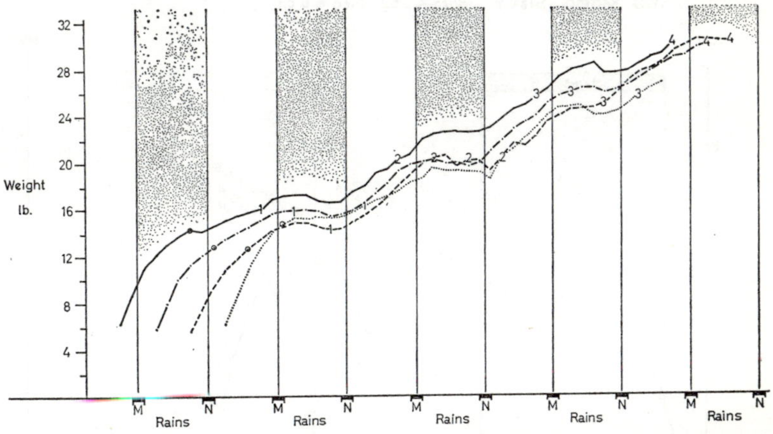

Fig. 3. Average growth curves of four cohorts of children born at different times of year, and measured at short intervals during the two years 1960—61. Ages are inserted on the curves

repeated each year at later ages. It may be noted that growth during the dry season is, on average, extremely rapid. The average increments are greater than those found in British children of the same age. The patterns of growth in height, which was measured every 3 months, are similar to those of weight.

The growth curves of individual children usually show the same kind of seasonal cycle, upon which short-term fluctuations are superimposed. The short-term fluctuations can usually be related to episodes of illness. Under the conditions of field work, we were seldom able to make a very precise diagnosis: and indeed it is possible that even with much greater clinical and laboratory facilities the exact diagnosis would often have remained in doubt. Most illnesses seemed to be of multiple aetiology. Investigation by qualified doctors was not continuously available, and laboratory resources were limited. Under these conditions, it was decided that all cases seeking or needing treatment should be helped, but that specific therapy, for example with penicillin or antimalarials, should not be given unless a reasonably accurate diagnosis could be made or unless the child was seriously ill.

In practice, parents were sometimes unwilling to co-operate even when a child was very ill indeed, preferring to rely on their traditional bush medicines, and on the advice of soothsayers.

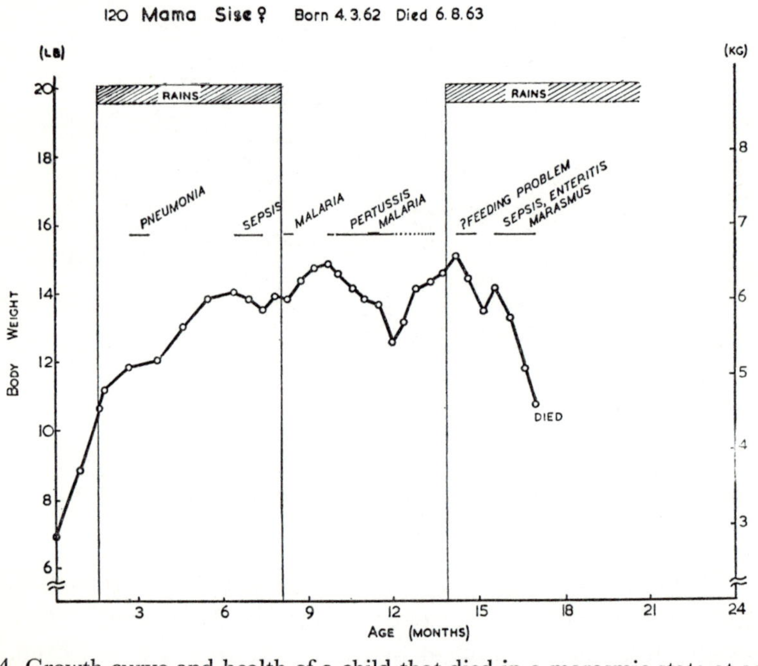

Fig. 4. Growth curve and health of a child that died in a marasmic state at age 17 months

During the first year of the survey, few cases of specific deficiency disease were seen, and probably no illnesses that could be confidently ascribed to a primary dietary defect. During the summer of 1963, however, there were several cases of marasmus and 'kwashiorkor'.

Food supplies were more plentiful in 1962 than in 1963, and it is possible that young children were fed in a less satisfactory manner in 1963. There was, however, no clear evidence of seriously defective food patterns among such children in 1963. A factor that may have more importance is that during the spring of 1963 there was an epidemic of whooping cough which affected most young children in the village, and which was associated with considerable loss of weight and with impairment of general health. Children so exposed may have been less able to withstand the further onslaught of disease during the rainy season.

Figs. 4 and 5 show the growth patterns and the more obvious illnesses of two children. One of them died with all the signs of severe

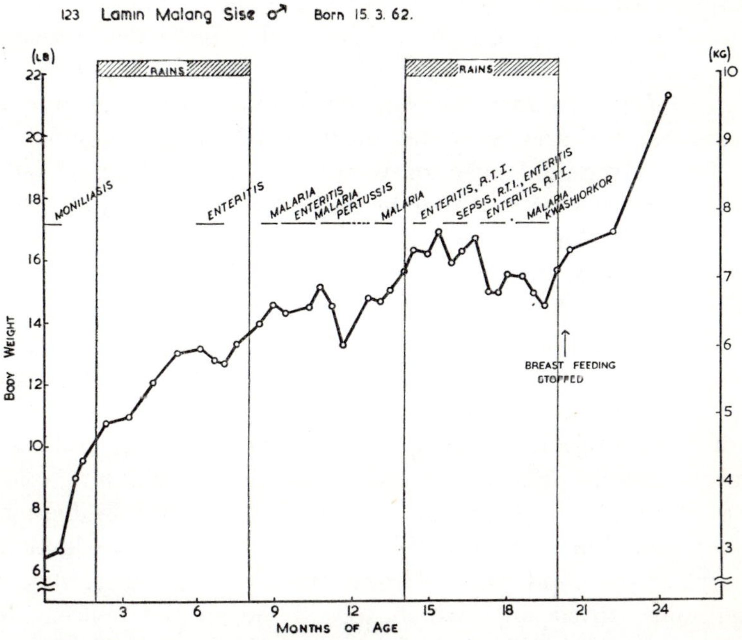

Fig. 5. Growth curve and health of a child that developed signs of kwashiorkor at about 20 months of age

marasmus. The other developed signs of kwashiorkor, but was recovering satisfactorily when last seen.

No. 120, Mama Sise, was being breast fed throughout. She grew very well during the first 6 months of life (mostly during the rains) apart from a severe respiratory illness, probably pneumonia, which responded to penicillin. Towards the end of the rains a setback to growth was associated with multiple superficial skin lesions which became septic. She began to grow well when the rains stopped, but in January 1963 developed whooping cough which persisted until about the end of April and caused considerable loss of weight. During this time, malarial parasites were frequently present in blood, sometimes in high density, but this was not obviously associated with acute illness. At the end of May 1963, she was noted to be vaguely ill and was refusing food other than breast milk. No specific diagnosis could be made. She seemed to be recovering during the later part of June, but early in July there was a severe episode of diarrhoea and vomiting, together with otitis media and other septic lesions. The mother was unco-operative and refused treatment on religious grounds. The child rapidly deteriorated and died in a marasmic state at 17 months of age.

No. 123, Lamin Malang Sise, was born about the same time as the previous case and grew very well until he was about 9 months of age, apart from a monilial infection of the mouth which interfered with feeding for a week or two after birth, and an episode of diarrhoea in October 1962. This recurred in January and February, 1963, and malarial parasites were found in the blood, in high density, about this time. When the child seemed to be recovering, he developed whooping cough, which was associated with a severe setback to growth. However, at the age of one year, a satisfactory recovery was being made. The onset of the 1963 rainy season was associated with a succession of attacks of enteritis, respiratory tract infections, and multiple superficial septic lesions. As fig. 5 shows, the child deteriorated steadily throughout the rainy season of 1963, and in September-October was thin and miserable with oedematous face and limbs. The care of the child was far from satisfactory, but it seemed to be getting some dried milk which we offered to the mother. Rapid recovery ensued with the end of the rainy season. It is of interest that breast feeding stopped just at this time.

Histories obtained from the mothers of such children are exceedingly unreliable. Had these two cases been seen by medical staff for the first time after admission to hospital at 17 and 20 months of age, respectively, a diagnosis of severe malnutrition would have been amply justified by the clinical findings, and it is most unlikely that histories obtained from the mothers would have uncovered the prolonged sequences of serious illness and setbacks to growth.

CONCLUSIONS

There seems to be little doubt that the repeated onslaught of infectious and parasitic diseases is the predominant cause of impaired growth and high mortality in these West African children. The effects of disease are probably reinforced by unsatisfactory feeding practices and by seasonal shortages of certain foods, but it is unlikely that the high prevalence and great severity of disease is primarily due to low immunity caused by undernitrution and malnutrition.

The abrupt onset of episodes of weight loss, together with such clinical and sociological information as is available, makes it more likely that serious forms of undernutrition and malnutrition were mainly due to anorexia, malabsorption and destruction of tissue caused by infectious disease.

To improve standards of growth and to reduce mortality among children in such communities, it is at least as important to prevent and to treat communicable diseases, as to improve food supplies and feeding practices.

REFERENCES

1. Gopalan, C. and B. Belavady, *Fed. Proc.* 20 (Part III, Suppl. 7): 177, 1961.
2. McGregor, I. A., W. Z. Billewicz and A. M. Thomson, *Brit. med. J.* 2: 1661, 1961.
3. Oomen, H. A. P. C. and S. H. Malcolm, *S. Pacific Comm. Techn. Paper*, No. 118, 1958.

GROWTH AND DEVELOPMENT OF OBESE CHILDREN

F. SCHWARZ

The statement of WILKINS (3), that 'more than 25 % of the patients seen at the Children's Endocrine Clinic have been referred because of obesity, which has caused the parents, physicians or nurses to suspect a 'glandular disorder' ', illustrates the frequency of obesity in children, and the general inclination to incriminate endocrine glands as the cause of it.

The group of children I want to discuss consists of 85 boys and 52 girls between the ages of 11 and 15 years. Many of them have been referred with a diagnosis of either adiposogenital dystrophy (Fröhlich's syndrome) or hypothyroidism. In 15 of the boys cryptorchidism was found, but there were no other endocrine disorders. Interrogation of parents and child usually disclosed emotional circumstances which could account for over-eating.

Table 1. *Percentage overweight in obese children 11—15 years old.*

Overweight	20-30%	31-40%	41-50%	51-60%	61-70%	>70%	total
boys	17	21	20	15	6	6	85
girls	3	14	16	3	11	5	52

The percentage of overweight has been calculated from the 50th percentile of weight for height according to DE WIJN and DE HAAS (5). Table 1 shows the results. There are relatively fewer girls in the group of 20 to 30 % overweight, probably because slight overweight does not cause as much concern in a girl as it does in a boy.

Figures 1 and 2 show the distribution of height by age for boys and girls. It is obvious that in both figures there are more points above, than below the 50th percentile, i.e. that the children tend to be above the height which is the average for their age.

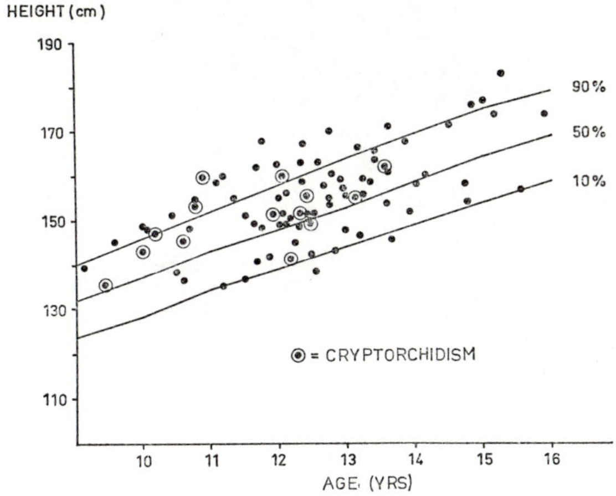

Fig. 1. Height of obese boys (percentiles from 5)

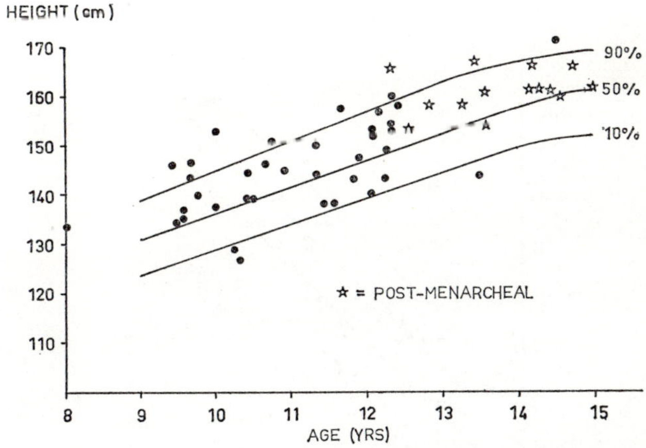

Fig. 2. Height of obese girls (percentiles from 5)

The bone age of the patients has been determined by use of the atlas of Greulich and Pyle (2). Parallel to the normal line in figures 3 and 4, two lines are drawn at a distance of one year. As the 'normal

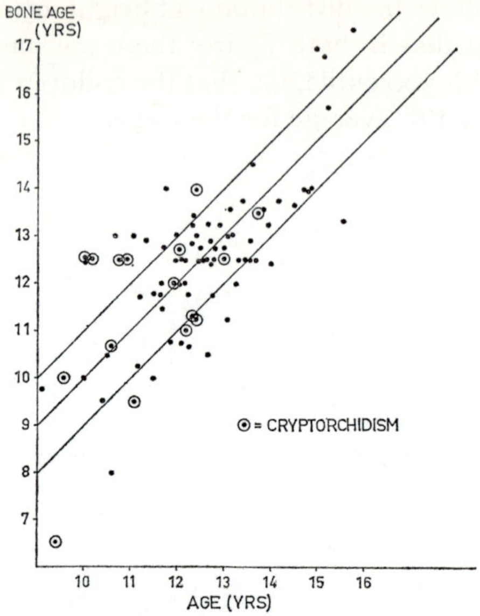

Fig. 3. Bone age of obese boys

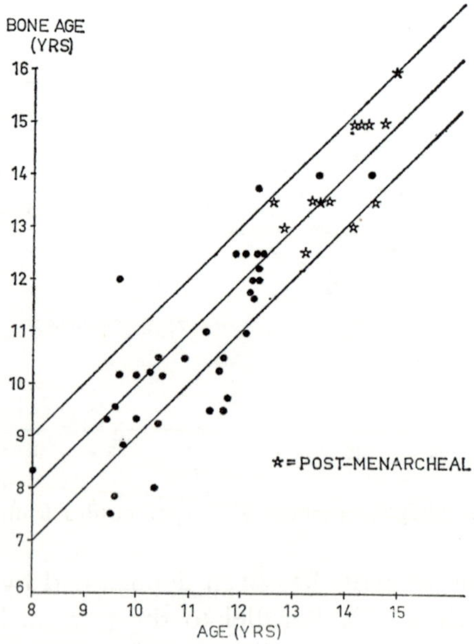

Fig. 4. Bone age of obese girls

distribution' for Dutch children is not known, this distance is chosen arbitrarily and for simplicity's sake. It is somewhat larger than the 1 standard deviation interval given by GREULICH and PYLE.

From figure 3 it can be seen that for boys the distribution is fairly symmetrical about the normal line. In girls the situation is different (fig. 4).

Up to the age of 12 years, most of the points lie below the normal average, while in the older children they are within the normal range.

The fact that obese children tend to be above average height, has been noted by numerous investigators. This could be explained by

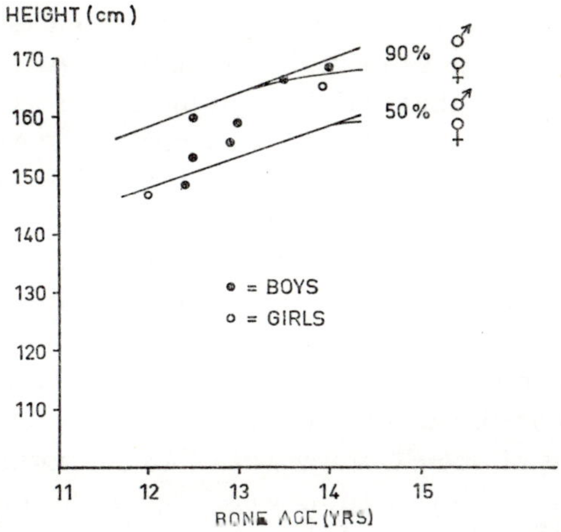

Fig. 5. Height versus bone age of 9 children who were tall and advanced in bone age

earlier ripening of the obese child, but then one would expect the bone age to be advanced also. This was not the case in our boys, and rather the reverse was found in the girls. If only the cases with a height above the 90th percentile are analysed, it appears that the bone ages of 16 of the 23 boys are within the 1 year limit, while 7 boys are more than one year advanced in skeletal maturation. The 2 tall girls also have bone ages above the 1 year limit. When the height of these 9 children is plotted against their bone age, instead of against their chronological age, it appears (fig. 5) that also by this standard they are tall, 7 of them being above the 50th percentile, though none above the 90th percentile.

According to WOLFF (4), pubic and axillary hair appear earlier in the obese than in the average boy. The menarcheal age of the girls he found to be between 12 and 13 years, the corresponding standard being 13.6 years. In the collection of our data we have unfortunately not used a uniform mode of description of the pubertal development. Therefore no statement about the time of puberty in the boys can be made. The fact whether a girl was menstruating at the time of examination, is shown in the figures 2 and 4. The menarcheal age can not be determined exactly from the small number of observations, but probably lies between 12.5 and 13 years. From figure 4, it can be seen that bone age at menarche lies in the same range. Since the average menarcheal age for Dutch girls has been estimated at 13.8 years, our data seem to support the findings of WOLFF.

This would suggest, that in obese girls menarche occurs at an earlier stage of skeletal development than in normals. The early menarcheal age and the excess of height without corresponding advance in bone age cannot be explained at the moment. We must now face the question whether over-eating can result in growth at a more than average rate without accelerating skeletal maturation. An alternative possibility would be, that a common genetic factor causes both obesity and tallness. Obesity often runs in families, but whether constitutional factors or eating habits are inherited, we do not know. WOLFF has compared the birth weights of obese children with those of normals and did not find any difference. If overfeeding were responsible, one would expect to find a correlation between height and overweight. In our material we did not find such a correlation. Finally, it would be interesting to know whether a reducing diet (which of course must contain sufficient proteins, vitamins and minerals) would slacken growth. WOLFF found this to be true in the follow-up of 82 obese children. We were not able to confirm his findings. Figures 6 and 7 show the longitudinal follow-up of 22 boys, 11 of whom lost more than 20 % of ideal body weight, 5 less then 20 %, and 6 lost no weight at all. There are no differences in the slopes of the growth curves. More detailed study of the growth velocity also gave negative results. Perhaps a study of children of a lower age group would give better results, as in our material the onset of the pubertal growth spurt may have blurred the picture.

Finally something ought to be said about the diagnoses under which many of the children were referred: hypothyroidism and adiposo-

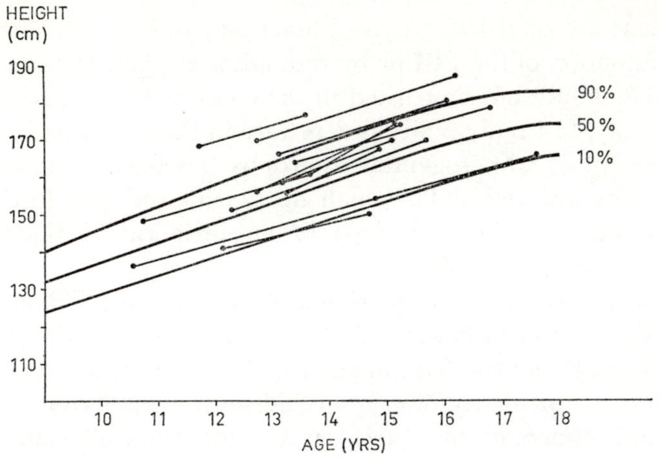

Fig. 6. Follow-up of boys who, on a reducing diet, lost more than 20 % of their ideal body weight

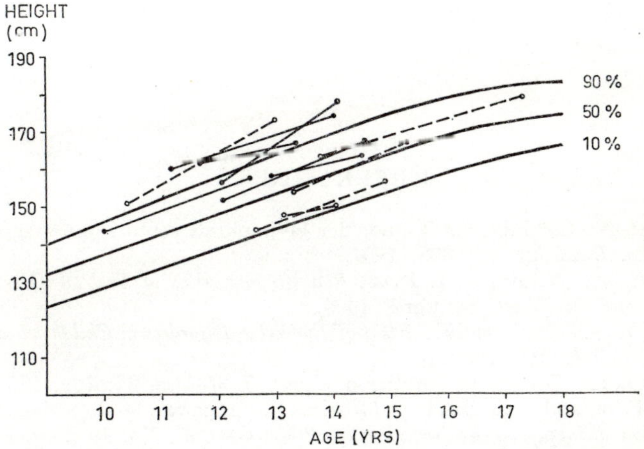

Fig. 7. Follow-up of boys who, on a reducing diet, lost no weight (drawn lines) or who lost less than 20% of their ideal body weight (interrupted lines)

genital dystrophy. About hypothyroidism we can be short. In an obese boy one must be aware of this possibility if growth and skeletal development are retarded. Thyroid function can be easily assessed by the determination of the PBI or by radioidine studies. Determinations of the BMR should not be trusted in these cases. A hypothyroid child may be stocky, but real obesity is very rare in this condition.

The concept of adiposogenital dystrophy has been derived from a publication by FRÖHLICH (1), which deals with the case history of a boy aged fourteen showing signs of an intracranial tumour and moderate obesity.

Many of the boys we have seen, had been erroneously diagnosed as cases of hypogonadism, because the penis was hidden in the pubic fat. We do not think that the high incidence of cryptorchidism in our boys reflects the true incidence of cryptorchidism in obese boys, but rather the fact that concomitant obesity and cryptorchidism caused more concern then either of these conditions alone. In figures 1 and 3 the cryptorchid obese boys do not seem to differ from boys who were obese only. On clinical observation and during the follow-up we could not find signs of hormonal dysfunction in these boys. We therefore think that the combination of both conditions is of no aetiological significance, and that the diagnosis adiposogenital syndrome or 'Fröhlich's syndrome' should be avoided.

REFERENCES

1. FRÖHLICH, A., Ein Fall von Tumor der Hypophysis cerebri ohne Akromegalie, *Wien. Klin. Rundschau* 15: 883, 1901.
2. GREULICH, W. W. and S. I. PYLE, *Radiographic Atlas of Skeletal Development of the Hand and the Wrist*, Stanford, 1959.
3. WILKINS, L., *Diagnosis and Treatment of Endocrine Disorders in Childhood and Adolescence*, Springfield Ill., 1959.
4. WOLFF, O. H., Obesity in childhood, *Quart. J. of Med.* 24: 109, 1955.
5. WIJN, J. F. DE and J. H. DE HAAS, Groeidiagrammen van 1—25 jarigen in Nederland, *Verhandelingen van het Ned. Inst. v. Praev. Geneesk.*, No. 49. Leiden, 1960.

EFFECTS OF ACUTE NON-ENDOCRINE DISEASE ON GROWTH

W. A. MARSHALL

Before any conclusions can be reached about the ultimate effect on stature of acute non-endocrine disease it is necessary to answer certain basic questions. Firstly, does the disease have any immediate effect on the child's rate of growth? If it does, does this effect persist; does the child's growth return to its normal rate on recovery from the illness; or does the child grow faster than before so that there is compensation for the effects of the illness? The same questions must then be asked in relation to skeletal maturity. If the maturation of the skeleton were delayed by exactly the same amount as growth in stature, and both stature and skeletal maturation progressed at the same relative rates after the illness, then there need be no effects on the ultimate height. If skeletal maturation were delayed more than growth in stature by the illness, the child could theoretically reach a greater final stature than he would have reached in the absence of illness. On the other hand if skeletal maturation were not affected while growth in stature was, then the child would have to grow more rapidly than normal after the illness in order to reach its normal adult height before the epiphyses fused. Thus the ultimate effect of the illness on stature will depend not only on its immediate effect on growth in stature and on skeletal maturation but also on the way that these two separate mechanisms behave after the illness has passed.

There is considerable doubt as to whether relatively mild acute illness can have any effect at all upon stature. Several attempts have been made to obtain information about this subject by comparing the growth of children who have suffered from illnesses with that of healthier children of the same age. In Great Britain the Ministry of Health Survey covering all social classes in England and Wales failed to show any difference in weight gain during the first three years between babies who had excellent, average or poor health records (9).

Drillien (4) found closer association with illness and length and weight gain in premature children, mostly born to families in poor circumstances, than in mature children born in better circumstances, but it is difficult to know the relative importance of the three factors illness, maturity and social class in producing these results. Acheson and his associates have shown that in the *Oxford Child Health Survey* children with illnesses were significantly shorter than those who had no illness during the same year of their lives. The effect on skeletal maturity was negligible. None of these children had been ill for more than a few weeks, even in the group whose illnesses were classified as 'severe'. The loss of stature involved was of the order of $\frac{1}{4}''$ for each year of 'severe' illness and there was no evidence of a subsequent acceleration (2, 7, 1). In any study which compares the amount of illness with the gain in weight or stature in two separate groups of children, it is impossible to say whether an increased amount of illness in one group caused them to grow less or whether children who grew less were more prone to illness. All the above observations could simply mean that illness occurs more frequently in children who do not grow very well, than in those who grow at a more satisfactory rate. This interpretation is supported by the fact that Acheson's survey also showed that the lower social classes had smaller stature for the same skeletal maturity, while no period of catch-up growth could be demonstrated following illness in small children. Prader, Tanner and Von Harnack (10) have shown that, where a severe illness produced a definite retardation of growth, cure of the illness is followed by a period of accelerated or catch-up growth. In the case of the Oxford children, those who suffered a severe illness in one year actually grew less in the following year than those who were free from illness in both years. Acheson (1) refers to data from a group of government controlled residential schools and orphanages in Ireland. These data show that girls who suffered from exanthemata showed a slight but significant spurt in growth after the illness. Apparently the spurt was not as great as the preceding slowing of growth and would not have compensated for the height loss. This however, would depend on the duration of the spurt and the corresponding effect on skeletal age. No information is given about these factors and Acheson points out that these preliminary findings may need revision in the light of a more extensive study which he was undertaking at that time. As TANNER (12) has pointed out, the only reliable method of determining whether or not minor illnesses really have an effect on growth is to study children longitudinally over a number of years and fit curves to the data obtained for each individual, omitting in the first place the points obtained following a period of illness. This curve serves as the individual's own control and the post-illness points can then be put in relation to the curve, so that it can be easily seen whether or not they are significantly depressed on the average. The presence of a significant catch-up afterwards can also be tested provided the measuring intervals are not more than six months apart. Even with this method it is possible that an illness producing little immediate effect but a slight long subsequent depression of growth might escape recognition. No studies of this nature have yet been published but TANNER (12) examined the data of the Harpenden Growth Study and the records of the Child Study Centre in London from this point of view and came to the conclusion that there is a great individual variation in reaction. Many children show no depression of growth following a severe attack of measles or pneumonia, others seem to show significant depressions without any illness at all being recorded. Several other workers have studied the growth curves of children whose illnesses had been carefully recorded, while their growth was followed longitudinally. Most of these studies have failed to reveal any retardation of growth over a six months' period in children who have suffered throughout it from colds, bronchitis, tonsillitis, measles and pneumonia, (5, 6, 8, 11). Most of these studies relate to well nourished and well cared for American children.

Some preliminary observations by MARSHALL (unpublished) on the longitudinally collected x-rays of children in the Harpenden Growth Study show that transverse lines in bone, which are believed to be associated with arrest in growth, occur more frequently during periods of time in which children have had illnesses than they do in similar periods in which there has been no illness, but nevertheless there are frequently illnesses which are not associated with development of lines and also it is not uncommon for lines to appear in the absence of recorded illness. The association with illness is however, statistically significant and is particularly marked in the case of the exanthemata.

There is no doubt that during severe and prolonged illness both growth and skeletal maturation may slow down. When recovery takes place there is usually a period of 'catch-up' growth during which growth may proceed at more than twice its normal rate for the age concerned. BAUER (3) studied the growth of 34 children with nephrosis. When the illness began, their growth was on the average 97 % of that of normal children of comparable age. After one year of illness this figure had sunk to 83 % and after 2 years to 71 %. The children with the greatest slowing of growth died. The length of children who recovered caught up to 90 % of that of normal children after 1 year and to 94 % after 18 months from the end of the illness. As they were not measured again, it is not possible to say whether they eventually caught up entirely.

PRADER, TANNER and VON HARNACK (10) have made a careful longitudinal study of the rate of growth and of skeletal maturity in five children suffering from various illnesses. Skeletal maturity was assessed according to the method of Tanner, Whitehouse and Healy (13). One of these children had two periods of severe anorexia before she was three years old. Growth was markedly slowed during each period of anorexia, but after each period the velocity of growth in body length reached more than twice the average for the chronological age. Skeletal age advanced at a little under twice the average rate when feeding became normal after anorexia. By the time the child was five years of age, the height, weight and the skeletal maturity were all well within normal limits and the height and weight velocities were average. Another case was a 2-year-old boy suffering from renal rickets. At the age of 6 years he developed severe renal acidosis which was treated with alkali. This caused a catch-up in growth and cured the rickets. The height velocity reached twice the average for the chronological age and was that of an average child of about 18 months. The skeletal maturity was retarded similarly to the height and weight and showed some catch-up. By the time the child was ten years old his skeletal maturity was at a percentile intermediate between the height and weight percentiles.

In conclusion, acute non-endocrine disease may not retard growth at all. If it does, the effect of this retardation on a child's ultimate height will depend on whether or not skeletal age is affected and whether there is any acceleration in either growth or skeletal maturation after the illness. In view of the catch-up which occurs after severe prolonged illness it is probable that there is a tendency for catch-up to occur if growth is delayed by acute illness. There is no reason to expect that this catch-up would not be complete unless the illness were to occur very late in adolescence or even after adolescence so that insufficient time would be available for the stature to return to normal before the epiphyses fused. A large number of acute illnesses in the same individual might perhaps produce a total amount of retardation in growth which would be sufficient to counteract part of the effect of the catch-up mechanism, but there is no evidence that this does in fact happen.

REFERENCES

1. ACHESON, R. M., Effects of nutrition and disease on human growth, *Human Growth*, Ed. J. M. TANNER, Oxford. Pergamon: (*Sym. Soc. Hum. Biol.* 3: 73—92) 1960.
2. ACHESON, R. M. and STEWART, Some bone scars of disease, *Quart. J. med. N. S.* 24: 415—416, 1955.
3. BAUER, H., Nephrosesyndrom und Körperwachstum, *Helv. paediat. acta* 9: 127—34, 1954.
4. DRILLIEN, C. H., A longitudinal study of the growth and development of prematurely and maturely born children. II. Physical development, *Arch. Dis. Childh.* 33: 423—31, 1958.
5. EVANS, M. E., Illness history and physical growth. II. A comparative study of the rate of growth of preschool children of five health classes, *Amer. J. Dis. Child.* 68: 390—94, 1944.
6. HARDY, M. C., Frequent illness in childhood, physical growth and final size, *Amer. J. Phys. Anthrop.* 23: 241—260, 1938.
7. HEWITT, D., C. K. WESTROPP and R. M. ACHESON, Oxford Child Health Survey. Effect of childish ailments on skeletal development. *Brit. J. prev. soc. Med.* 9: 179—86, 1950.
8. MARTENS, E. J. and H. V. MEREDITH, Illness history and physical growth. I. Correlation in Junior Primary children followed from fall to spring, *Amer. J. Dis. Child.* 64: 618—30, 1942.
9. Ministry of Health, Standards of normal weight in infancy, *Min. Hlth. Rep. Publ. Hlth.*, No. 99, London: H.M.S.O., 1959.
10. PRADER, A., J. M. TANNER and G. A. VON HARNACK, Catch-up growth following illness or starvation, *J. Pediat.* 62: 646—59, 1963.
11. SONTAG, L. W. and J. LIPFORD, The effect of illness and other factors on the appearance pattern of skeletal epiphyses, *J. Pediat.* 23: 391—409, 1943.
12. TANNER, J. M., *Growth at Adolescence*, 2nd. ed., Blackwell Sci. Publ., Oxford, England, 1962.
13. TANNER, J. M., R. H. WHITEHOUSE and M. J. R. HEALY, *A new system for estimating skeletal maturity from the hand and wrist, with standards derived from a study of 2,600 British Children*, Part II. The Scoring System: International Children's Centre, Paris, 1962.

DISCUSSION

Visser: What is the difference between males and females with regard to the effect of the sex steroids on the pubertal spurt Dr. Van der Werff ten Bosch?

Sex steroids, as you say, are responsible for the pubertal spurt in males and females. Do you mean oestrogens in the female and androgens in the male, or is it androgens also in the female?

Van der Werff ten Bosch: From the pharmacological point of view one can say that you can induce the spurt by both androgens and oestrogens. That is quite certain. How the androgens work and how the oestrogens work is not known. One possibility is that androgens act directly on the bone or through an increased secretion of growth hormone, while the action of oestrogens needs an extra earlier step i.e. that oestrogens induce the secretion of androgens by the adrenal cortex, and thus induce the same course of events.

Clignett: I have formerly heard that the thymus gland also acts as a growth promoting factor.

Van der Werff ten Bosch: The thymus gland had almost disappeared from the medical writing on growth until very recently, when the famous biochemist Szent-Györgyi took it up again (1963; p. 107 in *Man and his Future*, Ed. G. Wolstenholme, Churchill, London). He has isolated from the thymus gland of calves two separate factors, one of which stimulated the growth of young mice, while the other inhibited their sexual maturation. Such a mixture would seem to be the ideal thing to have during infancy. A high growth rate and no sexual maturation. When the thymus gland atrophies these two factors disappear, so that growth stops and sexual maturation proceeds. This is a very fascinating hypothesis. If the implications of these findings were true, in other words, if puberty were delayed because the thymus was secreting this substance, and puberty could only occur after the thymus has stopped producing this substance, then the sequence of events should be that the thymus gland atrophies first and that puberty begins subsequently. The evidence available at the moment indicates that the thymus gland atrophies, or can be made to atrophy, under the influence of sex steroids, and this fact suggests the opposite sequence of events.

Van Wersch: What are the relationships between the thyroid gland and pituitary growth hormone, with respect to their influence upon the growth of bone?

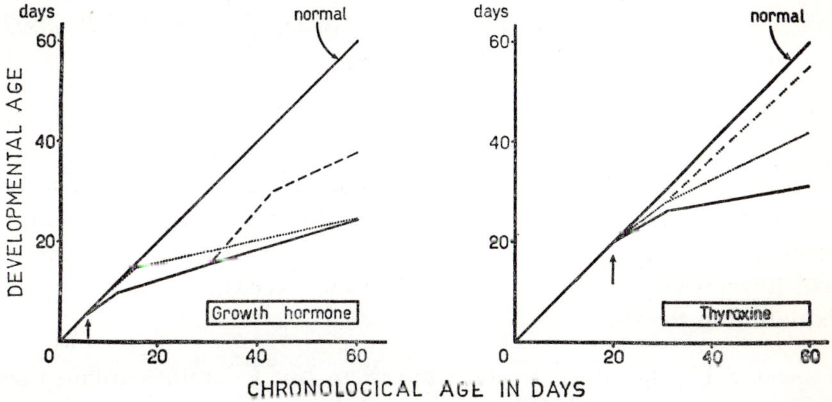

Fig. 1. Tibia growth (length age) and skeletal maturation (bone age) of rats following hypophysectomy (operation indicated by arrow), and the effects of treatment with either growth hormone (left) or thyroid hormone (right). - - - - - = lenght age; . . . . . = bone age; - - - - - = length age during treatment; . . . . = bone during treatment. Note the lack of an effect of growth hormone on the bone age, and of an effect of thyroxine on length age. (From data of SIMPSON, M. E., C. W. ASLING and H. M. EVANS, *Yale J. Biol. Med.* 23: 1, 1950, and of WALKER, D. C., C. W. ASLING, M. E. SIMPSON, C. H. LI and H. M. EVANS, *Anat. Rec.* 114: 19, 1952)

Van der Werff ten Bosch: Thyroidectomy in infancy results in retardation of linear growth and skeletal maturation (see opposite p. 38). The effect on linear growth seems to come about through three different mechanisms. Thyroid hormone deficiency causes: morphologica land functional changes in the pituitary gland (with a fall in growth hormone output), a lowering in the sensitivity of the skeleton to growth hormone, and a decrease in the food intake. The effects of thyroidectomy can be partially prevented by administration of growth hormone. Although the doses of growth hormone needed are relatively high, linear growth can be restored, while skeletal maturation is not stimulated by such treatment.

Hypophysectomy in infancy also results in retardation of both linear growth and skeletal maturation. In an animal thus operated there is deficiency of both thyroid hormone and pituitary growth hormone. The administration of thyroid hormone alone has very little effect on linear growth, but is followed by normal skeletal maturation, while growth hormone alone can bring about normal linear growth without appreciably altering the bone age (fig. 1). (see: VAN DER WERFF TEN BOSCH, J. J., Anterior pituitary function in infancy and puberty, in: *The Pituitary Gland*, Eds. B. T. DONOVAN and G. W. HARRIS, London, in the press.)

Van der Berg: The graphs that Dr. THOMSON showed, whichco mpared the weights of British children with African children, seem to suggest that the weights started to lag behind at about 6 months. The difference continued to increase until about 3 years or so, when the lines seem to become parallel, so that although the African children still had lower weights, the difference did not increase. Can you give an explanation for that.

Thomson: The facts are as you state them but I cannot explain them further. The pattern of faltering growth between about 6 months and 2 or 3 years of age has been reported from many parts of the world and is by no means peculiar to Africa. It should, however, be noted that the African pattern is a composite of different trends at different seasons: the wet season when weight increases much less than in Britain, and the dry season when it increases much faster.

These seasonal swings are real growth phenomena and are not merely due to dehydration in the summer months, since they are present in height as well as in weight.

Van Gelderen: I am surprised, Dr. THOMSON, that the children born in the village had about the same birth weight as English children. I should have expected the birth weights in this village, as in Nigeria, to be substantially lower than that of English children. Secondly, I think it is very difficult to separate the effects of multiple infections and malnutrition in these children.

In some areas, perhaps, malnutrition is more important while in other areas infections may be more important. One must assume that in areas where kwashiorkor is very common, almost all of the children are malnourished. Kwashiorkor may be only the small part of the iceberg which is visible, while much of the malnutrition lies just under the horizon. The fact that these children have so many infections, and that these infections influence growth to such a great extent, is in itself probably related to the lower grade of nutrition of these children.

Thomson: Birth weights in Africa are generally somewhat lower than in Britain, and there may be a seasonal variation in some areas. We have not yet completed the analysis of our own data.

The question whether malnutrition or infection comes first is of importance chiefly from the point of view of priorities in a programme of preventive medicine. In this particular area of Africa, which is probably fairly typical, there is no reason to believe that the ordinary diet is seriously defective. It is sufficient to support an extremely high standard of lactation, and during the healthier part of the year, the dry season, promote a rate of growth in children which is greater than the British average.

The adults are of good physique and are capable of doing a very hard day's work. In my opinion, the load of infections and parasitic disease is of greater significance than the quantity of the diet. But some children may not get sufficient food, especially when they are ill, because patterns of child care are extremely haphazard by Western standards.

Laron: Recently, with the help of Dr. VERED, we examined the relationship between obsesity, bone age and height. Figure 2 shows the difference (delta) between bone age and chronological age, plotted versus percent overweight in boys from 1 to 12 years old. It appears that in slightly obese children there is a lag in bone age, whereas with increasing degree of obesity, the bone age seems to advance. This relationship is not seen in the age group of 12 to 16, i.e. during puberty. It was further found that amongst children with a low degree of overweight there were many who were quite tall, whereas with increasing overweight the delta height age (height age minus chronological age) decreased. This was true for both boys and girls.

Schwarz: We have also looked for correlations between bone age, height age, and degree of obesity, but we could not find any.

Our children were between 9 and 15 years, so that perhaps the two groups that you distinguished have been mixed up.

Van der Vooren: I did not quite understand about the overweight of 20 %. Is it overweight for the standard weight at a certain age, or is it overweight for a standard weight at a certain height?

Schwarz: It is overweight for height, not for age.

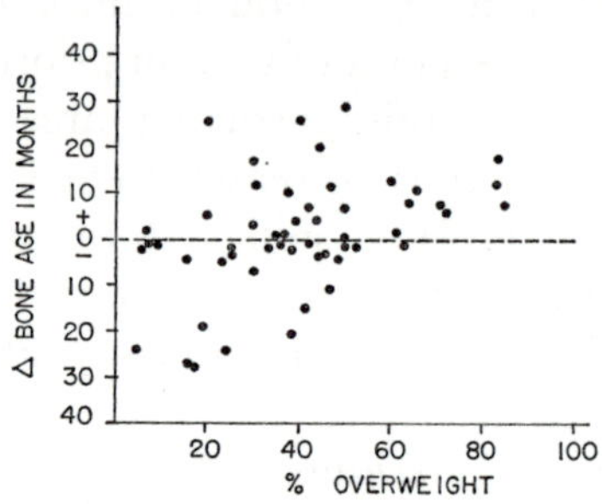

Fig. 2. Relationship between deviation of bone age and degree of obesity in boys 1—12 years old

Luyken: Dr. Marshall, for how long after an illness do the transverse lines remain visible?

Marshall: This is a very variable thing, and gives rise to one of the big technical problems in dealing with the lines. Some of them last for a very long time and are visible at least until maturity is reached, whereas others may disappear within a period of 6 months or so. There seems to be very little relationship between the severity of the illness and the length of time for which the lines remain.

This is a nuisance from the technical point of view, because you cannot identify a new line by simply counting the number of lines on the

X-ray. You have to go into much more complicated measuring techniques in order to decide whether or not a line has appeared or disappeared. In a given series of X-rays you may find that a very recent line is present and a very old line is present, but quite a lot of the lines in between have disappeared. So it is a very variable thing and the reason for the variation is not clear.

Prader: I think that the effects of disease on growth, on bone age and on final height may very well be age dependent. We have some insufficient evidence that if a disease is active during puberty, it may stop growth, but have no effect on the course of bone age, and could thereby lower final height.

I would like to ask Dr. MARSHALL: since we know so little about the effects of acute diseases, we must compare these with the effects of chronic diseases to guess what may happen in acute diseases. There is another situation which could give us some indication, and that is birth. I don't want to say that this is a disease, but it is an acute stress, just like some acute diseases. Could you comment on the influence of natural birth on growth and bone age?

Marshall: No, not really. One would need longitudinal information before, during and after birth, to reach any real conclusion and this would be somewhat difficult to obtain. There is insufficient neonatal data on growth, even immediately after birth, and certainly insufficient longitudinal data before birth, to give us a reliable comparison between the immediate pre-birth and the immediate post-birth states. It would be extremely interesting if we could get such information.

Prader: But does not birth lead to a growth line or a growth arrest line; I think it does usually.

Marshall: The earliest X-rays in the series which I am studying were taken at the age of 4 months, and certainly there were a lot of lines in the bones of some of the children, but in order to determine whether or not you have a new line, which has appeared in association with an illness or anything else, you must have an X-ray before the event and an X-ray after the event. It would be rather difficult to position the wrist before birth, to get the pre-birth X-ray to confirm this. I think lines have occurred before birth and it is quite a reasonable possibility that one might have appeared at birth, but one cannot prove that it did in fact appear then.

Polman: Can you find transverse lines in all the bones, and when they occur in one bone, can you find them also in other bones?

Marshall: This is one of the problems on which I am still working. There certainly are lines in the growing regions of all the long bones, and they may also appear in the bones of the skull and so on. As a general impression, if there are for example a lot of lines in the radius, there are also a lot of lines in the lower end of the femur. But I am engaged at the moment in comparing the actual incidence of the lines in the various regions and can't permit myself to comment yet.

Sobel: I would like to raise the question as to whether one could compare the growth lines of babies born by Caesarian section to those of babies born by natural delivery which, from the work of MIGEON, seems to be a greater stress. I realize that there would be problems even in this approach, since Caesarian section is selected as the method of delivery when there is some reason to suspect that there may be trouble with the infant.

Would it not be possible to use the lower limbs for such studies? Roentgenograms can be made without risk of irradiating the gonads of either boy or girl if one uses the lower limb.

Marshall: This is an interesting suggestion, but of course the reason for Caesarian section might already have proved a greater line producing factor than the normal birth would have been. I think there would be difficulties of interpretation, but by carefully considering and taking into account the reasons for Caesarian section in each case, something profitable might come of it.

Steendijk: I should like to go into Prof. PRADER's suggestion and look for growth arrest lines due to birth. This may not be easy, because they might disappear very quickly, in view of the tremendous rate of remodelling of the bone during the first year, which is about 100 times as high as in adults, and may be 10 times as high as during the following years of childhood.

Marshall: I agree there is a very rapid remodelling, but there is no doubt whatsoever that lines can and do persist from birth or before it, because at the age of 4 months, one can see on an X-ray many lines which, judging by their distance from the bone end must have been there before birth.

Querido: Is there any effect on the growth velocity of prolonged bedrest of children. If a child is bed-ridden for 3 or 6 months, and lies flat in bed, is there then an influence on velocity?

Marshall: I don't think we have any information on this. We certainly have none ourselves. We have not studied such cases, and I can't think at the moment of anything in the litterature.

CHAPTER VII

ABNORMAL BODY SIZE

ADULT STATURE

A. M. THOMSON

I propose to begin by comparing some characteristics of unusually tall and unusually short women in Aberdeen. These were selected from the obstetric records of all married women resident in the city who had a first single baby during the years 1948—63. There were over 16,000 such women, of whom 8.5 % have been called tall (at least 66 inches, 167.6 cm) and 10.3 % short (under 60 inches, 152.4 cm).

Over 90 % of the patients were delivered in hospital, and the data to be used are thus derived from a population which is for all practical purposes unselected. All the information required was not recorded in every case, but I am satisfied that the differences to be shown are real, and not due to incomplete recordings. Again, it may be noted that the patients were all primigravidae, and that multiple births are not included. An analysis based on a mixture of parities and types of pregnancy would undoubtedly blur the differences to be demonstrated.

Women in Aberdeen, with an average height of about 62.5 inches (158.8 cm) are appreciably shorter than those in the south of England or in Holland.

Age and geographical origin. The short women were slightly younger than the tall, 17 and 7 % respectively being under 20 years of age. Conversely 9 and 15 % were aged 30 years or more. This age differential should confer a slight obstetric advantage on the short group, since youth in primigravidae is associated with a relatively low incidence of pre-eclampsia and difficult labour (3).

Of the short women, 82 % were born and reared in the city, compared with 63 % of the tall. Ten per cent of the tall women were immigrants to Scotland, compared with 3 % of the short.

Social class and education (table 1). More than twice as many tall women as short were, or had been, in professional and clerical occupations, and nearly three times as many short women were in unskilled manual work. The occupations of the women were reflected in those of the men they married. Nearly half the tall women, and less than one-fifth of the short women had husbands in professional, technical and clerical occupations.

The educational background of the women shows differences in the same direction. Ten times as many tall women had been to University, and nearly four times as many continued full-time education beyond the minimum age for leaving school.

Table 1. *Occupational and educational distributions of tall and short primigravidae (percentages).*

	Tall	*Short*
Occupation	%	%
Professional, clerical	54.0	22.6
Shop assistants etc.	16.4	16.4
Skilled manual	16.3	26.5
Unskilled manual	13.3	34.5
	100.0 (1200 cases)	100.0 (1615 cases)
Education		
University	11.3	1.0
Vocational	4.2	2.2
Senior secondary	23.6	8.4
Minimum school	60.9	88.4
	100.0 (903 cases)	100.0 (1252 cases)

General health. It has been the custom of obstetricians in Aberdeen to grade every patient at her first antenatal visit in terms of general physique and health. Specific disabilities and diseases are relatively uncommon, and the grading depends mainly on the general impression gained of the patient's well-being and vitality. The gradings have all the defects of subjective judgements made by several different physicians, but they are not entirely meaningless, since it has been shown that patients given good gradings subsequently have lower rates of prematurity, operative delivery and perinatal death than patients with poor gradings (18). Table 2 shows that nearly seven times more tall than short women were considered to be in 'very good' health, and ten times more short than tall women were graded as being in poor general health. The differences persist even when the data are broken down by age and socio-economic status.

Table 2. *Assessment of general health and physique at first antenatal examination (percentages).*

	Tall	*Short*
Health		
Very good	34.2	5.4
Good	52.0	45.1
Fairly good	12.9	39.4
Poor	0.9	10.1
	100.0	100.0
	(1015 cases)	(1678 cases)

Complications of pregnancy. A comprehensive analysis could not be undertaken in the time available, but the records were analyzed for hypertensive complications of pregnancy and for antepartum haemorrhage. The short women should have a slight advantage, due to their younger average age. Despite this, they had a slightly higher incidence of antepartum haemorrhage, and of pre-eclampsia (defined as hypertension accompanied by protcinuria). The differences tend to persist within age groups and socio-economic classes and are probably 'real', but their significance is doubtful.

The duration of antenatal care in the two groups is similar. We previously found no appreciable association between stature and weight-for-height (6) or weight gain during pregnancy (17).

Type of labour. The main difference between the two groups was that 2.8 % of the tall women were delivered by Caesarean section, compared with 10.8 % of the short. None of the sections in the tall women were undertaken on account of cephalo-pelvic disproportion: the main indications were uterine inertia, foetal distress, age and infertility justifying elective section and toxaemia. By contrast, more than half the sections in short women were undertaken primarily because of cephalo-pelvic disproportion.

Reference may be made to BERNARD's (5) analysis of pelvic shape and size in tall and in short women. He showed that short women not only tend to have a generally contracted pelvic brim, but also frequently show evidence of antero-posterior flattening, with a relatively small obstetric conjugate.

Length of gestation and birth weight. As would be expected, the short women had smaller babies than the tall women (fig. 1). The average difference is about 0.9 lb (400 g). Fig. 2 shows that average birth weights were lower in the short women at every stage of gestation. In the short women 13.5 % of the babies weighed 2500 g or less and were therefore 'premature' by the conventional definition, compared with 4.2 % in the tall women. An excess of true prematurity was in fact present in the short women, 10.5 % being delivered at least 3 weeks before term, compared with 5.9 % in the tall women.

Perinatal deaths. The stillbirth and first week death rates per 1000 births were respectively, 11.2 and 14.4 for tall and 29.8 and 18.4 for short women. Table 3 gives a breakdown of perinatal deaths according to the clinico-pathological classification of causes used by BAIRD, WALKER and THOMSON (4). The short group shows an excess of death, in all cause groups except antepartum haemorrhage and unexplained deaths in mature babies (which are usually asphyxial in nature, and occur more frequently in postmature pregnancies). It is perhaps noteworthy that in these two exceptional groups, advancing maternal age is a predisposing factor.

Table 3. *Perinatal death rates per 1000 births, by clinico-pathological cause.*

Main cause	*Tall*	*Short*
Malformations	3.7	10.1
Mechanical causes	1.4	6.0
Toxaemia	3.0	6.6
Antepartum haemorrhage	4.5	3.0
Unexplained (premature)	6.0	11.3
Unexplained (mature)	5.2	5.4
All other causes	1.4	5.4
All causes	25.4 (34 deaths)	47.7 (80 deaths)

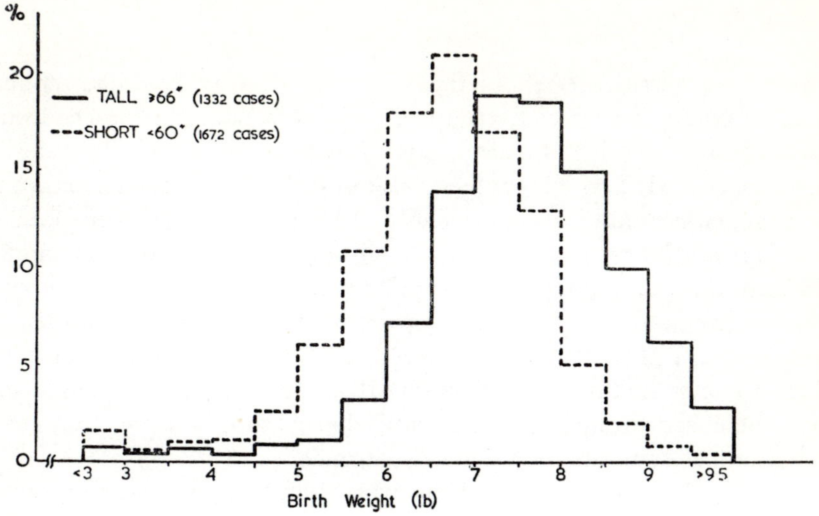

Fig. 1. Distributions of birth weights in tall and short primiparae

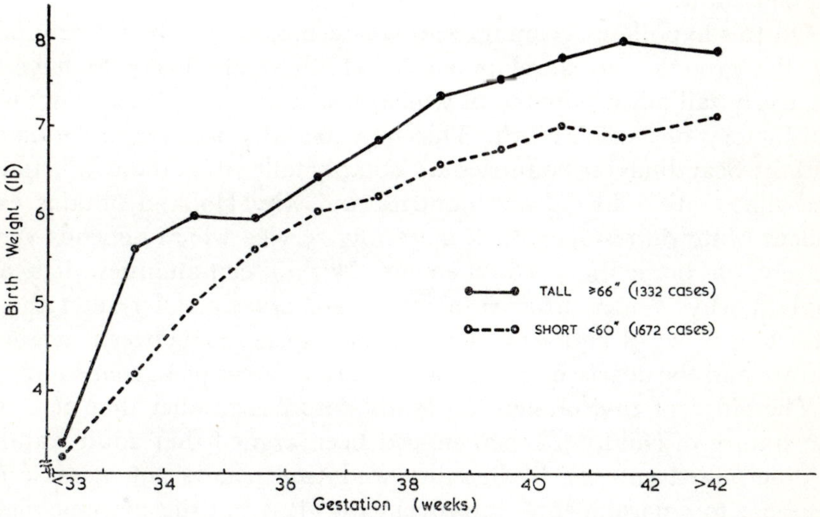

Fig. 2. Mean birth weights by length of gestation in tall and short primiparae

DISCUSSION

The evidence presented shows that short women are not smaller replicas of tall women. Taken as a group, they have a poorer socio-economic background, are less healthy, and have a conspicuously inferior obstetric record. There is evidence also that they give inferior scores in intelligence tests (14), are more likely to have illegitimate pregnancies and pre-nuptial conception (15), less likely to have twin pregnancies (2) and that they go on to have larger families and more closely-spaced pregnancies, with a disproportionately large number of mentally and physically-handicapped children (9). They are also less likely to migrate than tall women (10). I should perhaps emphasize that these are group characteristics; there are of course, numerous individual exceptions to the general trends.

The simplest hypothesis and the most useful in practice, to account for the social, physical and obstetric inferiority of short as compared with tall women, is that a high proportion of the short group are not genetically short, but have been stunted by a poor environment and poor nutrition during growth. A child whose growth is impaired by an unsatisfactory diet, a poor environment, or disease — or by all three — becomes a socially, anatomically and physiologically handicapped adult.

On this hypothesis, communities which provide the best conditions for the growth and development of children are likely to have a relatively tall adult population which, *inter alia*, will have a relatively satisfactory obstetric record. This may be why women in Holland and the Scandinavian countries are notably taller than those in Britain and many other European countries and why Holland obtains excellent obstetric results with a maternity service which depends very largely on domiciliary confinement. Within communities, it may explain why women from rural areas are usually taller than those who live in cities and why there is an association between average stature and the degree of prosperity in various areas of a given country.

The effect of environment on adult stature is smaller than it is on the stature of children. It has indeed been argued that adult stature is determined entirely by heredity and that it does not increase in response to environmental improvements (12); but this extreme view cannot be sustained in face of clear evidence of rising adult stature paralleling socio-economic and nutritional improvements during the past century (7, 8).

We may accept then, that adult stature does respond to changes in the conditions of growth, but there is still much uncertainty about the period of growth that is important. The indications are that it is impairment of growth at a very early stage that is significant; a set-back to growth after the earliest years is followed by 'catch-up' which restores growth to its original channel (1, 7, 13). Experiments with animals point to the same conclusion, though there seems to be a good deal of difference between species (11).

We in Aberdeen have been 'environmentalists' for many years. Most mothers in the city have been measured since 1948, and we have been looking for some secular increase in average stature, since socio-economic and nutritional conditions have undoubtedly improved dramatically since the great industrial depression of the early 1930's. There has been no evidence of significant change so far, and if adult stature is 'fixed' at a very early stage of growth, it is perhaps too soon to expect change. We have also become increasingly aware of the complexities of the subject. With a trend towards earlier marriage and childbearing, the youngest mothers in the city are not directly comparable, in socio-economic terms, with women of similar age in earlier years. Again, out-migration selectively skims off a relatively tall section of the population, which may not be fully compensated by in-migration (10). Heights of women in the poorer socio-economic strata do not show greater variance, perhaps with some skewing, when compared with heights in the well-to-do strata, though this might be expected if the poorer women, but not the wealthier, contain a high proportion of stunted individuals. We have not succeeded in isolating any socio-economic group in which stature has no influence, or relatively little influence, upon obstetric performance.

For these reasons, I am beginning to doubt whether the environmental hypothesis alone is sufficient to explain the different characteristics of tall and short women. A genetic difference may be involved (16). Yet I am bound to agree with my sociological colleagues that it is very difficult to conceive of an effective degree of genetic segregation between the social strata in a single city, in view of the very large degree of social and geographic mobility that has prevailed during recent generations.

A genetic difference is more easily accepted when comparisons are made between groups of widely different geographical or ethnic origin. It would indeed be interesting to know how far the greater stature of Dutch and Scandinavian women is due to superior environment and how far to different genetic origin. The difference of average stature between, say, European and Chinese is doubtless largely genetic in origin. But even then, it seems remarkable that in international comparisons average stature seems to reflect fairly well the historical levels of living of the populations concerned. Perhaps ethnic differences of stature are not so firmly based in genetics as we have usually believed. Alternatively, it seems possible that natural selection, in a Darwinian sense, brings about an adaptation of adult body size to the customary level of subsistence. Selection of such a kind would presumably improve survival value by tending to match nutritional needs with nutritional supplies.

REFERENCES

1. Acheson, R. M., In: *Human Growth*. Symposia of the Society for the study of human biology, Vol. III, p. 73, Ed.: J. M. Tanner, Oxford: Pergamon Press, 1960.
2. Anderson, W. J. R., *J. Obstet. Gyn. Brit. Emp.* 63: 205, 1956.
3. Baird, D., F. E. Hytten and A. M. Thomson, *J. Obstet. Gyn. Brit. Emp.* 65: 865, 1958.
4. Baird, D., J. Walker and A. M. Thomson, *J. Obstet. Gyn. Brit. Emp.* 61: 433, 1954.
5. Bernard, R. M., *Edinb. med. J.* 59: 1 Proc., 1952.
6. Billewicz, W. Z., W. F. F. Kemsley and A. M. Thomson, *Brit. J. prev. soc. Med.* 16: 183, 1962.
7. Boyne, A. W., In: *Human Growth*. Symposia of the society for the study of human biology, Vol. III, p. 97, Ed.: J. M. Tanner, Oxford: Pergamon Press, 1960.
8. Boyne, A. W. and I. Leitch, *Nutr. Abstr. Rev.* 24: 255, 1954.
9. Fairweather, D. V. I. and R. Illsley, *Brit. J. prev. soc. Med.* 14: 149, 1960.
10. Illsley, R., A. Finlayson and B. Thompson, *Millbank Mem. Fund Quart.* 41: 115, 217, 1963.
11. McCance, R. A., In: *Nutrition Proc. 6th Internat. Congr. Nutr.*, p. 74, C. F. Mills and R. Passmore, editors, Edinburgh: Livingstone.
12. Morant, G. M., *Proc. roy. Soc. B.* 137: 443, 1950.
13. Prader, A., J. M. Tanner and G. A. V. von Harnack, *J. Pediat.* 62: 646, 1963.
14. Scott, E. M., R. Illsley and A. M. Thomson, *J. Obstet. Gyn. Brit. Emp.* 63: 338, 1956.
15. Thompson, B., *Brit. J. prev. soc. Med.* 10: 75, 1956.
16. Thomson, A. M., *Eugen. Rev.* 51: 3, 1959.
17. Thomson, A. M. and W. Z. Billewicz, *Brit. med. J.* 1: 243, 1957.
18. Thomson, A. M. and W. Z. Billewicz, *Proc. Nutr. Soc.* 22: 55, 1963.

SHORT STATURE, A SYMPTOM*

EDNA H. SOBEL

It is evident from much of the previous discussion that many things can interfere with growth in height. We know that adult stature depends on both the rate of growth and the duration of growth, and that both of these components of adult stature are subject to regulation by genetic constitution and by somatic and environmental factors (3; 6; 7; 9).

Short stature can be considered a sign of a disorder that may be treatable, rather than a disorder in itself even though it may be very unpleasant for the patient to be short. This point of view can be illustrated by two different problems leading to growth failure: one an endocrine disorder and the other a disorder of a major organ. Endocrine disease is the least common cause of short stature (2; 12, p. 167). Disorder of a major organ system is a more frequent cause of growth failure, and may be much more difficult to detect (7; 8).

1. *Hypothyroidism* more often begins in prenatal life or in infancy than in childhood (10, p. 29; 12, p. 88). When fully-developed it is not easily confused with any other condition. It is most unusual now to see children with early onset of hypothyroidism who have escaped medical attention and treatment. Two such children are shown in figure 1. Figure 2 shows the growth chart of a 10-year-old girl in whom the diagnosis was more difficult. The complaints included moderately short stature, pallor and easy fatigue. At the age of 10 her height was just below the 10th percentile. Fortunately, records of previous measurements were available from her school. Although such measurements are not made with the precision used by investigators, they are really invaluable for evaluating the growth progress of a child.

* Funds for this project were supplied by the Public Health Service, National Institutes of Health (NIH HD 00139) and by the G. D. Searle Company, Chicago, Ill.

In this instance, it is evident that the child had been at the 50th percentile for height at 5 years of age, and had gradually lost ground so that she was below the 10th percentile at 10 years of age. Her height was within normal limits, but her growth was abnormal. More subtle signs of abnormality led to the correct diagnosis of hypothyroidism. She was a little puffy, her skin was a little dry, her pallor was due not to anemia but to poor peripheral circulation. When she was treated with desiccated thyroid, she had a growth spurt.

Figure 3 A shows another patient whose major complaint was short stature, accompanied by obesity. The photograph on the left shows her at age 12: height-age 7 11/12; weight-age more than 16 years; bone-age 7 4/12. Among the diagnoses considered was Cushing's syndrome; this hypothesis was reinforced by the radiographic finding of an enlarged sella turcica. As Dr. SCHWARZ mentioned, most overweight children are tall, and do not have any endocrine disease. In Cushing's syndrome obesity may be associated with retarded growth, but not with pallor and puffiness about the face, which our patient had. Enlargement of the sella turcica does occur in long-lasting juvenile hypothyroidism (1; 5) so that this observation neither indicates the diagnosis of Cushing's disease, which would be in disagreement with the clinical findings, nor of a pituitary tumor with secondary hypothyroidism. Figure 3 B shows the same patient after 6 months of thyroid therapy: much taller, in mid-adolescence, rosy, no longer hypothyroid but still obese. Her growth chart is shown in figure 4; figure 5 shows growth velocity as well as height achieved.

2. Short stature may be the chief sign of serious *disorder of a major organ*. A 13-year-old girl presented with the chief complaints of growth failure and anorexia of four years' duration (8, patient 1). The family history included short stature in the mother, and diabetes on both sides of the family. A family history of diabetes always raises the possiility of endocrine disease in the patient. The girl's personal history included increased sensitivity to cold weather, which raised the possibility of hypothyroidism. She assured us that she had normal bowel function, with no constipation or diarrhea. She had fleeting abdominal pain when she ate, which she herself thought was emotional. Her behavior was hostile and very immature: she still sucked her fingers and preferred to play alone with dolls. She had previously been treated with desiccated thyroid, to which she had not responded, and

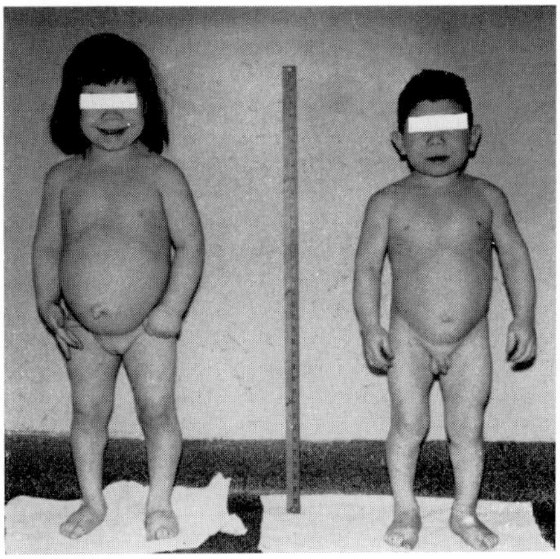

Fig. 1. Two hypothyroid children who had never been treated. Measuring stick 91 cm; girl aged 12 years, height-age 2 years 10 months; boy aged 9 years; height-age 2 years 6 months. Patients of the Cincinnati General Hospital, Cincinnati, Ohio

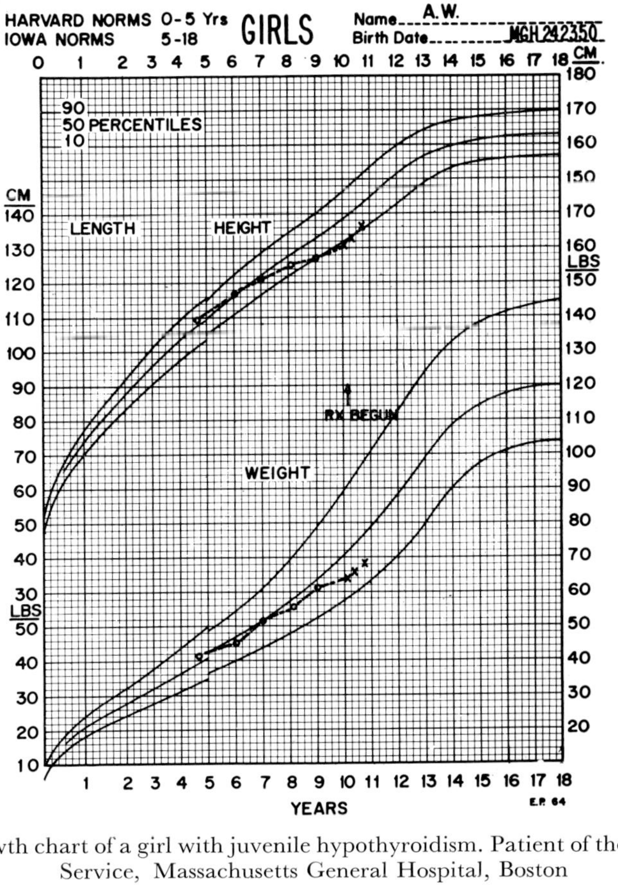

Fig. 2. Growth chart of a girl with juvenile hypothyroidism. Patient of the Children's Service, Massachusetts General Hospital, Boston

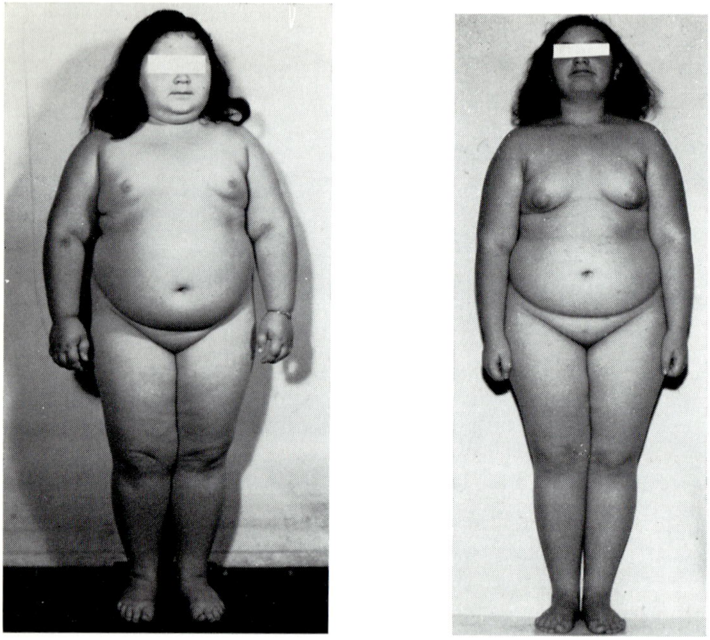

A B

Fig. 3. Photographs of a girl with juvenile hypothyroidism. Patient of the Children's Hospital, Cincinnati, Ohio

A. Before treatment, age 12, height-age $7^{11}/_{12}$, weight-age more than 16, bone-age $7^{4}/_{12}$ years

B. The same patient, 6 months later

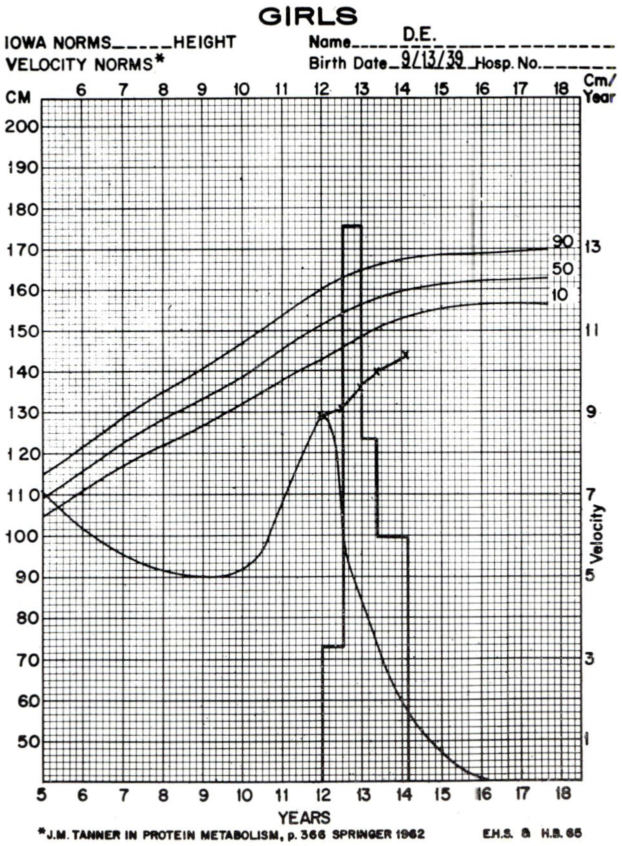

Fig. 4. Height achieved and growth velocity of patient with juvenile hypothyroidism whose photographs are shown in fig. 3

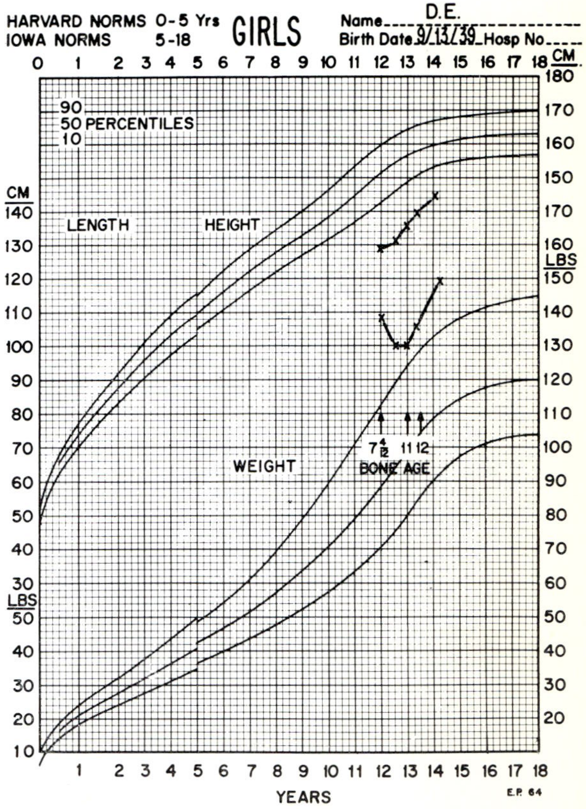

Fig. 5. Growth chart of patient with juvenile hypothyroidism whose photographs are shown in fig. 3

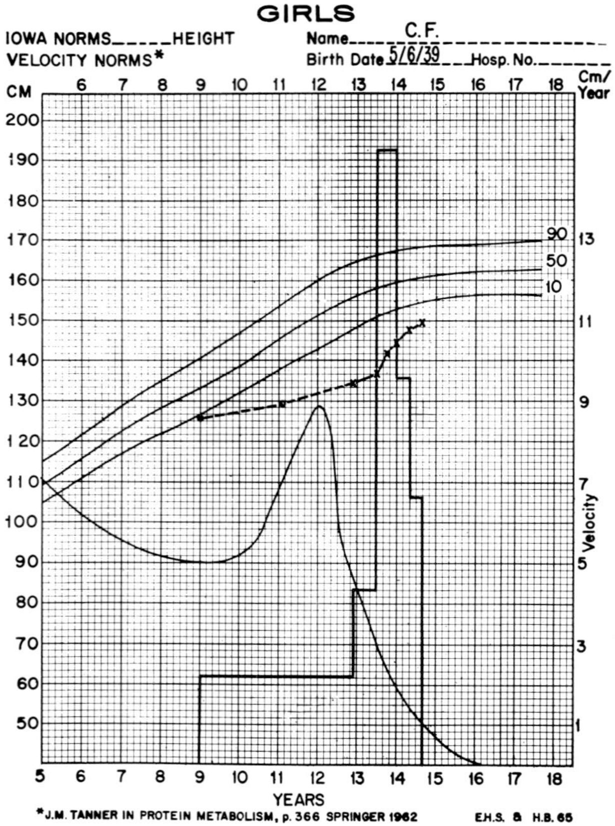

Fig. 6. Height achieved and growth velocity of patient with chronic regional enteritis in relation to time of corrective surgery

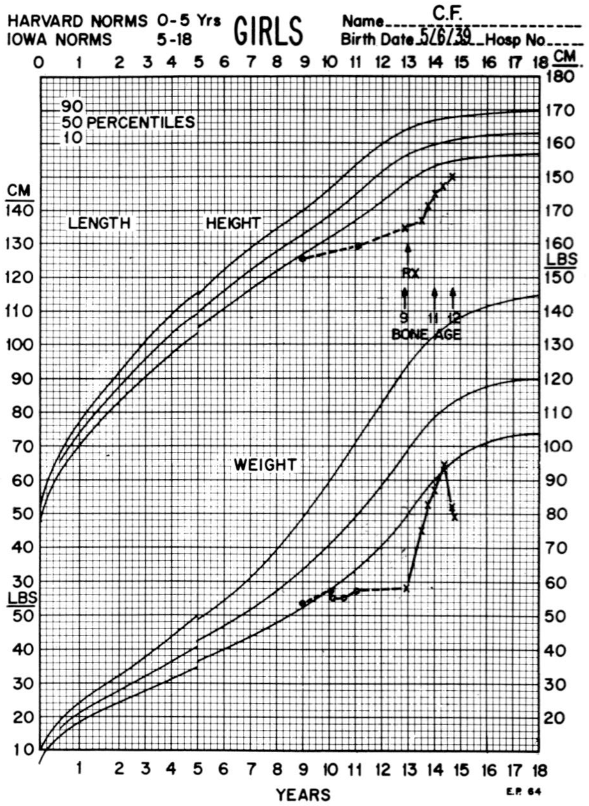

Fig. 7. Growth chart of patient with chronic regional enteritis, showing progressive failure of growth and weight gain from 9 years of age until surgery (Rx); thereafter, steady weight gain and growth spurt until weight loss occured with reactivation of disease. Adapted from ref. 8, fig. 2

with pituitary extract by mouth, to which she could not have responded even if she had been hypopituitary because, as we now know, such therapy is not effective.

The patient seemed sad and was lacking in spontaneity. She appeared much thinner than would have been expected from her weight-age of 8 6/12 and height-age of 8 9/12. Skeletal maturation as judged from the hand and wrist was 9 years; such marked retardation does not necessarily indicate endocrine disease. Dental development was normal for her age as judged from the emerged teeth. She was sexually immature, which is not abnormal for a girl of 13, and to be expected for a girl whose bone-age was 9 years. The abdomen was somewhat full for such a thin person, but otherwise not abnormal. The first impression was anorexia nervosa or disorder of a major system, possibly intestinal because of the abdominal fullness.

The laboratory studies included those we have found helpful in the initial investigation of patients with short stature, and radiologic examination of the gastrointestinal tract. Some of the results were entirely normal: urinalysis, complete blood count, plasma non-protein nitrogen, pH, bicarbonate, chloride, cholesterol, inorganic phosphate, calcium, and alkaline phosphatase activity. The hormone content of the urine was also considered normal (17-ketosteroids 4.0 mg, 17-ketogenic steroids 9.8 mg and gonadotrophins less than 3 mouse uterine units per 24 hours). One of the chemical findings was abnormal: the plasma proteins were only 5.3 grams per 100 ml, consistent with the clinical impression of malnutrition. The explanation lay in a jejunocolic fistula, demonstrated in the radiologic examination undertaken on the slender clinical clue of abdominal fullness. Treatment was surgical. The obstructed jejunum was resected; the fistula was excised and repaired. The pathologic diagnosis was active regional enteritis, which was consistent with the patient's emotional problems even though the relationship of emotional disorders to this disorder is far from clear.

Figure 6 is the growth chart of this patient. The earliest measurements available were those at nine years, when she was already short but not underweight for height. Her growth became progressively slower. Between 9 and 10 years she lost weight and then failed to gain, so that she was indeed thin at the first examination. Following surgery there was a dramatic gain in weight, followed by a growth spurt.

Unfortunately active disease recurred. In 4 months she lost 5.7 kg while the rate of growth slowed to 6.66 cm/year in comparison to the velocity of 10.67 cm/year in the preceding 15 months and that of 2.2 cm/year in the four years before treatment (figure 7). Some of the post-operative catch-up growth probably can be attributed to her adolescent growth spurt as breast development began within 2 months. However, the peak velocity of 15.24 cm/year is almost twice that expected of average girls (11, p. 1) and even greater in relation to that of girls with maximal growth at age 14 6/12 (4). It is surely comparable to the velocity achieved by children in whom an endocrine disorder can be corrected (3); see also figure 5.

In this particular patient the disease, which had manifested itself almost exclusively by growth failure, had a fatal outcome. Other serious diseases that interfere with growth may be equally difficult to detect (3; 7; 8). In this particular patient growth failure was the major symptom of a life-threatening disease. Investigations were directed not to the endocrine system, but to her general health. Endocrine therapy would have been entirely inappropriate.

REFERENCES

1. Bellini, M. A. and I. Neves, The skull in childhood myxedema: its roentgen appearance, *Am. J. Roentgenol.* 76: 495, 1956.
2. Martin, M. M. and L. Wilkins, Pituitary dwarfism: diagnosis and treatment, *J. Clin. Endocrin.* 18: 679, 1958.
3. Prader, A., J. M. Tanner and G. A. von Harnack, Catch-up growth following illness or starvation, *J. Pediat.* 62: 646, 1963.
4. Shuttleworth, F. K., The physical and mental growth of girls and boys age 6 to 19 in relation to age at maximum growth, *Monographs Soc. Res. Child. Dev.* 4: 237, 1939, Table 26.
5. Silverman, F. N., Roentgen standards for size of the pituitary fossa from infancy through adolescence, *Am. J. Roentgenol.* 78: 451, 1957.
6. Sobel, E. H., Factors regulating growth. In: *Mechanisms of Regulation of Growth*, Report of the Fortieth Ross Conference on Pediatric Research, G. M. Owen, ed., 55—56, Columbus, Ross Laboratories, 1962.
7. Sobel, E. H., School Age: Growth Problems. In: *Biologic Basis of Pediatric Practice*, R. E. Cooke, ed., McGraw-Hill, New York, In Press.
8. Sobel, E. H., F. N. Silverman and C. M. Lee, Jr., Chronic regional enteritis and growth retardation, *A.M.A. J. Dis. Child.* 103: 569, 1962.

9. TALBOT, N. B. and E. H. SOBEL, Endocrine and other factors determining the growth of children, *Advances in Pediatrics* 2: 238, 1947.
10. TALBOT, N. B., E. H. SOBEL, J. W. MCARTHUR and J. D. CRAWFORD, *Functional endocrinology from birth through adolescence*, The Commonwealth Fund, Harvard University Press, Cambridge, Mass. 1952.
11. TANNER, J. M., *Growth at adolescence*, Charles C. Thomas, 1955.
12. WILKINS, L. *The diagnosis and treatment of endocrine disorders in childhood and adolescence*, Charles C. Thomas, Springfield, 2nd ed. 1957.

DISCUSSION

Croughs: Dr. Thomson, was the distance from the mean of your large women as large as the distance from the mean of the short women? Secondly. It is known that many genetic malformations are accompanied by short stature. This is not seen with large stature. Could it be that short women fall in two groups, one group with the same genetical potencies as large women and completely normal, and another group with congenital malformations associated with short stature. Could it be that the latter group causes all the bad findings you obtained?

Thomson: Heights have a normal distribution, and in the series reported the tall and the short women were approximately the same distance from the mean. Our main hypothesis is that the short women consisted of a mixture of the genetically short and the physically stunted. But if this is the sole explanation, one would expect the distribution of heights in the poorer socio-economic classes, where many women may be stunted, to be different from the distribution in the upper classes, where most women will be well-grown. But we have found no evidence of a change in the shape of the distribution curve in the poorer and wealthier classes.

Congenital malformations of the central nervous system are more common among the babies of short women than among those of tall women, but I doubt if this is a genetically-determined phenomenon.

Smit: Dr. Thomson, is there a difference between the ratios of the lower and the upper measures between the groups of tall and short women, and has this any significance or does it give an information?

Thomson: Our routine clinical measurements do not give any information on body proportions, but I know from other material that tall women have legs which are longer in proportion to total height than those of short women. In other words, tallness is largely produced by greater growth of the lower limbs. During growth from foetal life into adult life, the legs become relatively longer and longer, and the relatively longer legs of tall women probably means greater perfection of growth, or more complete growth. ISABELLA LEITCH has pointed out that artists seeking to depict the most perfect type of human body always portray subjects with relatively long legs.

De Wijn: Dr. THOMSON, what about the prematurity rates, perinatal mortality, and obstetrical deaths among the tall women who belong to the lowest socio-economic classes?

Thomson: Unusually tall women in the poorer socio-economic classes seem to have slightly increased rates of prematurity and perinatal mortality. It may be that women with a relatively low growth potential are better adapted to a poor environment than those who grow fast and become tall. It is interesting to speculate that there may be some degree of natural selection, in the Darwinian sense, which over many generations tends to adapt growth rate and adult body size to the habitual level of subsistence.

Visser: Dr. THOMSON has given very good evidence for an effect of the environment on ultimate height. I did not understand why he has to wait another one or two years for women to become pregnant in Scotland. If there is something of a secular trend, why don't you measure girls of 16 or 18 years and compare them with girls of 20 years ago. I think that this effect must then become clear.

Thomson: A paper from the Rowett Institute (LEITCH and BOYNE, *Nutr. Abstr. Rev.* 30: 1173, 1960) has shown that adolescents in a wealthy school in England have not increased in average stature during the last 30 years. Presumably they have always been adequately fed, and have always attained the genetic limits of their growth. But such circumstances are exceptional, and it is reasonable to presume that for most people the nutritional and environmental improvements that have taken place during the past 50 years or more, have caused some increase in average adult stature. But we do not know how quickly or by how much adult stature responds to changes of the environment during growth. If adult size is affected only by alterations to the very earliest stages of growth, a delay of up to 20 years would be expected before a change of adult stature became apparent. I think that the greatest change in the growth of children in Britain probably occurred during the war years, when pregnant and lactating women, and children, were treated as priority groups in the national food programme. Children born during the war are now about 20 years old, and so will have reached their full adult height. But women having babies at 16 or 17 years of age are mostly from the poorest and worst-educated classes, and therefore represent the social group which is likely to respond least to social improvements. To ascertain the full effect of the wartime and post-war environmental improvements, we must wait until the women having babies now are an approximately random sample of babies born then.

Incidentally, the problem of secular trends is further complicated by differential migration, since tall people tend to migrate more freely than short; and by the changing pattern of age at marriage and childbearing. Women having babies at 20 or 21 years of age now, are not necessarily comparable in socio-economic terms with women having babies at such an age 10 or 20 years ago, when average age at marriage was later.

CHAPTER VIII

SOME TYPES OF ABNORMAL GROWTH

GROWTH-LIMITING FACTORS IN RENAL DISEASE

H. A. W. M. TIDDENS

Chronic renal disease is one of the organic disorders frequently accompanied by retarded statural growth (7, 14, 29, 30). The term 'renal dwarfism' found rapid and general acceptance after its introduction by BARBER in 1920 (1). Many papers have since been published under this heading. The majority is concerned with the classification of infrequently occurring syndromes in which severe skeletal disease and multiple aberrations of tubular function play a major part (7, 26). The nature of the dependence of growth on kidney function has received only little attention. The possibilities of preventing dwarfism in renal disease have received hardly any attention at all.

WEST and SMITH (30) have tried to elucidate the relationship between growth retardation and common renal disease. They defined the part played by each of the disturbances of renal function involved by comparing the frequency of occurrence in dwarfed and normally growing patients. In this paper a different approach was chosen. Taking chronic pyelonephritis as a model, a short survey is given of what is known of the effects that each of four common functional disorders may have on statural growth. A study of this kind does not lead to definite conclusions. It rather indicates possibly profitable lines for future research and casts a doubt upon the inevitability of growth disturbance in renal disease.

Pyelonephritis has been defined by KIMMELSTIEL (15) as an infectious disease of the kidney characterised by a primary inflammatory reaction of pelvis and parenchymal interstices to invading organisms with secondary effects on the tubular, glomerular and vascular apparatus. Pyelonephritis is a common disease of infancy. The exact incidence is unknown. Rigid criteria for the diagnosis are being developed. It will be necessary to correlate the results of quantitative bacteriological studies, quantitative studies of cellular elements in unsedimented urine, qualitative studies of urinary pus cells and casts, studies of renal function with the accent on concentrating ability and excretion of phenol red and similar substances, and proper evaluation of case histories (bacteriaemia). Congenital abnormalities of structure or function of the urogenital tract and the nature of the primary lesion are important factors in the development of chronicity (27). Again it is as yet impossible to estimate the incidence of chronic pyelonephritis. It certainly is the most important single cause of renal insufficiency in childhood (3, 23).

As a common disease, and with its peak incidence in a period of rapid growth, chronic pyelonephritis constitutes a suitable model for the study of the effects of renal disease on growth. Longitudinal studies of young patients with chronic pyelonephritis, and possibly short-term growth studies of infants suffering from acute forms of the disease, are definitely indicated. Even without studies of this kind it is possible to say on the available evidence, that a high proportion of patients with chronic pyelonephritis are more or less dwarfed (18).

It is not probable that *chronic infection* contributes to growth failure in an appreciable way (30). It will be shown that the resulting *disorders of kidney function* offer a more likely explanation. Chronic pyelonephritis may lead to a confusing number of functional disturbances (4). Four of these are of sufficient importance to warrant special interest. They result in the following signs: polyuria, acidosis, azotaemia and bone disease. The underlying causes of these signs and the possible effect they may have on statural growth will be discussed.

POLYURIA

The regulation of the amount of body fluid and the osmolality of body fluid depends largely on a feed-back mechanism which regulates the amount of circulating anti-diuretic hormone. ADH production is stimulated by increased osmolality or decreased fluid volume. The effects of ADH on the renal end-organ is an increase in medullary tonicity and the production of more concentrated urine. A normal medullary architecture and an adequate supply of salt and urea to the tubules, are necessary for the correct function of the renal end-organ (2). In *chronic pyelonephritis* damage to the medulla in general, and to the collecting ducts in particular, leads to inadequate ADH response through impairment of concentrating ability (2, 4). This in turn limits the variations in fluid and solute intake that are possible without endangering the constancy of body fluid volume and osmolality. In more simple terms: the patient will have to drink more water than a healthy child both during the day and the night. If he does not meet this requirement, osmolality and body fluid volume will be disturbed as in patients who suffer from diabetes insipidus.

It is a well-established fact that children with diabetes insipidus of central and renal origin are retarded in growth (6, 16, 35). Studies of Hillman et al. (12) have shown the influence of polyuria and polydipsia on the daily activities of these children. Fig. 1 shows the effect

RENAL DIABETES INSIPIDUS

	PERCENT OF OBSERVATION PERIODS	AVERAGE VALUES FOR					
		FLUID INTAKE			URINE OUTPUT		
	ACTIVITY OF PATIENT D.K. 939560 15 mo. 6.6 kg.	VOLUME PER HOUR ml.	INTERVAL BETWEEN DRINKS min.	VOLUME PER DRINK ml.	VOLUME PER HOUR ml.	INTERVAL BETWEEN VOIDINGS min.	VOLUME PER VOIDING ml.
WHOLE COW'S MILK	SLEEP (51%) DRINK (28%) PLAY (21%)	247	24	120	135	50	112
DILUTE FORMULA	SLEEP (45%) DRINK (6%) PLAY (49%)	120	66	141	77	66	102
DEXTROSE & WATER	SLEEP (37%) DRINK (7%) PLAY (56%)	89	66	127	74	90	132
	ACTIVITY OF NORMAL 15 mo. 12 kg.						
WHOLE COW'S MILK	SLEEP (29%) DRINK (7%) PLAY (64%)	50	288	240	25	240	100

Fig. 1. Daily activities during representative 8-hour periods while ingesting diets with different contents of solutes, of a 15 months' old boy with congenital renal diabetes insipidus. Data obtained from a normal infant of the same age are included for comparison (data from 12)

on the pattern of behaviour. This experiment clearly illustrates how the need to drink excessive quantities may profoundly upset a child's life. A direct result that can be studied quantitatively is a decrease in the food intake. Studies of Vest and his co-workers (28) concerning the effect of untreated central diabetes insipidus on caloric intake suggest that the stunted growth in diabetes insipidus may be considered to be hypocaloric dwarfism.

If fluid intake falls below the acceptable minimum, changes in the osmolality of the body fluid will result.

It has been shown that patients with congenital nephrogenic diabetes insipidus do not gain weight or height as long as their serum electrolyte levels are too high (8, 35). Increase of the intake of water or decrease of

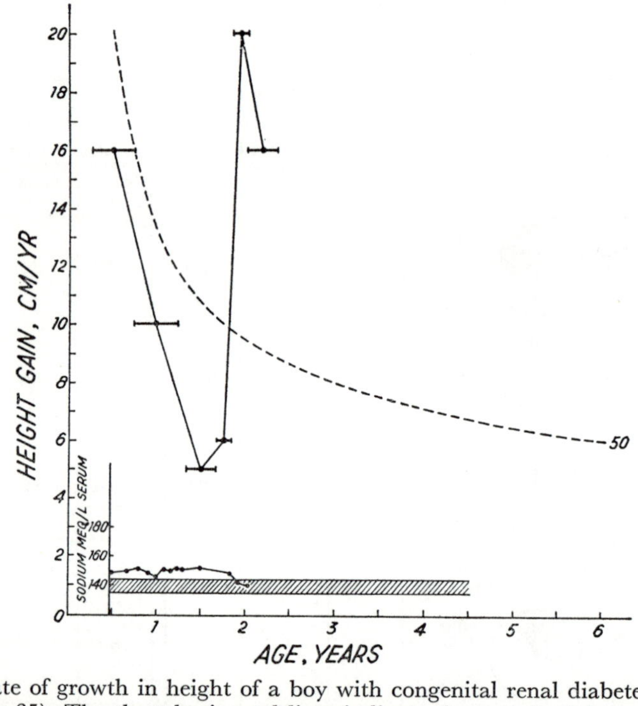

Fig. 2. Rate of growth in height of a boy with congenital renal diabetes insipidus (data from 35). The short horizontal lines indicate the period of time over which the velocity represented was measured. (The 50th percentile has been copied from 22)

the solute load by adjustment of the diet, may lower the serum electrolytes to normal values and result in normal growth. Fig. 2 illustrates this point. The growth velocity chart has been constructed with the kind permission of the author, from data supplied in WIJFFELS's thesis on diabetes insipidus (35). For the sake of simplicity, sodium levels only are indicated. Other serum electrolyte values moved in the same direction (35). GAUTHIER has discussed the available data on solute changes, and found that there is probably an increase (9).

It is clear that the reduced concentrating ability may have an adverse effect on growth, through decreased food intake and hyper-osmolality.

ACIDOSIS

The oxidation of ingested food yields varying amounts of non-volatile acids, in excess of base, that must be excreted if acidbase balance is to be maintained. The metabolism of sulphur-containing amino acids is mainly responsible for this (13). The normal kidney is perfectly capable of excreting hydrogen ions at a rate that prevents an increase of hydrogen ion concentration in the body. In chronic pyelonephritis hydrogen ion excretion is often impaired. Two mechanisms play a role: the minimal attainable urinary pH is higher than in normal subjects, and in more advanced stages there is a deficient secretion of ammonium. The first mechanism, failure to produce an adequate lowering of urinary pH, seems to be related to tubular damage; the second mechanism is related to a decrease in the number of properly functioning nephrons (2, 4, 17, 33).

There is evidence that acidosis may lead to defective growth. West and Smith (30) studied growth in 41 children with chronic renal disease, 21 of which showed marked growth retardation. While chronic acidosis occurred in 76 % of the retarded children, it was never found in normally growing children. Cooke et al. (5) studied the effects of acidosis on growth in rats, and they concluded that acidosis bears a relationship to retardation of growth. All their acidotic animals stopped growing with the notable exception of one group, made acidotic by the addition of 0.4 % acetozolamide to the diet.

Znamensky and Tiddens (36) reported a patient suffering from renal acidosis and rickets. Minimal attainable urinary pH was 6.3 and ammonia secretion was reduced. Under treatment with alkali (at the age of 6 years) rickets healed promptly. In the first 6 months of treatment height increased from 89 to 96 cm. Prader, Tanner and Von Harnack (22) in their paper on catch-up growth demonstrated a boy who underwent implantation of both ureters in the colon because of ectopia of the bladder. At the age of 6 years, he had severe acidosis and rickets. Treatment with alkali cured the rickets and resulted in catch-up growth. This is demonstrated very well in fig. 3, reproduced from the original publication by kind permission of Prof. PRADER.

The reduced capacity for hydrogen ion excretion that is often found in chronic pyelonephritis may lead to acidosis. Experimental work on the relation between acidosis and growth has not led to unequivocal results. Clinical studies support the idea that acidosis may play a role in the impairment of growth associated with pyelonephritis.

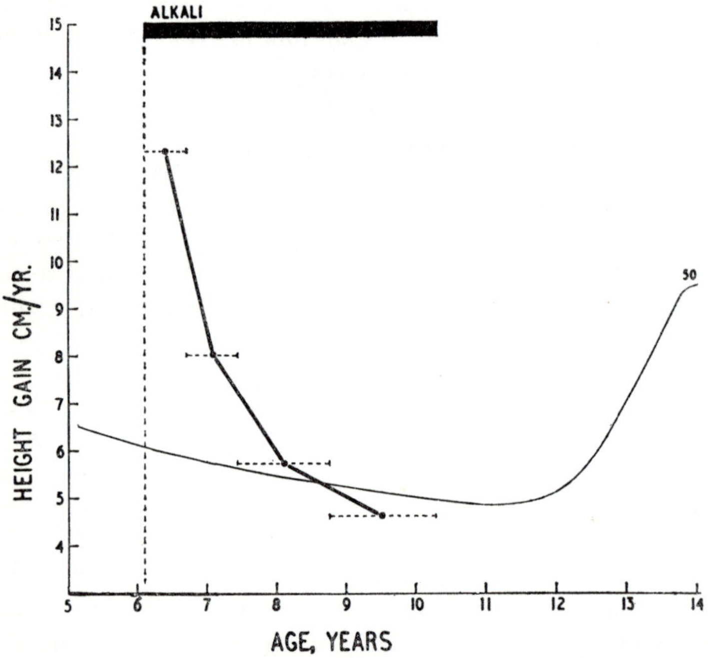

Fig. 3. Catch-up growth following alkali treatment of a boy with severe renal acidosis and rickets (reproduced from 22)

AZOTEMIA

In the functional disturbances discussed so far, damage to tubuli and other medullary structures played an important role. Azotemia as expressed by high blood urea levels is, of course, indicative of diminished glomerular filtration, provided urea production is normal. As such it is seldom an early symptom of pyelonephritis.

Sooner or later, however, a diminution of the number of functioning nephrons becomes apparent in pyelonephritis (4). A loss of filtering surface will lead to retention of nitrogenous substances and create a state of osmotic diuresis in the remaining nephrons. Retention of anions is a typical feature. In other respects homeostasis is reasonably well maintained by the osmotic diuresis mentioned above (2). Diminution of the amount of glomerular filtrate may aggravate difficulties in the control of body-fluid volume and osmolality and in the control of hydrogen ion balance. Altogether this stage of chronic renal failure constitutes a very complex problem which is very difficult to relate to retardation of growth. To my knowledge no studies have been published on the relationship between GFR and statural growth, all other factors being equal. It is possible to say something, however, on the influence growth-arrest may have on the blood urea concentration. Urea production is the result of deamination in the liver of the excess amino acids derived from protein consumption and protein breakdown. The greater the amount of protein that is being incorporated in the body, the less urea will be produced when a constant amount of building substances is eaten. McCance (19) concluded from studies in neonates that stability in the new-born animal depends on integration of food, growth and renal function. The role growth plays in homeostasis will, of course, be maximal in the period in which growth velocity is maximal, and this coincides with the period in which different kidney functions have not yet matured. The importance of growth for the maintenance of a constant internal environment diminishes with the maturation of kidney function. It is clear that its significance will increase as soon as disease limits kidney function again. This applies to all aspects of kidney function mentioned up to now. It finds its clearest expression in blood urea levels. If a child stops growing, more protein will be catabolised and more degradation products will have to be excreted. This does not mean that more urea must be excreted only, but also e.g. more hydrogen ion. A vicious circle may then ensue. Inability to excrete a normal hydrogen load may lead to further increase of this load.

In adults high urea levels in renal disease may indicate that the protein intake is too high, provided the patient receives sufficient calories. This is not necessarily so in children. Protein intake in a child with growth-arrest on account of some of the factors mentioned, may very well lead to appreciably higher urea levels than the same protein intake produces in the same child when it grows again, after a vicious circle has been interrupted by adequate symptomatic treatment. The younger the child and consequently the higher the growth velocity to be expected, the greater the homeostatic influence of growth will be.

The one influence that certainly does play a part in growth retardation in patients with high urea levels is the anorexia that may result. Uraemia may lead to gastro-intestinal disturbances which influence the food intake (23).

SKELETAL DISORDERS

Chronic pyelonephritis may lead to the same 'bony complications' that may result from advanced glomerulonephritis, nephrosis, and other types of renal disease (25). All early descriptions of renal dwarfism concerned patients with a severe form of one of these complications, i.e. renal rickets. The effect of this type of skeletal disease on growth is probably identical to the effect on growth of other types of severe rickets. The relationship between renal and skeletal disease has been partially clarified in the brilliant work of STANBURY (25), who has postulated 'an acquired resistance to or conditioned deficiency of vitamin D' as the basic abnormality responsible for the bony complications. This supposedly leads to impaired calcium resorption, changes in citrate metabolism, impaired mineralisation of bone and functional hypoparathyroidism. All these functional changes can be corrected by adequate doses of vitamin D, adequate in this case meaning higher and sometimes considerably higher than the doses normally employed. We do not know which anatomical or functional changes in the kidney lead to these profound metabolic changes and in which stage of the disease they begin to operate. It is possible that the metabolic changes may affect growth long before skeletal changes become noticeable. This paediatric aspect of STANBURY's work certainly calls for further investigations.

Fig. 4 is presented as an incentive to studies of this kind. It shows the apparent influence on growth of vitamin D in a patient with overall renal insufficiency studied by ROYER and associates (24), although it is impossible to accept a direct relationship between treatment and the marked increase in the growth rate without data on the caloric intake.

The biochemical signs associated with altered vitamin D activity in renal disease closely resemble the biochemical picture in pseudo-nutritional rickets, a syndrome first recognised by PRADER, ILLIG and HEIERLI (21). Patients with pseudo-nutritional rickets can be cured by administration of moderately high doses of vitamin D. Under treatment growth in height proceeds at a normal rate, in contrast to what happens in classical resistant rickets. Study of these patients could provide additional information on the relationships between calcium metabolism and growth.

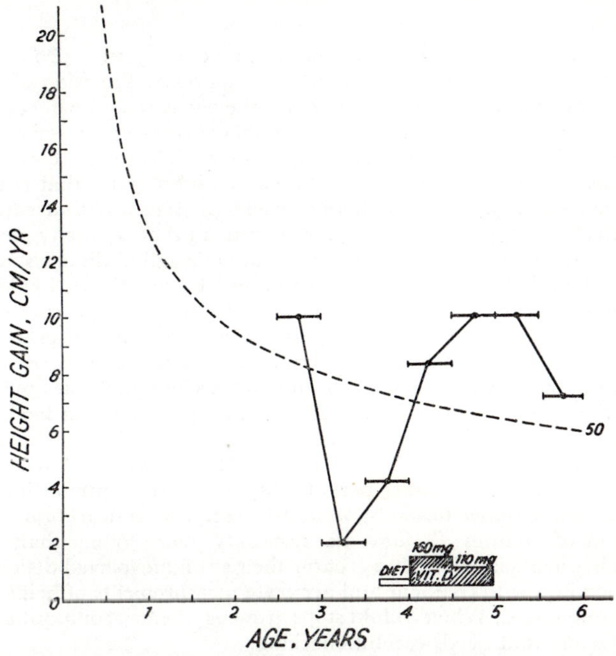

Fig. 4. Catch-up growth following treatment with low-solute diet and vitamin D, of a boy with chronic renal insufficiency of unspecified cause (data from 24)

In chronic pyelonephritis other functional disorders may also be found. The disease may even lead to multiple tubular defects combined with diminished glomerular filtration, a picture identical to the disorders often found in cystinosis (see below). The abnormalities that have been discussed may be considered to constitute the common picture of chronic pyelonephritis. The evidence suggests that growth retardation in chronic pyelonephritis is mainly the result of two factors:

a. decreased caloric intake,
b. failure of homeostatic mechanisms.

Growth retardation in pyelonephritis, and in other forms of acquired renal disease, should therefore not be accepted as inevitable, but rather be considered as a challenge to the paediatrician that can be met by proper symptomatic treatment.

The essence of such treatment is the selection of a diet that is in every way adapted to the limited homeostatic abilities of the patient.

The food should contain sufficient *calories* to prevent excessive protein catabolism, in a palatable form to prevent aggravation of anorexia. Provision of *protein of high biological value* in an amount sufficient to cover the needs of a growing child is another important point. The minimum protein intake necessary for growth is usually overestimated. However, customary low-protein diets often contain relatively high amounts of proteins of low biological value and may for that reason give disappointing results (10). The diet should provide a *solute load* that can be excreted with a relatively normal water intake, a requirement that is usually met more easily in pyelonephritis than in patients suffering from congenital diabetes insipidus. The *hydrogen load* should not exceed the limits imposed by the diseased kidney; addition of alkali is sometimes necessary. It is impossible to judge the correct amount of protein or any of the other dietary factors correctly as long as severe homeostatic disturbances exist. Correction of hyperosmolality and acidosis, if necessary, by parenteral fluid therapy or dialysis, will interrupt vicious circles as mentioned above and create the best conditions for an efficient interplay between food, growth and renal function. Evidence is accumulating that short-term administration of anabolic steroids may sometimes be helpful (11, 20, 32). It is not yet clear whether administration of these drugs over longer periods may aid hypertrophy of intact nephrons (11). The calcium balance has to be watched closely. Administration of higher than average doses of vitamin D may be necessary more often than is generally believed. Fairly artificial diets always carry the risk of unexpected deficiencies. Good medical supervison with frequent and accurate measurements of height and weight are the best safe-guard. When a child stops growing, dietary composition is certainly one of the factors that needs careful checking.

Some of the points raised are illustrated by the following case.

Figs. 5 and 6 show the height and weight distance charts, and fig. 7 the growth velocity curve, of a patient with severe and progressive renal disease. She demonstrated a perfectly normal pubertal growth spurt and reached a height of 160 cm at the age of 16 years.

Table I shows some data.

This patient was only seen occasionally until the age of 7 years. Intensive dietary treatment was started at 10 years. In addition, she received occasional antibiotic treatment for exacerbations of her pyelonephritis. She learnt to micturate in two tempi as advised by Williams (31). From the age of 10 years a low dose of Deca-Durabolin

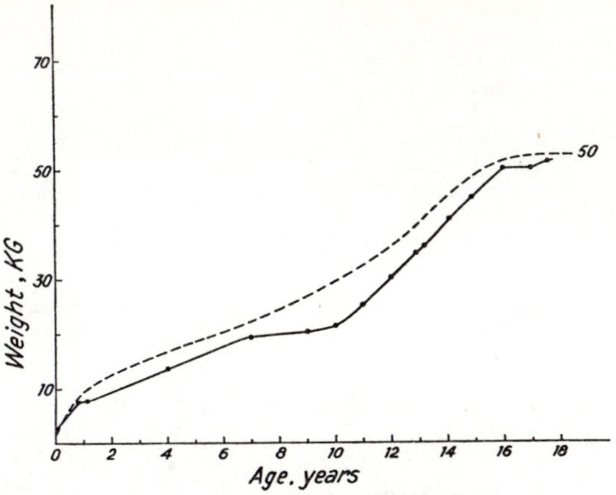

Fig. 5. Weight-distance chart of patient W. with megacystis-megaureter syndrome who developed pyelonephritis at the age of 8 months. Intensive dietary treatment was started at 10 years

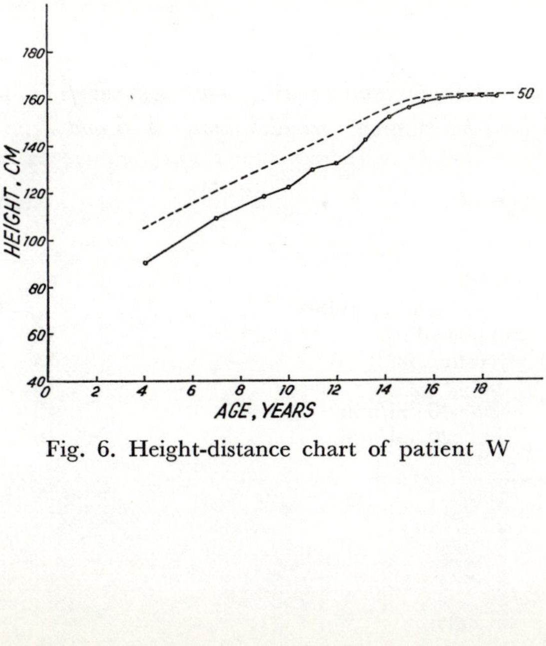

Fig. 6. Height-distance chart of patient W

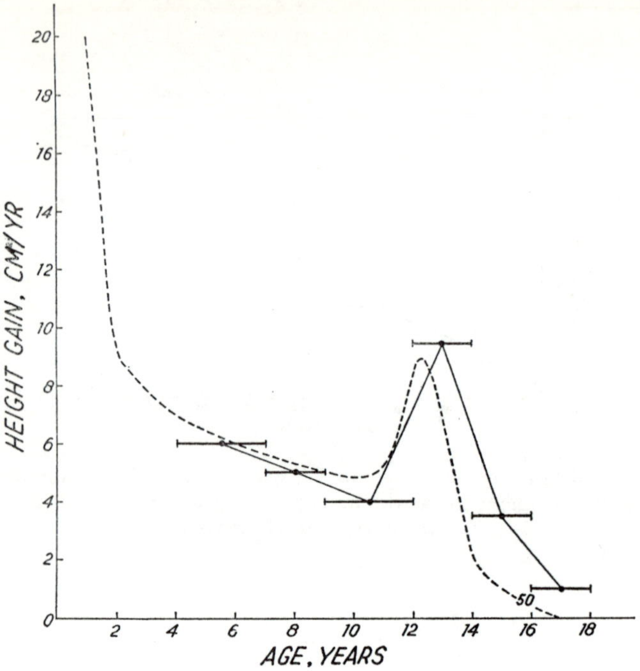

Fig. 7. Rate of growth in height of patient W, showing normal adolescent growth-spurt

Table I. *Some data on patient W., who suffered from the megacystic-megaureter syndrom (see also figures 5, 6 and 7).*

Onset of:	At age:
Pyelonephritis	$^{8}/_{12}$ years
Loss of concentrating ability	2—3 years
Hyper aminoaciduria	10—12 years
Renal glycosuria	13—14 years
TRP < 60 %	15 years
GFR 30—40 ml/min	10 years
GFR < 20 ml/min	16 years

was administered at 4 weeks' intervals. Hyperamino-aciduria occurred in the presence of normal alpha-amino-N levels in the blood. $\frac{\text{Alpha amino N} + 100}{\text{total N}}$ varied. Values of 3 were reached repeatedly. The amino-acid pattern was pathological. Minimal pH reached under acid-loading was 5.6 (at 10 years). This patient never had acidosis, possibly because of the low hydrogen ion load under strict dietary treatment. Normal growth in this child with chronic progressive renal disease, which eventually resulted in a secondary de Toni-Fanconi syndrome, certainly contrasts with the pessimistic finality that the term renal dwarfism implies.

It supports the theory that the adverse effects renal disease may have on growth can often be prevented.

REFERENCES

1. Barber, H., The bone deformities of renal dwarfism, *The Lancet* I: 18, 1920.
2. Black, D. A. K., The kidney and electrolyte homeostasis, in: *Renal disease*, ed. by D. A. K. Black, 3rd ed. 1964, Oxford, Blackwell. p. 76.
3. Brod, J., Chronic pyelonephritis, *The Lancet* I: 973, 1956.
4. Brod, J., Chronic pyelonephritis, in: *Renal disease*, ed. by D. A. K. Black, 3rd. ed. 1964, Oxford, Blackwell, p. 279.
5. Cooke, R. E., D. G. Boyden and E. Haller, The relationship of acidosis and growth retardation, *J. Pediat.* 57: 326, 1960.
6. Ellborg, A. and H. Forssman, Nephrogenic diabetes insipidus in children, *Acta Paediatrica* 44: 209, 1955.
7. Fanconi, G. and A. Prader, Renaler Zwergwuchs, *Schweiz. med. Wschr.* Bd. 83: 186, 1953.
8. Gautier, E. and M. Simpkiss, The management of nephrogenic diabetes insipidus in early life, *Acta Paediatrica* 46: 354, 1957.
9. Gautier, E., Neonatal hyperosmolality, an instance of unresponsiveness to antidiuretic hormone, *Maandschr. Kindergeneesk.* 32: 283, 1964.
10. Giovannetti, S. and G. Maggiore, A low-nitrogen diet with proteins of high biological value for severe chronic uraemia, *The Lancet* I: 1000, 1964.
11. Hess Thaysen, J., Anabolic steroids in the treatment of renal failure, in: *Protein meta bolism*, ed. by F. Gross, 1962, Berlin, Springer Verlag, p. 450.
12. Hillman, D. A., O. Neyzi, P. Porter, A. Cushman and N. B. Talbot, Renal (vasopressin-resistant) diabetes insipidus. Definition of the effects of a homeostatic limitation in capacity to conserve water on the physical, intellectual and emotional development of a child, *Pediatrics* 21: 430, 1958.
13. Hunt, J., The influence of dietary sulfur on the urinary output of acid in man, *Clin. Sci.* 15: 119, 1956.
14. Kaplan, S. A., *Growth disorders in children and adolescents*, 1964, Springfield, Ch. C. Thomas, p. 140.

15. KIMMELSTIEL, P., Significance of chronic pyelonephritis, in: *Biology of pyelonephritis*, 1960, London, J. & A. Churchill, p. 215.
16. KIRMAN, B. H., J. A. BLACK, R. H. WILKINSON and P. R. EVANS, Familial pitressin-resistant diabetes insipidus with mental defect, *Arch. Dis. Childh.* 31: 59, 1956.
17. KLEEMAN, C. R., W. L. HEWITT and L. B. GUSE, Pyelonephritis, *Medicine* 39: 3, 1960.
18. LINNEWEH, F., Pyelonephritis, *Mod. Probl. Pädiat.* Bd. 6: 251, 1960.
19. MCCANCE, R. A., Age and renal function, in: *Renal disease*, ed. by D. A. K. BLACK, 3rd ed., 1964, Oxford, Blackwell, p. 157.
20. PARSONS, F. M., Dietary treatment and anabolic steroids in acute renal failure, in: *Water and electrolyte metabolism II*, ed. by J. DE GRAEFF and B. LEYNSE, 1963, Amsterdam, Elsevier, p. 204.
21. PRADER, A., R. ILLIG and E. HEIERLI, Eine besondere Form der primären vitamin-D-resistenten Rachitis mit Hypocalcämie und autosolmaldominantem Erbgang: die hereditäre Pseudo-Mangelrachitis, *Helv. paediat. Acta* 16: 452, 1961.
22. PRADER, A., J. M. TANNER and G. A. VON HARNACK, Catch-up growth following illness or starvation. An example of developmental canalization in man, *J. Pediat.* 62: 646, 1963.
23. ROSENHEIM, M. L. and E. J. ROSS, Chronic renal failure, in: *Renal disease* ed. by D. A. K. BLACK, 3rd ed., 1964, Oxford, Blackwell, p. 335.
24. ROYER, P., H. MATHIEU and S. GERBEAUX, Explorations biologiques du métabolisme calcique chez l'enfant, in: *Rein et foie*, maladies de la nutrition, symposium international sur la lithian calcique, Juin 1962, Vittel.
25. STANBURY, S. W., Bony complications of renal disease, in: *Renal disease*, ed. by D. A. K. BLACK, 3rd ed., 1964, Oxford, Blackwell, chapter 22.
26. TIDDENS, H. A. W. M., *The renal de Toni syndrome with dwarfism*, 1957, Amsterdam, Diligentia, p. 14.
27. TIDDENS, H. A. W. M., *Pyelonephritis en pediatrie*, 1963, Oratory lecture university Utrecht.
28. VEST, M., N. B. TALBOT and J. D. CRAWFORD, Hypocaloric dwarfism and hydronephrosis in diabetes insipidus, *Amer. J. Dis. Child.* 105: 175, 1963.
29. WATSON, E. H. and G. H. LOWREY, *Growth and development of children*, 1958, Chicago, The Year Book Publ. Inc., p. 314.
30. WEST, C. D. and W. C. SMITH, An attempt to elucidate the cause of growth retardation in renal disease, *Amer. J. Dis. Child.* 91: 460, 1956.
31. WILLIAMS, D. I., The diagnosis and treatment of obstructive uropathy in childhood, *Mod. Probl. Padiät.* 6: 458, 1960.
32. WOLTHUIS, F. H., Protein-sparing action of androgenic steroids, in: *Water and electrolyte metabolism II*, ed. by J. DE GRAEFF and B. LEYNSE, 1962, Amsterdam, Elsevier, p. 193.
33. WRONG, O. M., Test of renal function, in: *Renal disease*, ed. by D. A. K. BLACK, 3rd ed., 1964, Oxford, Blackwell, p. 446.
34. WRONG, O. M. and H. E. F. DAVIES, The excretion of acid in renal disease, *Quart. J. Med.* 28: 259, 1959.
35. WIJFFELS, J. C. H. M., *Nephrogene diabetes insipidus*, Thesis, 1959, Leiden, H. E. Stenfert Kroese.
36. ZNAMENSKY, P. Y. and H. A. W. M. TIDDENS, Een geval van idiopathische renale acidose, *Maandschr. Kindergeneesk.* 24: 193, 1956.

RICKETS AND GROWTH

R. STEENDIJK

Considering the short stature encountered in patients suffering from rickets, the question arises whether the reduced height is the result of the rachitic process at the metaphyses of the long bones — i.e. incomplete and disorganised ossification of the cartilage septa — or of the deformities of the long bones such as bending, coxa vara, genu varum, or of both. In addition, as it has been known for a long time that rickets is more severe during periods of rapid growth than during periods of slow growth, it would be interesting to find out whether an increase in the rate of growth might be counteracted by an increase in the severity of the deformities and/or the metaphyseal lesions.

These problems can best be studied in chronic rickets. Primary vitamin D-resistant rickets is most suitable in this respect because the disease cannot be cured completely even when the highest possible doses of vitamin D are given, and because the patients are perfectly healthy apart from the rickets.

In an attempt to answer these questions, 4 patients with primary vitamin D-resistant rickets were studied: 2 boys (P.V., aged 17, and P.N., aged 16 years) and 2 girls (A.V., aged 14, and M.M. aged 14 years). In the boys and in the girl M.M., therapy with high doses of vitamin D had been instituted several years prior to the investigation. These patients had severe deformities of the legs. The girl A.V. had hypophosphataemia but no visible deformities at the time of the investigation. Signs of active rickets and slight deformities of the legs had been present in the first 4 years of life during which time the girl had been treated with vitamin D in doses up to 8.000 I.U. per day. Between ages 4 and 11 no therapy had been given and there were no signs of active rickets on X-ray photographs of knee and wrist. During her 12th year, slight genu valgum developed on both sides and signs of active rickets, which were slight but unmistakable, were visible on

X-ray photographs. With vitamin D in doses up to 120.000 I.U. per day, these signs and the deformities slowly disappeared. Data on the growth and development of this girl are presented in fig. 1. It can be seen that the recurrence of visible signs of rickets (indicated by 'R' in fig. 1) coincided with the pubertal growth spurt.

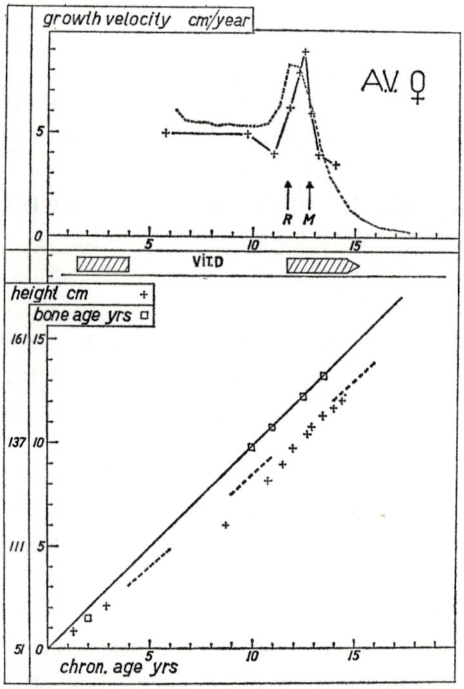

Fig. 1. Growth and growth rate in A.V. 'R' indicates onset of deformities; 'M' indicates time of first menstrual period. The dotted line in the upper part of the figure represents normal growth velocity for girls having their peak velocity at approx. 12½ years. The interrupted dotted line in the lower part of the figure represents the 10th percentile for height in Dutch children (from 2)

The other 3 patients always had some X-ray signs of active rickets during the period they were treated with high amounts of vitamin D, whereas the deformities persisted. In P.N. and M.M., the deformities of the legs increased during the growth spurt. In P.V., this was not noted.

It should be mentioned that an attempt to check the increasing deformities in P.N. and M.M. by an increase in the dose of vitamin D was curtailed by the onset of hypercalcaemia.

These observations confirm that the severity of rickets increases with an increased growth rate. As a pubertal growth spurt was observed in all patients studied (2), it appears that the effect of the higher growth rate was not completely balanced by the effect of increased deformities. Although it may be assumed that the growth rate would have been higher in the absence of rickets, it is impossible to obtain quantitative information on this point in a longitudinal study of this kind.

To find out whether the deformities or the rachitic lesions at the metaphyses were mainly responsible for the short stature of the patients, several measurements were taken: height, span, lower segment (distance between the upper edge of the symphysis pubis and the floor) and upper segment (difference between height and lower segment) (3) were determined. For comparison, the same measurements were done on 10 normal boys and 10 normal girls of similar developmental age as the patients. This particular choice of measurements was decided

Table 1. *Body measurements expressed in centimeters. The values for the normal range and the average of each measurement have been derived from 10 normal control subjects in each group.*

	height	span	lower segment	upper segment	span/ height	lower segment/ height
Boys						
Normal range	156—180.5	161—182	80—95	74—88.5	0.99—1.05	0.49—0.55
average	170	173	88	82.6	1.02	0.52
P.N.	152	160	71	81	1.05	0.47
P.V.	151.5	160	71	81.5	1.05	0.47
Girls						
Normal range	154—168	153-171.5	77—87	74—87.5	0.97—1.04	0.48—0.54
average	161	163	81.6	79.5	1.00	0.51
A.V.	149	153	72	77	1.03	0.48
M.M.	145.5	152.5	66	79.5	1.05	0.45

upon since in P.V., P.N. and M.M. deformities were only conspicuous in the legs; the spinal column of these patients was perfectly straight on clinical examination. The long bones of the arms were slightly deformed; this was evident only on X-ray examination. A.V. had no deformities on clinical or X-ray examination. The results of this study are presented in table 1. The data indicate that the effect of rickets on growth was not equal in all parts of the body: the legs (lower segment) were too short in comparison with height and the spine (upper segment) appeared to have reached a normal length. The ratio span/height was high, indicating that the arms were less involved than the legs. Even in the girl A.V., who no longer had any deformities, the lower segment was relatively short.

As the metaphyseal rachitic lesions are generalized and not limited to the legs, whereas the deformities in these patients were mainly present in the legs, it can be concluded from these data that the short stature was mainly due to the deformities. In A.V., the short lower segment may have been the result of the slight deformities which were present during the first years of life. Although the legs appeared to be straight at the time of the investigation, a complete catch-up may not have taken place.

Whether in addition a genetic effect and/or a direct growth retarding effect of rickets was present cannot be concluded from these data. WINTERS and his co-workers (4) concluded from an extensive study on many patients that hypophosphataemia without apparent skeletal disease may lead to stunting of growth. However, some of the patients with subclinical rickets known to the author appear to grow quite normally. The main problem here, as in so many other cases of slight to moderate stunting of growth is, of course, that one never knows how the particular patient would have grown if he or she had not suffered from the disease which appears to be the cause of the short stature.

Finally, there appears to be a positive correlation between the serum-phosphate level and the retardation of growth in primary vitamin D-resistant rickets. In the cases described here, the serum-P level, though still subnormal, had been higher in A.V. than in the other patients (table 2). This has also been noted by FRASER and SLATER (1). An obvious explanation for this is the negative correlation which exists between the serum-P level and the extent and severity of the deformities.

Table 2. *Serum-phosphate levels in the patients without and with treatment.*

	Serum-phosphate levels (mg %)	
	Without vitamin D	With vitamin D
Subject		
P.N., P.V., M.M.	2.0—2.6	2.5—3.8
A.V.	2.7—3.1	2.8—3.9

SUMMARY

In 4 patients with primary vitamin D-resistant rickets a longitudinal and cross-sectional growth study was made. It appeared that: 1. the rachitic deformities increased in severity during the pubertal growth spurt in 3 cases and, 2 the short stature was to a large extent caused by the deformities of the legs.

REFERENCES

1. Fraser, D. and R. B. Slater, The diagnosis and management of various types of rickets, *Pediatric Clin. North America* 5: 417, 1958.
2. Steendijk, R., Studies on growth in refractory rickets, *J. Ped.* 60: 340, 1962.
3. Wilkins, L., *The diagnosis and treatment of endocrine disorders in infancy and childhood,* 2nd ed., 1957, Springfield, Ill.
4. Winters, R. W., J. B. Graham, T. F. Williams, V. W. McFalls and C. H. Burnett, A genetic study of familial hypophosphataemia and vitamin D resistant rickets with a review of the literature, *Medicine* 37: 97, 1958.

DWARFISM IN MENTAL DEFICIENCY

H. H. VAN GELDEREN

Growth of mentally defectives has seldom been studied. Recently a study of growth and maturation has been carried out in a large institution for mentally defectives near Leiden (1, 2). It is my purpose to present here some data of the first part of this study. Only some general conclusions about growth shall be given and details of body measurements and sexual maturation shall be omitted. As mental deficiency may occur in numerous syndromes and diseases, many of which are of unknown origin, the nature of the information gained very much depends on the classification of the patients. Our classification (table 1) has been based mainly on the time at which the cerebral defect or anomaly arose. The findings to be discussed here, are from the first 600 patients studied at ages between 3 and 16 years, of whom nearly

Table 1. *Classification.*

A. Prenatal
   1. mongolism (Down's syndrome)
   2. multiple congenital anomalies
   3. specific syndromes
   4. lues, toxoplasma and other foetopathies
   5. familial severe oligophrenia
      a. with hyperaminoaciduria
      b. without hyperaminoaciduria

B. Perinatal
   1. with cerebral palsy, including kernicterus
   2. without cerebral palsy

C. Postnatal brain damage

D. Subcultural, mild mental retardation

70 % could be classified. A small number of children had to be excluded because of severe malnutrition, chronic illness, thyroid deficiency, thyroid medication, or inability to be measured.

It is essential to mention that the classification bears little or no relation to the severity of the mental defect, apart from the group of subculturals. This also means that living conditions in the institution, nutrition, exposure to illness etc. is in no way correlated with the classification used. The group of mildly mental defectives (subculturals) forms a useful group for comparison, as they live in the same institution and differ from the other patients mainly in that they have no serious cerebral abnormality.

To minimize the difficulties in assessing height in these patients all measurements were performed by the author.

Bone age also was always determined by the author according to Greulich and Pyle (3). In the author's experience the Greulich and Pyle atlas seems to be 6 months advanced over normal Dutch children in the age range studied. The height standards used for the calculation of height ages are the data on Dutch children collected in 1955 (4). Table 2 shows the mean ratios of height age and skeletal age to chronological age; the ratio is expressed as a percentage in the same way as we express the I.Q. These ratios have been used for easy comparison though they are influenced by such factors as age and stage of sexual maturation.

Table 2. *Mean height age and bone age as percentage of normal for age.*

	Height age	Bone age
mongolism	71	91
multiple congenital anomalies	77	92
familial oligophrenia with hyperaminoaciduria	82	82
familial oligophrenia without hyperaminoaciduria	88	91
perinatal with palsy	80	84
perinatal without palsy	94	97
postnatal brain damage	98	99
subcultural	101	95

The table shows distinct differences between the diagnostic groups. In general, three patterns of growth can be distinguished:

a. dwarfism with near-normal skeletal maturation
b. dwarfism with skeletal retardation
c. normal growth.

The differences found between the groups with the two types of dwarfism and the normally growing patients are highly significant.

Of special interest are the cases of mongolism, as they form a homogeneous group (fig. 1). They show severe retardation in height and almost normal bone age. It is of interest that this pattern is also found in the group with multiple congenital anomalies (fig. 2), in whom we may expect chromosomal disorders or damage in early foetal life.

Figures 3 and 4 demonstrate that in the perinatally injured, growth retardation occurs mainly among the children with cerebral palsy. In these children, however, bone age is retarded nearly as much as height age. Figure 5 shows that children with postnatal brain damage, many of whom have cerebral palsy, usually grow normally. Among the few dwarfs are all the cases with basal brain damage, i.e. tuberculous meningitis and fracture of the base of the skull. Notwithstanding the fact that the subcultural mildly retarded have been admitted mainly because of the poor social background, this group as a whole shows normal growth (fig. 6).

In the early prenatal cases and in the patients with chromosomal abnormalities, the pattern of dwarfism would be consistent with an intrinsic growth defect or growth hormone unresponsiveness. Only part of these children had a low birth weight, though as a group birth weight was below the normal average. The lower growth rate might be considered as one of their congenital anomalies. In children with multiple congenital defects who are not mentally deficient (not reported here), growth retardation is also frequent.

The fact that the perinatally injured cases with palsy are dwarfed, while those without cerebral palsy are not, suggests a direct relation between the cerebral damage and the growth retardation. The type of dwarfism: reduction in stature as well as in bone age, is also seen in other chronic illnesses and in chronic malnutrition.

The normal growth in children with cerebral palsy in whom the

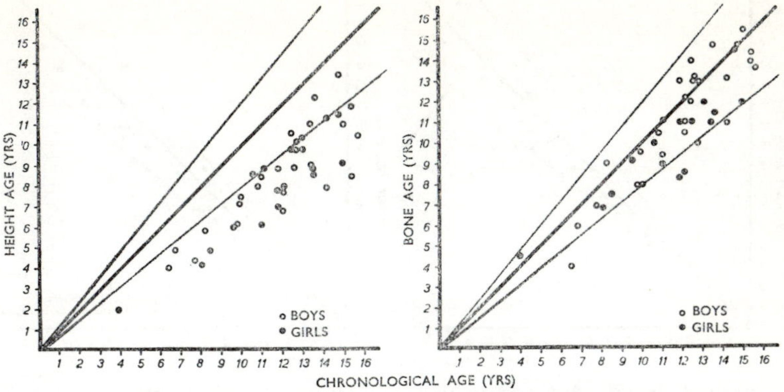

Fig. 1. Height age and bone age in mongolism

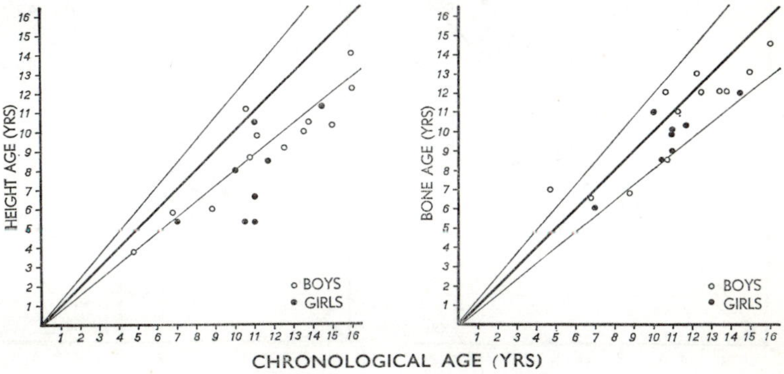

Fig. 2. Left: height age in multiple congenital anomalies; right: bone age in multiple congenital anomalies

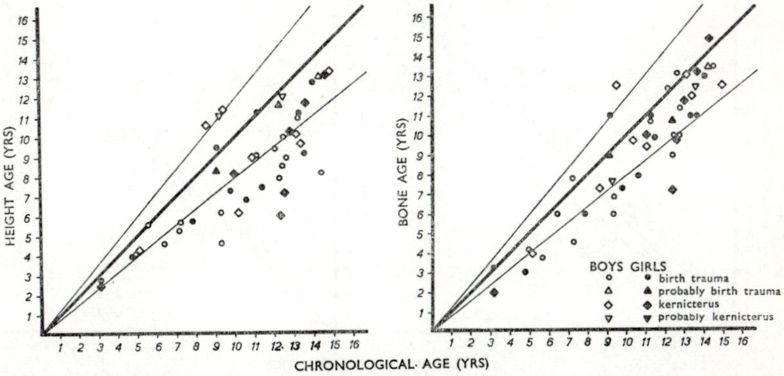

Fig. 3. Height age and bone age in perinatal group with cerebral palsy

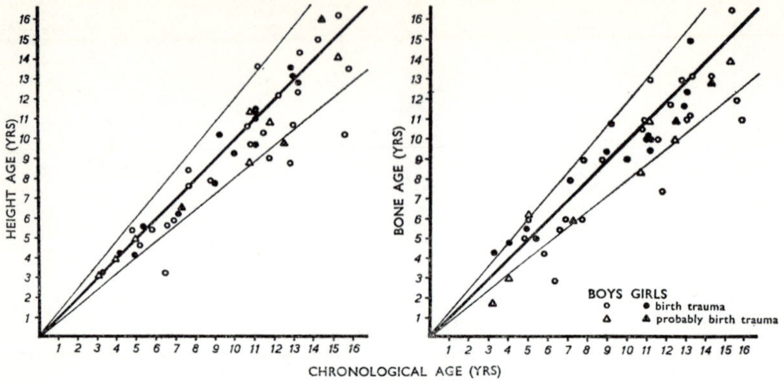

Fig. 4. Height age and bone age in perinatal group without palsy

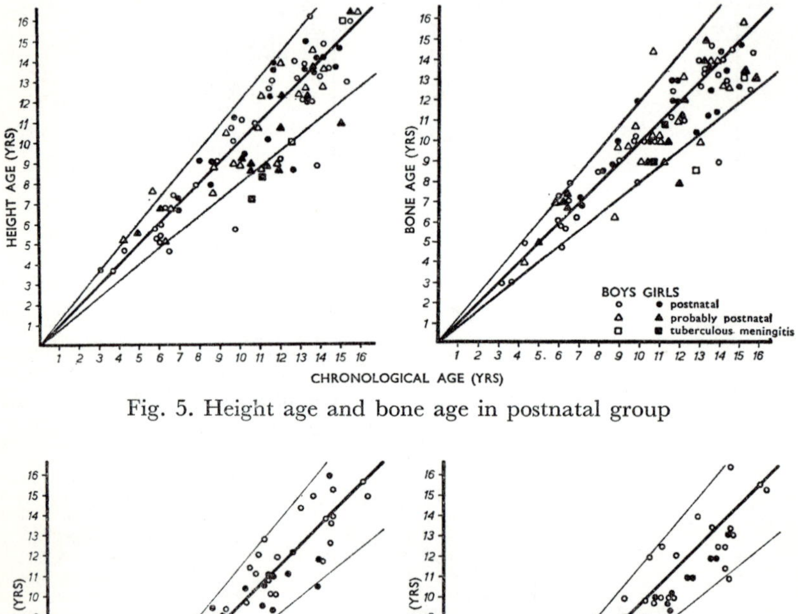

Fig. 5. Height age and bone age in postnatal group

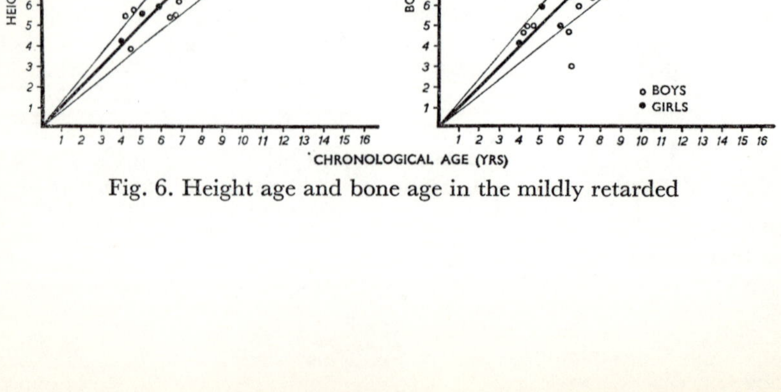

Fig. 6. Height age and bone age in the mildly retarded

damage occurred after the first months of life, suggests that this cerebral growth-stunting factor operates only during a certain critical period of brain development.

The number of known cases of damage after the first foetal months is too small for analysis; however, it seems that these children are not usually dwarfed. Data on a group of congenital toxoplasmosis patients, studied in the Children's Department, confirm this impression. The familial severely deficient group is still too heterogeneous for analysis.

REFERENCES

1. GELDEREN, H. H. VAN, Studies in Oligophrenia I, *Acta Paed.* 51: 643, 1962.
2. GELDEREN, H. H. VAN and L. J. DOOREN, Studies in Oligophrenia III, *Acta Paed.* 52: 557, 1963.
3. GREULICH, W. W. and S. I. PYLE, *Radiographic atlas of skeletal development of the hand and wrist,* 2nd. ed., Stanford, 1959.
4. DE WIJN, J. F. and J. H. DE HAAS, Biologische ontwikkeling van de adolescent, *Nederlands Leerboek der Interne Geneeskunde,* Amsterdam, 1960, p. 710.

THE TALL CHILD

J. J. VAN DER WERFF TEN BOSCH and R. ENTHOVEN

The definition of a tall child is quite as arbitrary as the definition of a short child, and is best made with reference to the percentiles for height of the population to which the child belongs. Tall children are nearly always healthy, and usually have one or two tall parents.

Some children are tall for a limited period of time only. The clearest examples are cases of sexual precocity, true (secretion of sex steroids by gonads which mature early, through early secretion of pituitary gonadotrophins) or pseudo (sex steroids present although gonads are still immature, e.g. in untreated congenital adrenal hyperplasia), and such cases usually end up as short adults in consequence of the early fusion of the epiphyses (fig. 1). Less conspicuous are children who come in puberty at an early time within the normal age range, and who may for some time be tall in comparison with their age peers who have not yet started to mature sexually.

Tallness is an inconstant (9, 11) feature of Marfan's syndrome, an hereditary collagen disease (10, 7) characterized by elongated long bones, cardiovascular, ocular and other defects (8).

True gigantism, with adult height over 210 cm, is always due to a pituitary eosinophilic adenoma. Such tumours secrete large amounts of growth hormone. In adults, with calcified epiphyseal discs, the ensuing periosteal growth results in acromegaly. In children such tumours may cause gigantism through two co-operating factors: firstly, the growth rate is stimulated (see fig. 2), whereby more height gain occurs per unit of time, and secondly, the tumour causes gonadotrophin deficiency, so that the pubertal rise in sex hormone output which is responsible for epiphyseal fusion in normal individuals, does not occur, and growth may continue into the third decade.

While true gigantism results from the combined effects of an increase in the rate of growth and an increase in the length of the period of growth, male hypogonadism may lead to tallness through the latter of the two effects alone. If the testes are removed before puberty, as in eunuchs, or if they remain inactive, as in hypogonadotrophic hypogonadism, the period of growth is greatly extended. Examples of

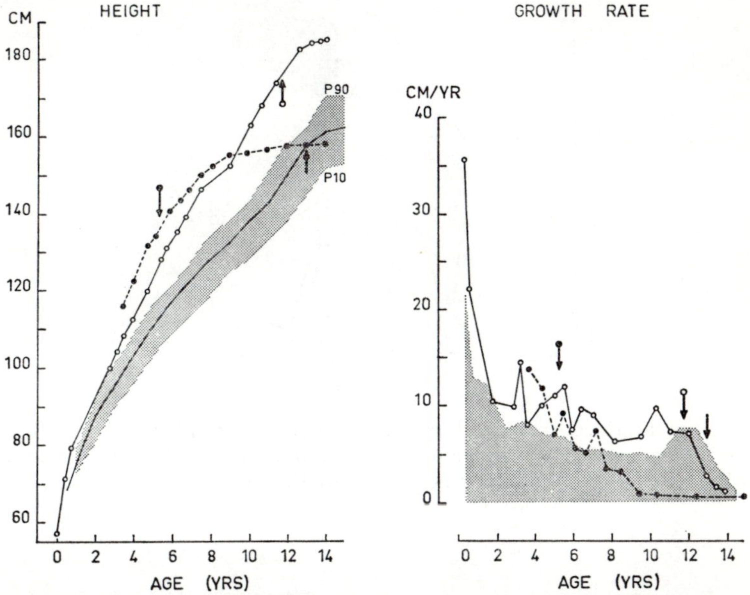

Fig. 1. Height attained (left) and growth velocity (right) of a girl with true sexual precocity (•—•) and of a healthy tall girl with tall parents (○—○). Note the difference in the ages at menarche (↓ and ↑). At about 9 years the two girls have identical statures, but the former has almost stopped growing, whereas the latter has just started her pubertal spurt. The shaded area in the left figure delimits the 10th and 90th percentiles for height in a cross-sectional study of Dutch girls (from 12). The drawn line in the left figure is the growth curve of a normal average girl (menarche at ↑) described by Bayer and Bayley (2); the shaded area in the right figure indicates the growth velocity of this girl

growth in height after the age of 19 years are depicted in fig. 3. It can be seen that considerable increase in size may occur when growth is allowed to continue, even at a relatively slow rate.

HEALTHY TALL CHILDREN

From the aetiological point of view the tall child nearly always belongs to Albright's (1) category of 'what endocrinology is not'. We have

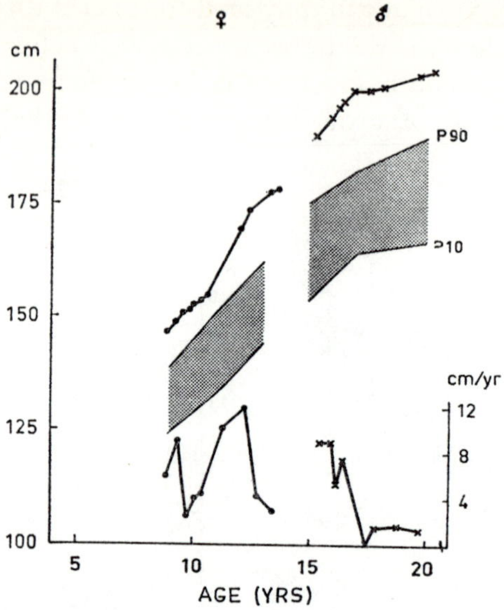

Fig. 2. Height attained (top) and growth velocity (bottom) of a girl (left) and a boy (right) with a pituitary eosinophilic adenoma. The shaded areas delimit the 10th and 90th percentiles for height (from 12) for the corresponding sex

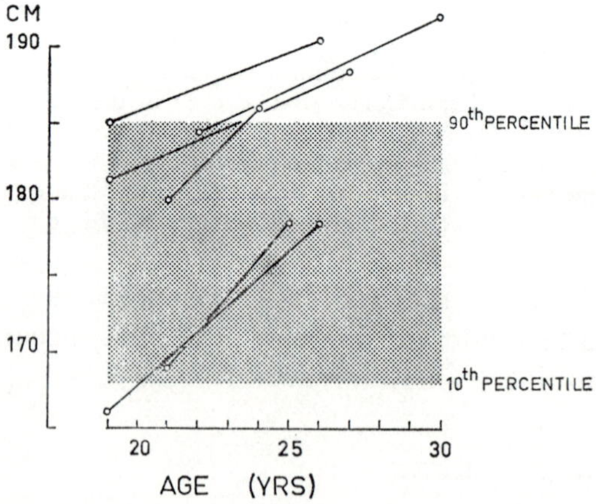

Fig. 3. Height attained at subsequent ages beyond the age of 19 years, of six men with hypogonadotrophic hypogonadism. Percentiles from 12

recently made a survey of all the children with a height of over the 90th percentile for their age, which occur in the files of our department. Excluded from this follow-up were individuals who have suffered from a known endocrine disorder, and cases of Marfan's syndrome. All of these normal individuals for whom relevant information was available, are included in the data which will be discussed. None of the children had received hormone preparations.

Height and weight standards used, are for Dutch children and were collected in 1955 (12). Bone ages of hand and wrist were estimated

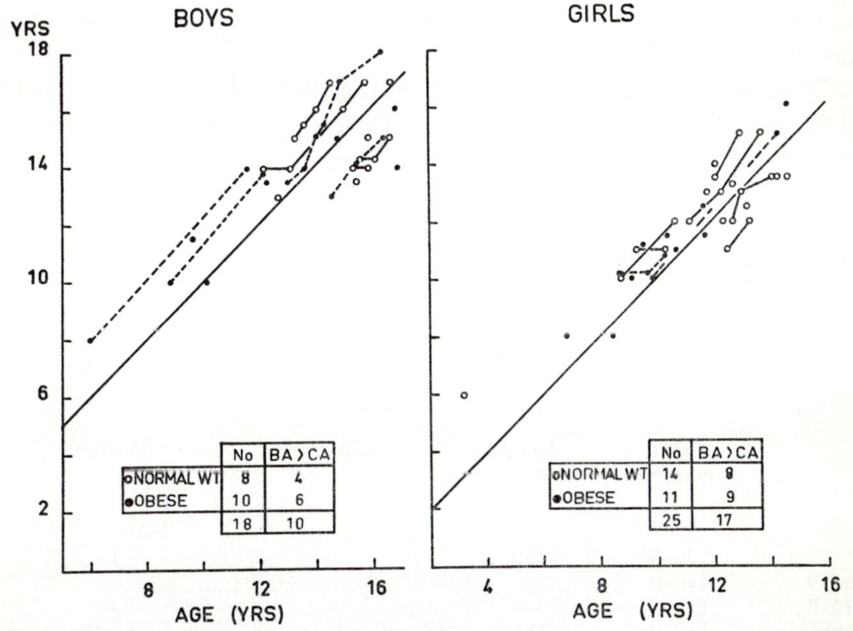

Fig. 4. Bone ages of children whose height exceeded the 90th percentile, plotted against their chronological ages. Lines connect multiple observations on single individuals. For explanation of inset, see text. BA = bone age. CA = chronological age

independently by the two authors (Greulich and Pyle method, 4) after randomization of all the films, and without knowing the age at which they had been made. Observer differences were dealt with by independent re-examination and, where necessary, by joint inspection and compromise. Adult heights were predicted with the tables, and following the instructions, of Bayley and Pinneau (3). 'Observed adult heights' are identical measurements obtained repeatedly at an interval of at least six months, or measurements obtained when the skeleton was mature.

Skeletal maturation. Values for single or repeated bone age estimations of 43 tall children are shown in fig. 4 In 2/3 of all the children the bone age was higher than the chronological age. Subdivision into 'obese' children (weight above the 90th percentile of the weight appropriate for the height) and children of 'normal' body weight, showed that skeletal maturity was advanced in nearly all the obese tall girls (see also fig. 6). At prepubertal ages nearly all children were advanced in skeletal maturity.

Sexual maturation. The average age at menarche of Dutch girls was 13 8/12 years in 1955 (5). Thirteen of 15 tall girls were younger than average when their menstrual periods began (table 1).

Table 1. *The age at menarche and post-menarcheal growth of tall girls.*

Case	At menarche		Growth after menarche (cm)	
	Age (yrs.-months)	Height (cm)	Observed	Predicted
MEI	10—3	159	—	16
SCO	11—0	—	—	—
TDB	11—6	—	—	—
HAL	11—9	171	8.5	8—10
SLO	11—10	176	—	11
MEE	11—11	161	7.0	7.5
PAV	12—0	179	—	7.0
REU	12—8	168	7.5	4.5
BIK	12—8	172	—	11—0
MDB	13—0	182	9.0	—
GRO	13—4	—	—	—
DYK	13—6	180	7.5	11—12.5
SCM	13—7	175	4.0	8.0
GEN	13—10	175	7.0	—
SWA	15—7	172.5	0	0.5

Predicted adult height. For 12 children a comparison was possible between predicted and observed adult height. It was found that the predicted height of these tall children nearly always exceeded the observed height (table 2). The greatest differences occurred in girls with a bone age of 11—13 years, and in boys with a bone age of 13—15 years, when the prediction was made (fig. 5). The latter findings probably indicate that during puberty the spurt in height slightly precedes, in time, the spurt in skeletal maturation in terms of X-ray changes.

Table 2. *The error in adult height prediction in tall children.*

Sex	Case	For height prediction			Adult height (cm)		
		Age (yrs.-months)	Bone Age (yrs)	Height (cm)	Observed	Predicted	Difference
Girls	SWA	9—10	10	149	172.5	173	0.5
		14—4	15	171		173	0.5
	HAL	11—3	12	167	179.5	181	1.5
		12—4	13	174		181	1.5
		13—9	15	176.5		179	—0.5
	REU	11—10	13	163	175.5	172.5	—3.0
	DYK	12—7	11	175	187.5	191	3.5
		13—4	12	179		192.5	5.0
	SCM	14—8	13½	178.5	179	183	4.0
	MEE	14—8	16	168	168	168.5	0.5
Boys	GRO	6—1	8	132	183.5	190	6.5
		11—8	14	169		187	3.5
	WAC	13—0	13½	183	199	202.5	3.5
		13—8	14	189		204	5.0
		14—1	15	192		198.5	—0.5
	COE	13—4	15	188	191.5	191.5	0
		13—8	15½	189		191.5	0
		14—2	16	190.5		192	0.5
	WYK	14—10	15	185	190	192.5	2.5
	BAK	15—0	14	186	200	205.5	5.5
		15—11	14	194.5		215	15.0
	KRA	15—6	13½	187	198.5	206	7.5

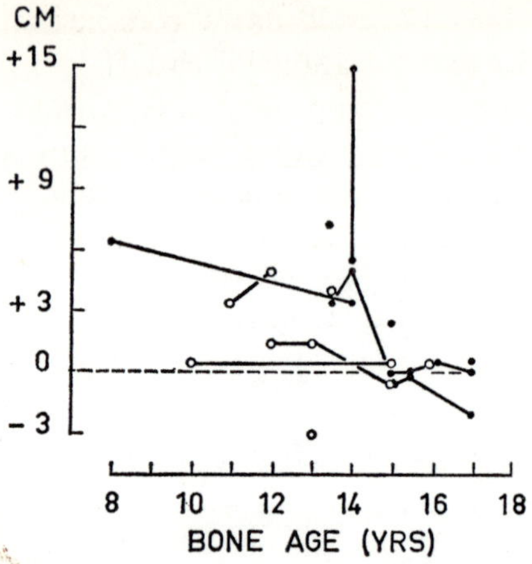

Fig. 5. The difference between predicted and observed adult height, of 5 tall girls (○) and 7 tall boys (•), plotted against the bone ages from which the predictions were made

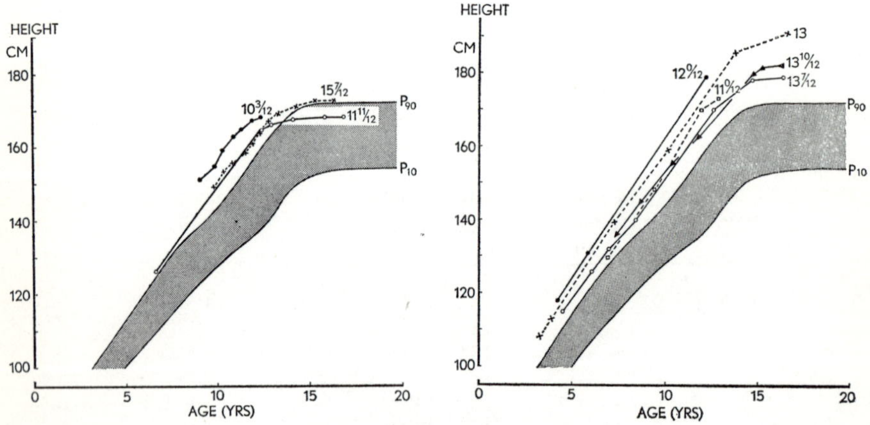

Fig. 6. Growth curves of tall girls who: 1. have experienced menarche (see ages along the graphs), 2. have been measured at least once before the age of 10 years. Right: girls with normal weight for their height.
Left: girls whit weight above the 90th percentile of the weight appropriate to their height. Shaded areas delimit the 10th and 90th percentiles (from 12). Note that in this sample the obese tall girls will be smaller adults than the tall girls of normal weight (see also 6)

A general characterization of the development of healthy tall children (see the girl in fig. 1, and fig. 6) is, that they tend to be long at birth, at all times grow at a faster rate than average children, tend to be advanced in skeletal maturity before puberty, and come in puberty relatively early. The prediction of adult height with the Greulich and Pyle atlas and the Bayley and Pinneau tables yields overestimates for tall children.

REFERENCES

1. ALBRIGHT, F., Introduction (to chapter 'Diseases of the ductless glands'), *Textbook of Medicine*, Eds. R. L. CECIL and R. F. LOEB, Philadelphia, 1951, p. 1215.
2. BAYER, L. M. and N. BAYLEY, *Growth Diagnosis*, Chicago, 1959, p. 101.
3. BAYLEY, N. and S. R. PINNEAU, see 4.
4. GREULICH, W. W. and S. I. PYLE, *Radiographic atlas of skeletal development of the hand and wrist*, 2nd ed., Stanford, 1959.
5. LAND, G. M. VAN 'T and J. H. DE HAAS, Menarche-leeftijd in Nederland, *Ned. T. Geneesk.* 101: 1425, 1959.
6. LLOYD, J. K., O. H. WOLFF and W. S. WHELEN, Obesity in childhood — a long term study of the height and weight, *Brit. med. J.* 2: 145, 1961.
7. LOVEMAN, A. B., A. M. GORDON and M. T. FLIEGELMAN, Marfan's syndrome. Some cutaneous aspects, *Arch. Dermatol.* 87: 428, 1963.
8. McKUSICK, V. A., *Heritable Disorders of Connective Tissue*, 2nd ed., St. Louis, 1960.
9. PAPPAS, E. G., D. MASON and C. DENTON, Marfan's syndrome. A report of three patients with aneurysm of the aorta, *Am. J. Med.* 23: 426, 1957.
10. SJOERDSMA, A., J. D. DAVIDSON, S. UDENFRIEND and C. MITOMA, Increased excretion of hydroxyproline in Marfan's syndrome, *Lancet* 2: 994, 1958.
11. WILSON, R., Marfan's syndrome: description of a family, *Am. J. Med.* 23: 434, 1957.
12. WIJN, J. F. DE and J. H. DE HAAS, Biologische ontwikkeling van de adolescent, *Nederlands Leerboek der Interne Geneeskunde*, Amsterdam, 1960, p. 710.

GROWTH OF CHILDREN WITH CONGENITAL ADRENAL HYPERPLASIA

H. K. A. VISSER, M.D.*

INTRODUCTION

Congenital adrenal hyperplasia is the most important cause of the so-called adrenogenital syndrome in infancy and childhood. It is an 'inborn error of metabolism', caused by hereditary enzymatic defects in the biosynthesis of hydrocortisone. At least three, and possibly four, of those defects have been described sofar.

Figure 1 shows schematically the biosynthetic pathways for hydrocortisone and aldosterone in the adrenal cortex. Cholesterol is a precursor for all adrenocortical steroids. By splitting off the side chain at C_{21} Δ_5-pregnenolone is formed. The next step consists in the shift of the double bound from the Δ_{5-6} to the Δ_{4-5} position and oxidation of —OH to = O at C_3. These changes, requiring the activity of an isomerase and a dehydrogenase, result in the formation of progesterone. This steroid is subsequently hydroxylated at the positions C_{17}, C_{11} and C_{21} to hydrocortisone (cortisol) and at C_{21}, C_{11} to corticosterone. This last compound then is converted to aldosterone via 18—OH corticosterone (requiring the activity of an hydroxylase and dehydrogenase).

Adrenal androgens are synthetized either directly from cholesterol or via Δ_5-pregnenolone by splitting off the side chain (dehydroepiandrosterone, DHA) or via progesterone or DHA (Δ_4-androstenedione). It is very likely that both DHA and Δ_4-androstenedione are then transformed to testosterone.

Three hereditary enzymatic defects in the biosynthesis of adrenocortical steroids have been described sofar. An impaired synthesis of

* Supported in part by a PHS returning research fellow grant (RF-41) from the Public Health Service, National Institutes of Health, Bethesda, Md. U.S.A., and a grant from the Netherlands Organization for the Advancement of Pure Research (Z.W.O.)

hydrocortisone explained by a relative lack of 21-hydroxylation, 11-hydroxylation or 3β-ol-dehydrogenation, will ultimately lead to com-

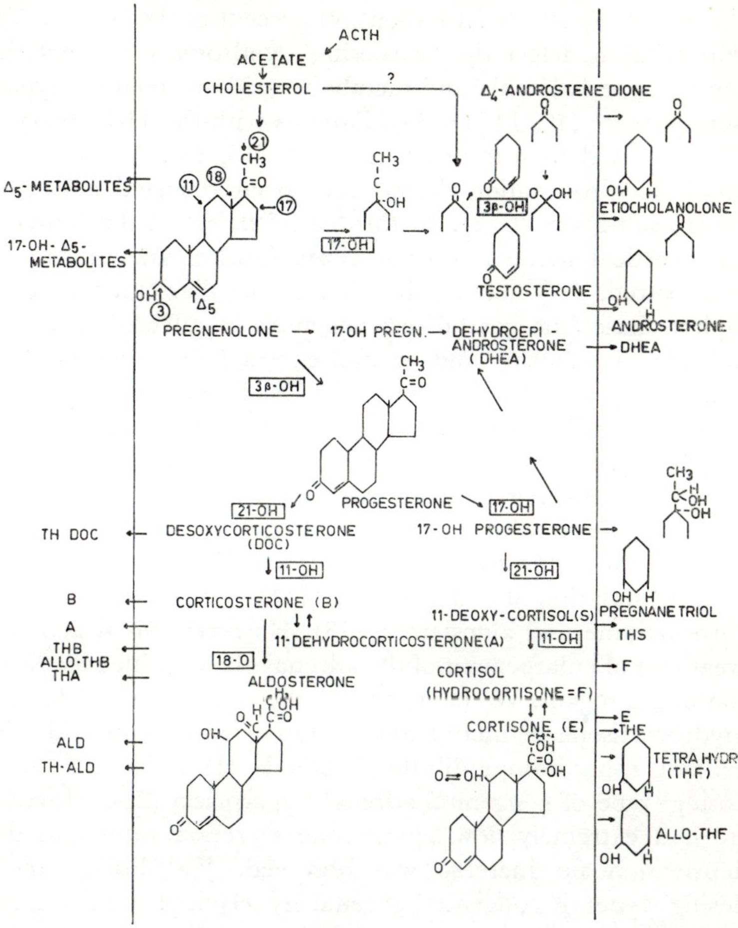

Fig. 1. Schematic presentation of adrenocortical biosynthesis of aldosterone, hydrocortisone and androgens. The most important steroids (hormones and metabolites) excreted in the urine are mentioned at the left and right side. Hereditary enzymatic defects are known for 3 —OH, 21 —OH, 11 —OH, 18 —O

pensatory hypertrophy of the adrenal cortex by excessive corticotrophin secretion via the negative feedback action between the anterior pituitary gland (ACTH) and the adrenal cortex (hydrocortisone).

The increased elaboration of androgenic substances results in the characteristic pictures of the adrenogenital syndrome in infants and children, particularly in the female patient (female pseudohermaphroditism) (1, 7, 18, 33). In about 30 percent of the patients with a 21-hydroxylation defect the 'salt-losing' syndrome is present: hyponatraemia, hyperkalaemia and metabolic acidosis, changes typical of Addison's disease (10, 14, 17, 33). Patients with the 11-hydroxylation defect generally demonstrate hypertension (15, 27). A few cases with the 3β-ol-dehydrogenation defect have been reported and most of them were salt-losers (6, 7). In this 'early' defect in the biosynthesis of adrenocortical steroids also the biosynthesis of androgens is more or less impaired. This may result in a very peculiar clinical picture of incomplete masculine genital organogenesis in affected males (male pseudohermaphroditism) and normal external genitalia in affected females. A clinically similar form as the 3β-ol-dehydrogenation defect has been described by PRADER and co-workers as 'lipoid adrenal hyperplasia' (23, 24). This form may be due to a very early defect, between cholesterol and Δ_5-pregnenolone (see figure 1).

In many patients with congenital adrenal hyperplasia the defects in the biosynthesis of adrenocortical steroids are compensated by the increased stimulation of endogenous ACTH with normal production of hydrocortisone and aldosterone (13). However this is achieved at the great cost of enlargement of the adrenal glands with excessive production of androgens. We have studied the production of aldosterone and hydrocortisone in infants and children with congenital adrenal hyperplasia, using isotope dilution methods (13). Patients with the 'salt-losing' type of congenital adrenal hyperplasia (21-hydroxylation defect) had extremely low aldosterone secretion rates and during salt-deprivation no increase was observed. 'Salt-losing' and non 'salt-losing' types of congenital adrenal hyperplasia are two different genotypes (11, 25). Our findings of differences in the production of aldosterone (and hydrocortisone) suggest that both groups of patients also biochemically represent two different types of the same disorder. This could be explained by two different genetically controlled changes in the 21-hydroxylation process (13).

Genetic studies indicate a recessive autosomal heredity for the defects in the biosynthesis of adrenocortical steroids (11, 25, 29).

The diagnosis of a specific defect is greatly facilitated by studying the increased production and excretion of steroid precursors (and their metabolites), which accumulate before the enzyme block.

WILKINS and co-workers reported in 1950 that the administration of cortisone, in relatively small dosage to patients with congenital adrenal hyperplasia led to a decrease of the urinary 17-ketosteroids (33). Since then it has been demonstrated by many investigators that this effect of suppression can be maintained by doses of glucocorticoids which are not in excess of the physiologic requirements of the body and produce no abnormal metabolic effects.

Therapy with hydrocortisone does not only suppress pituitary ACTH secretion and as a result the production of adrenal androgens, but in view of the biochemical pathogenesis of congenital adrenal hyperplasia it supplies the deficient hormone, particularly under conditions of stress.

Therapy with hydrocortisone also permits normal somatic growth and osseous development. It corrects (in combination with mineralocorticoids) salt-water loss in the 'salt-losing' patients, and hypertension in the patients with 11-hydroxylation defects. Sexual development in girls and boys has been regulated with this treatment and in a number of treated female patients pregnancies have occurred. Several normal children born of these pregnancies have been described (21, 28).

GROWTH IN UNTREATED PATIENTS

Generally patients with congenital adrenal hyperplasia show clinical manifestations of increased secretion of androgens from birth on. However, on rare occasions the genitalia of the female infant may be normal and the symptoms of virilization become evident in later infancy, childhood or adolescence, and even in adulthood. Several older girls are described with normal external genitalia at birth but with signs of virilization in later life and with the biochemical findings of congenital enzyme defects (9, 12, 19, 22). A female infant with normal external genitalia, but with pubic hair and progressive virilization during early life is reported by MARIE and co-workers (22a). They described this infant as having congenital adrenal hyperplasia and suggest that excessive secretion of androgens did not occur until after the fifth month of foetal life, when development of the external genitalia is complete. It is difficult to say if these patients, with symptoms of virilization in later life and normal external genitalia at birth, have 'mild' forms of congenital adrenal hyperplasia or truly acquired forms of adrenocortical hyperplasia or adrenocortical tumours.

In the untreated female patient with congenital adrenal hyperplasia somatic growth and osseous development become far advanced for the age of the patient. By the fifth year of life, height age may be eight years and bone age ten years. Epiphyseal fusion occurs early and will lead to a dwarfed adult, who was excessively tall during childhood. It is very interesting that infants with congenital adrenal hyperplasia do not show signs of advanced osseous development at birth, although changes of the external genitalia indicate the excessive secretion of androgens during foetal life.

Usually pubic hair appears by the age of two to four years, followed shortly by axillary hair. Other symptoms of progressing virilization are acne, deepening of the voice, further enlargement of the clitoris, with frequent erections, and later on coarse masculine facial hair and even baldness. There is increased muscular development and although the untreated female patients in early childhood may look feminine, later on these patients look more masculine, particularly when at the age of puberty development of the breasts fails to occur.

In males congenital adrenal hyperplasia cannot usually be diagnosed clinically in early infancy, except when symptoms of the salt-losing syndrome occur. Embryologic organogenesis has not been disturbed by the increased secretion of androgens. However, the penis of young male infants with this disorder may be enlarged and hyperpigmentation of the scrotum may occur. After birth there is rapid somatic growth and osseous development. The penis becomes large and pubic hair appears. Patients often reach the age of two or three years before the symptoms of virilization attract attention. In boys this syndrome has been called macrogenitosomia praecox or pseudosexual precocity. It is important to recognize that the testes remain infantile in size, and this enables to distinguish the disease from true sexual precocity (the idiopathic form or due to an intracranial lesion) in which the testes are enlarged at an early age. Other symptoms of virilization in the male patient are acne, deepening of the voice and strong muscular development. Epiphyseal fusion occurs early and the patients may reach their adult height at a young age. Mostly they are then 'short

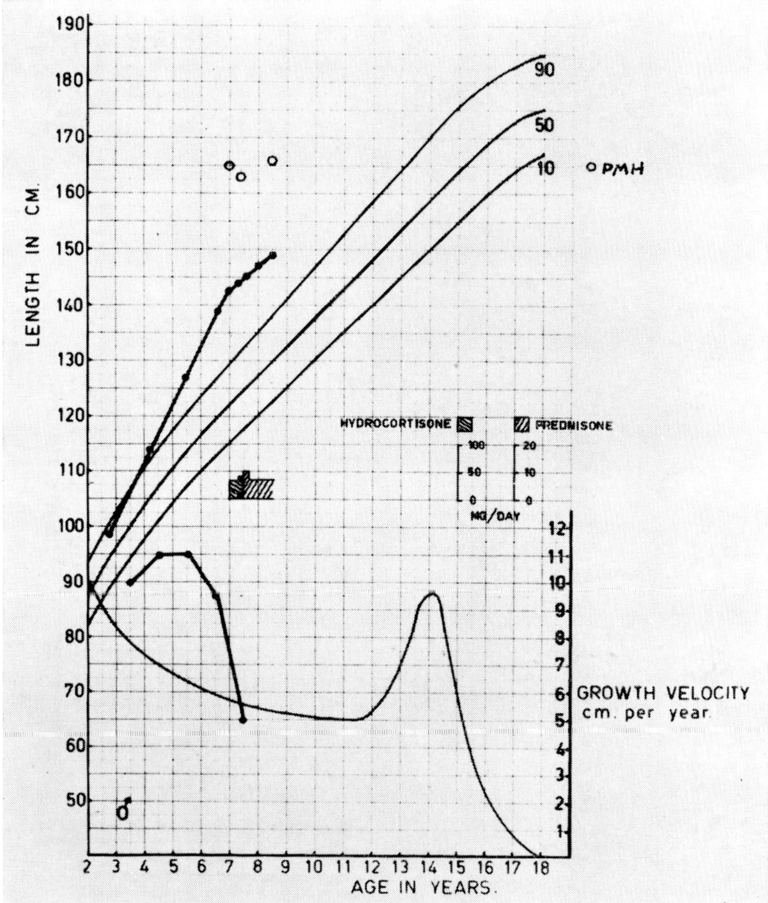

Fig. 2. Length (cm) and growth velocity (cm per year), plotted against chronological age, of a boy with congenital adrenal hyperplasia (21-hydroxylation type) before and after treatment with glucocorticoids (chron. age 7, bone age $13^{6}/_{12}$; chron. age $8^{6}/_{12}$, bone age 14). PMH = predicted mature height. See text

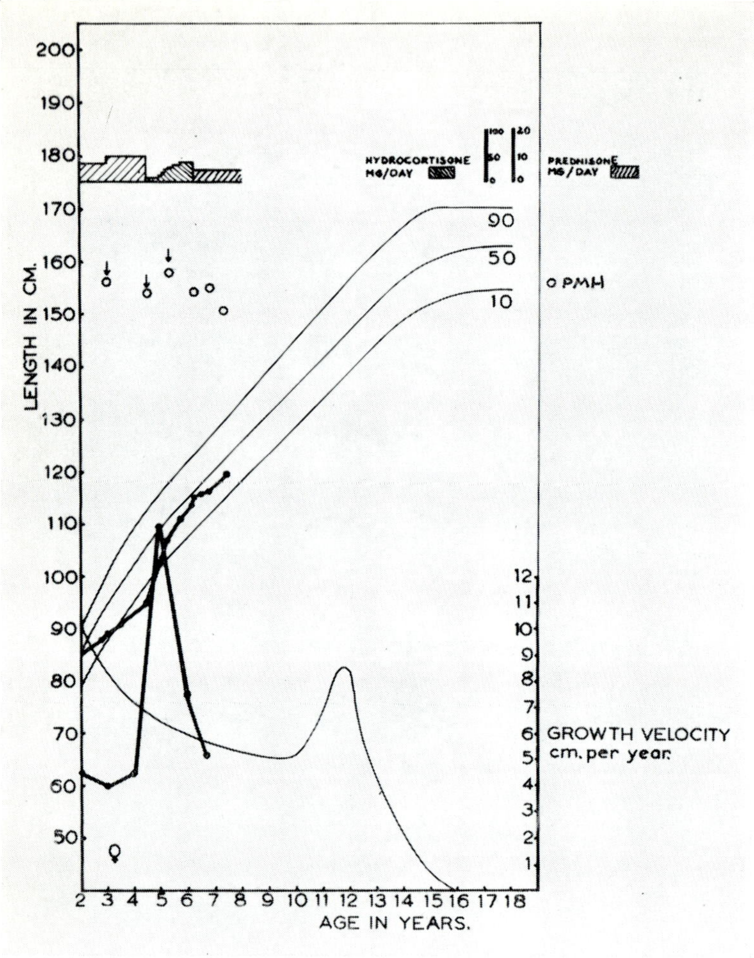

Fig. 3. Effect of overtreatment with glucocorticoids on length and growth velocity, plotted against chronological age, of a girl with congenital adrenal hyperplasia (21-hydroxylation type). PMH = predicted mature height. See text

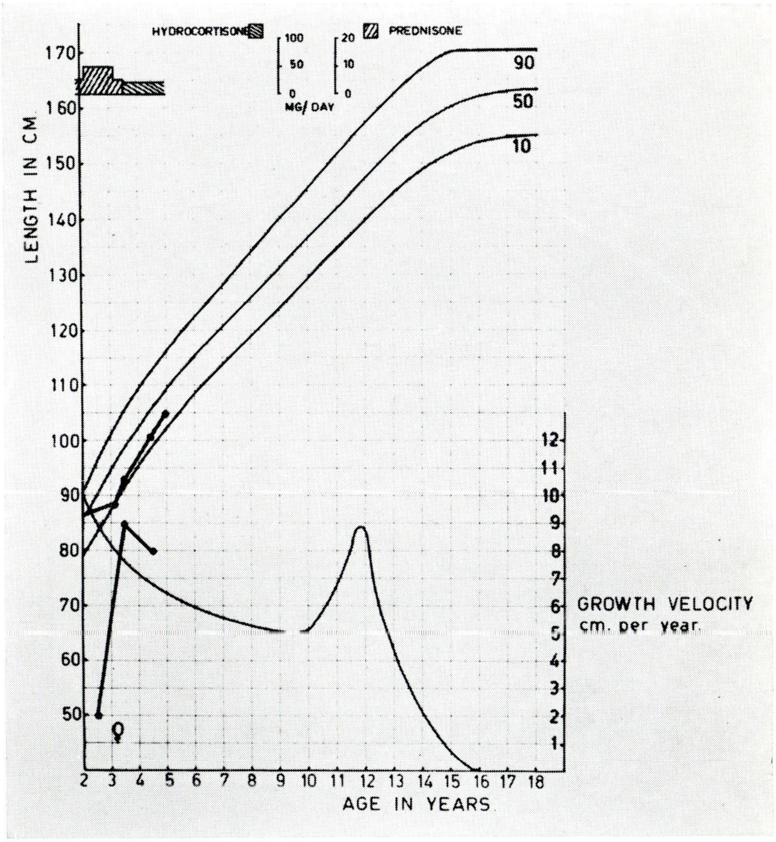

Fig. 4. Same as fig. 3. Girl with congenital adrenal hyperplasia (21-hydroxylation type). Chron. age $3^{6}/_{12}$, bone age 2; chron. age $4^{11}/_{12}$, bone age $3^{3}/_{12}$

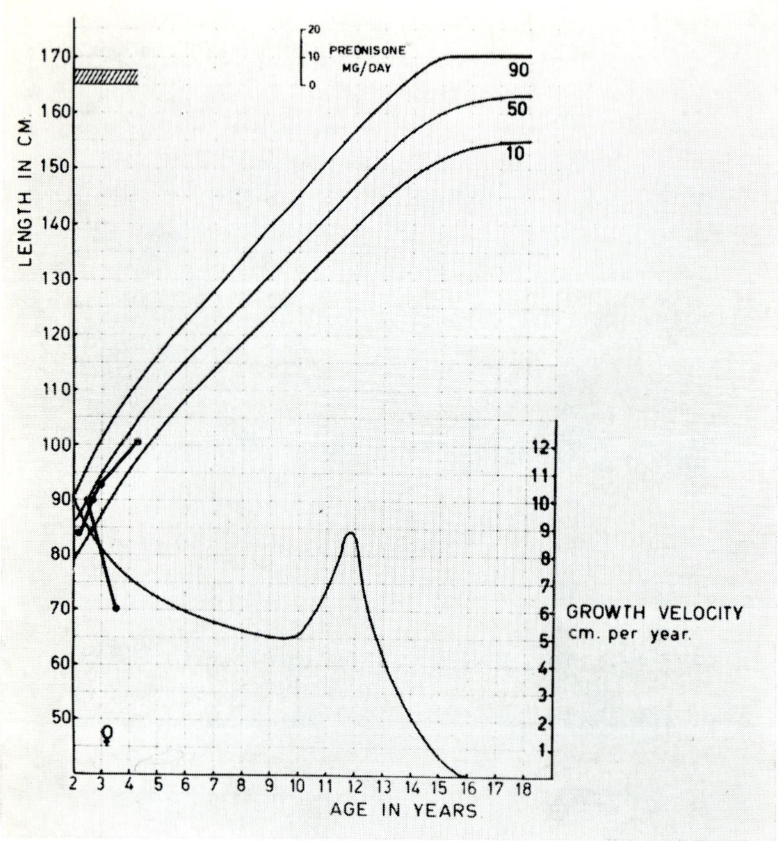

Fig. 5. Normal growth pattern of a girl with congenital adrenal hyperplasia (21-hydroxylation type, salt-losing type) during treatment with prednisone. Length and growth velocity are plotted against chronological age

adults', but this is not always the case. We recently observed two brothers, 9 and 13 years of age, with congenital adrenal hyperplasia (21-hydroxylation type). Length was 154 and 168 cm, bone age 13 and 15 years respectively. In both boys symptoms of increased growth rate and of virilization did not attract the attention before the age of 5 years.

It seems to us that ultimate height in patients with conditions of increased production of androgens depends on the 'quality' and the 'quantity' of the androgenic substances. In this regard children with congenital adrenal hyperplasia take an intermediate position between children with so-called premature adrenarche on the one hand and those with true sexual precocity on the other. This will be discussed in more detail in our paper on effects of androgens and anabolic steroids on growth rate and height (pag. 290).

GROWTH DURING TREATMENT WITH GLUCOCORTICOIDS

Congenital adrenal hyperplasia is a unique 'experiment of nature'. Studies of patients with this disorder have enriched considerably our knowledge on the metabolism of adrenocortical steroids, the psychosexual orientation and maturation in man and the effects of androgens on growth and skeletal maturation.

Since the classical studies of WILKINS and co-workers (33), it has become possible to treat patients with congenital adrenal hyperplasia in such a way that a normal pattern of growth and development can be maintained. When treatment with glucocorticoids has begun in early life and is adjusted properly, the patient will reach normal adult height.

When treatment with glucocorticoids is started greater doses of steroids are required to suppress the excessive endogenous ACTH secretion than later on. It should be emphasized however that adequate suppression can be maintained by doses of glucocorticoids which are not in excess of the physiologic requirements of the organism. Excessive amounts of glucocorticoids inhibit protein anabolism and retard growth. Patients overtreated with glucocorticoids show ultimately all aspects of Cushing's syndrome.

The drugs of choice are hydrocortisone or cortisone acetate for oral or intramuscular use. Prednisone has been used with good results

(1 mg prednisone is equivalent to 5 mg hydrocortisone) but there is no need for other synthetic glucocorticoids and indeed side reactions of some of these drugs make their use even undesirable.

Hydrocortisone secretion rates in normal young infants, when corrected for body surface, are the same as in normal older children and adults. BERTRAND et al. found a mean value of 12.4 $mg/m^2/24$ hour in normal individuals between 5 and 52 years of age, in infants they found 17.1 $mg/m^2/24$ hour (5). KENNY et al. report 11.3 ± 1.6 $mg/m^2/24$ hour in adults and 15 $mg/m^2/24$ hour in young infants (20).

Maintenance doses of hydrocortisone for patients with congenital adrenal hyperplasia vary and individualization of therapy is necessary. Useful criteria are the response of the urinary 17-ketosteroids, the long-term clinical response, particularly statural growth and skeletal maturation and the possible appearance of side effects of glucocorticosteroids. Recommended maintenance doses for hydrocortisone are 5—25 mg/day for age 0—5 years, 25—50 mg/day for 5—10 years, 50—75 mg/day for 10 years and above. Hydrocortisone when prescribed orally should be given in 3—4 doses per day and as alcoholic hydrocortisone, not as hydrocortisone acetate which is less well absorbed in the gastro-intestinal tract.

Patients with congenital adrenal hyperplasia should be periodically examined, growth rate and skeletal maturation carefully checked and urinary excretion of 17-ketosteroids regularly determined.

For an extensive discussion on the medical and other treatment of congenital adrenal hyperplasia the reader is referred elsewhere (7, 8, 31).

One aspect of medical treatment is of considerable interest in regard to the correlation of the onset of puberty with bone age rather than with chronological age. When treatment with glucocorticosteroids is started at a later age and bone age is considerably advanced, symptoms of gonadal maturation may occur in a very short time. Thus adrenal suppression permits an appropriate function of the gonads at puberty, but puberty is highly correlated with bone age. A girl of six years, with a bone age of thirteen may show development of the breasts and the beginning of menses within a few weeks after treatment has started.

The following growth charts may illustrate some of the problems of medical treatment in regard to statural growth and skeletal maturation, as just discussed. In these charts the 10, 50 and 90 percentiles for length are those for Dutch children of De Wijn and De Haas (30). The standard curves for growth velocity (cm per year) were constructed using data from the growth velocity curves of Bayer and Bayley (3) for North-American children, and of Prader, Tanner and Von Harnack (26) for West-European children. Predicted mature height (PMH) was calculated using the radiographic atlas of Greulich and Pyle (16) (for estimation of bone age) and the tables of Bayley and Pinneau (4).

Fig. 2 shows the growth curves of a boy with congenital adrenal hyperplasia (21-hydroxylation type, no salt-loss) before and after treatment. Although he was seen by several doctors and the parents were concerned about his rapid growth, the definite diagnosis of congenital adrenal hyperplasia was not made before the age of 7 years, when other symptoms of virilization were evident. At this time bone age was 13½ years. His growth velocity decreased sharply after treatment was started. His predicted adult height is calculated as 165 cm. With prednisone 7.5 mg per day in two doses (2.5 mg in the morning, 5.0 mg in the evening) growth velocity is now normal for the boy's age. It can be expected that he will reach his adult height at an age of about 13 years. Theoretically the dose of glucocorticoids in the evening should be greater than in the morning, in regard to the diurnal rhythm of the secretion of ACTH and hydrocortisone.

Fig. 3 shows the course of growth in a girl who is treated with glucocorticosteroids from the age of 1½ years on (21-hydroxylation type, no salt-loss). Between the ages of 2 and 4½ years she was treated with prednisone 7.5—10 mg per day. Her bone age in this period increased only from 2 to 3 years and her length increased from 85 to 95 cm, a growth velocity much too low for this period of age. There were other symptoms of overtreatment with glucocorticoids at the age of 4½ years: obesity, moon face and hypertension. She complained of headache and the fundi of her eyes showed papillary oedema. Treatment was stopped for some period and these symptoms of overtreatment disappeared rapidly. During this period and later, on hydrocortisone treatment 10—20 mg per day, a catch-up growth was observed with a growth velocity of more than 13 cm in a year. From the age of 6 3/12 years (bone age 6 years) she is treated with prednisone 2 × 2.5 mg per day and the growth velocity is now normal for age. It is of interest that her predicted adult height did not change markedly during the whole period of treatment and this would indicate that bone maturation and growth in length were inhibited by glucocorticoids to the same extent. However, height predictions before the age of 6 years had to be calculated using a table from Bayley (2) as the tables of Bayley and Pinneau (4) start at a bone age of 6 years, and as a result all PMH values cannot be strictly compared.

Fig. 4 illustrates the same course of events as in fig. 3 in a girl (21-hydroxylation type, no salt-loss). Between her 2nd and 3rd year of age growth velocity was not more than 2 cm, but after changing to hydrocortisone 4 × 5 mg per day a normal growth velocity for age and an equivalent increase of bone age occurred.

Fig. 5 shows the results of treatment in a girl (21-hydroxylation defect, salt-losing type), who is treated from birth on. Since her 2nd birthday (bone age 2) normal growth velocity and bone maturation are observed with prednisone 2 × 2.5 mg per day. Up to now she is treated with deoxycorticosterone acetate (DOCA) and a recent salt balance study indicated that this treatment could not be discontinued.

SUMMARY

Congenital adrenal hyperplasia is a unique 'inborn error of metabolism' to study the effects of androgens and glucocorticoids on growth and development. In the untreated child somatic growth and osseous development become far advanced for the age of the patient. When treatment with glucocorticoids is started in early life and is properly adjusted, a normal pattern of growth and development can be maintained.

REFERENCES

1. Bartter, F. C., F. Albright, A. P. Forbes, A. Leaf, E. Dempsey and E. Carroll, The effects of adrenocorticotropic hormone and cortisone in the adrenogenital syndrome associated with congenital adrenal hyperplasia: an attempt to explain and correct its disordered hormonal pattern, *J. Clin. Invest.* 30: 237, 1951.
2. Bayley, N., The accurate prediction of growth and adult height, *Mod. Probl. Paediat.*, 7, p. 234, Karger, Basel/New York, 1962.
3. Bayer, L. M. and N. Bayley, *Growth diagnosis*, The University of Chicago Press, Chicago, Ill., U.S.A., 1959.

4. BAYLEY, N. and S. R. PINNEAU, Tables for predicting adult height from skeletal age, revised for use with the Greulich-Pyle hand standards, *J. Pediat.* 40: 423, 1952.
5. BERTRAND, J., B. LORAS, R. GILLY, A. ROUX, J. M. SAEZ and A. FREDERICH, Determination de la secretion cortico-surrenale en hydrocortisone par une technique de dilution isotopique, *Arch. franç. Péd.* 20: 299, 1963.
6. BONGIOVANNI, A. M., Unusual steroid pattern in congenital adrenal hyperplasia: deficiency of 3β-hydroxy-dehydrogenase, *J. Clin. Endocrinol. and Metab.* 21: 860, 1961.
7. BONGIOVANNI, A. M. and A. W. ROOT, The adrenogenital syndrome, *New Engl. J. Med.* 268: 1283, 1342, 1391, 1963.
8. BRETON, A., B. GAUDIER, C. PONTÉ, P. SAINT-AUBERT and P. DEBRUXELLES, Indications thérapeutiques au cours des intersexualités somatiques, *Méd. Infant.* 68: 69, 1962.
9. BROOKS, R. V., D. MATTINGLY, I. H. MILLS and F. T. G. PRUNTY, Post-pubertal adrenal virilism with biochemical disturbance of congenital type of adrenal hyperplasia, *Brit. Med. J.* 1: 1294, 1960.
10. BUTLER, A. M., R. A. ROSS and N. B. TALBOT, Probable adrenal insufficiency in infant: report of case, *J. Pediat.* 15: 831, 1939.
11. CHILDS, B., M. M. GRUMBACH and J. J. VAN WYK, Virilizing adrenal hyperplasia: genetic and hormonal study, *J. Clin. Invest.* 35: 213, 1956.
12. DECOURT, J., M. F. JAYLE and E. BAULIEU, Virilism cliniquement tardif avec excrétion de prégnanetriol et insuffisance de la production de cortisol, *Ann. Endocrinol.* 18: 416, 1957.
13. DEGENHART, H. J., H. K. A. VISSER, R. WILMINK and W. CROUGHS, Aldosterone and hydrocortisone secretion rates in infants and children with congenital adrenal hyperplasia suggesting different 21-hydroxylation defects in 'salt-losers' and 'non salt-losers', *Acta Endocrinol* 48: 587, 1965.
14. DIJKHUIZEN, R. K. and E. BEHR, Adrenal hypertrophy in infants: a new clinical entity of the neonatal period, *Acta Pediat.* 27: 279, 1940.
15. EBERLEIN, W. R. and A. M. BONGIOVANNI, Plasma and urinary corticosteroids in hypertensive form of congenital adrenal hyperplasia, *J. Biol. Chem.* 223: 85, 1956.
16. GREULICH, W. W. and S. I. PYLE, *Radiographic atlas of skeletal development of the hand and urist,* Stanford Univ. Press, Calif., U.S.A., 1959.
17. IVERSEN, I., Congenital adrenocortical hyperplasia with disturbed electrolyte regulation, 'dysadrenocorticism', *Pediatrics* 16: 875, 1955.
18. JAILER, J. W., Virilism, *Bull. New York Acad. Med.* 27: 377, 1953.
19. JAYLE, M. F., S. H. WEINMAN, E. BAULIEU and Y. VALLIN, Virilisme post-pubertaire discret par deficience de l'hydroxylation en C_{21}, *Acta Endocrinol.* 29: 513, 1958.
20. KENNY, F. M., P. MALVAUX and C. J. MIGEON, Cortisol production in newborns and infants, *Pediatrics* 31: 360, 1963.
21. LARON, Z., Observations on baby born to mother with congenital adrenal hyperplasia, *Am. J. Dis. Child.* 98: 162, 1959.
22. LIPSETT, M. B. and B. D. RITER, Urinary steroids in postnatal adrenal hyperplasia with virilism, *Acta Endocrinol.* 38: 481, 1961.
22a. MARIE, J., S. KOSTICH-JOKSITCH, H. BRICARE, J. SALET, G. CSEE and B. LEVÈQUE Hyperplasie congénitale des surrénales ne compartant pas de sinus urogénital et s'accompagnant de développement prémature des seins, *Sem. d' hôp. de Paris* 33: 1594, 1957.

23. Prader, A. and H. P. Gurtner, Das Syndrom des Pseudohermaphroditismus masculinus bei kongenitaler Nebennierenrinden — Hyperplasie ohne Androgenüberproduktion (Adrenaler Pseudohermaphroditismus masculinus), *Helv. Paediat. Acta* 10: 397, 1955.
24. Prader, A. and R. E. Siebenmann, Nebenniereninsuffizienz bei kongenitaler Lipoidhyperplasie der Nebennieren, *Helv. Paediat. Acta* 12: 569, 1957.
25. Prader, A., G. J. P. A. Anders and H. Habich, Zur Genetik des kongenitalen adrenogenitalen Syndroms (virilisierende Nebennierenrindenhyperplasie), *Helv. Paediat. Acta* 17: 271, 1962.
26. Prader, A., J. M. Tanner and G. A. von Harnack, Catch-up growth following illness on starvation, *J. Pediat.* 62: 646, 1963.
27. Shepard, T. H. and S. W. Clausen, Case of adrenogenital syndrome with hypertension treated with cortisone, *Pediatrics* 8: 805, 1951.
28. Swyer, G. I. and D. G. Bonham, Successful pregnancy in female pseudohermaphrodite, *Brit. Med. J.* 1: 1005, 1961.
29. Visser, H. K. A. and W. S. Cost, A new hereditary defect in the biosynthesis of aldosterone: urinary C_{21}-corticosteroid pattern in three related patients with a salt-losing syndrome, suggesting an 18-oxidation defect, *Acta Endocrinol.* 47: 589, 1964.
30. De Wijn, J. F. and J. H. de Haas, *Groeidiagrammen van 1—25 jarigen in Nederland*, Nederlands Instituut voor Praeventieve Geneeskunde, Leiden, The Netherlands, 1960.
31. Wilkins, L., *The diagnosis and treatment of endocrine disorders in childhood and adolescence*, C. Thomas Publ., Springfield, Ill., U.S.A., 1957.
32. Wilkins, L., W. Fleischmann and J. E. Howard, Macrogenitosomia praecox associated with hyperplasia of androgenic tissue of adrenal and death from cortico-adrenal insufficiency: case report, *Endocrinology* 26: 385, 1940.
33. Wilkins, L., R. A. Lewis, R. Klein and E. Rosemberg, The suppression of androgen secretion by cortisone in a case of congenital adrenal hyperplasia, *Bull. John Hopkins Hosp.* 86: 249, 1950.

DISCUSSION

Laron: It has been stated in the literature that children who develop diabetes are tall for their age. On the other hand, it is known that amongst children with diabetes there is a group which is short. I think one should not make general statements. We have reviewed

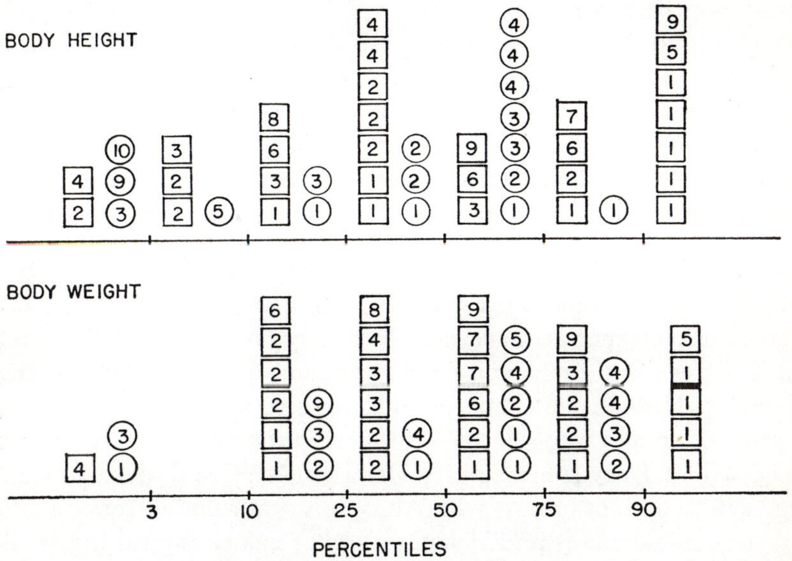

Fig. 1. Distribution of height and weight in diabetic children. The figures denote the duration of the disease in years

□ = boys ○ = girls

42 children with diabetes mellitus (fig. 1 shows their distribution among the percentiles for height and weight). It is noteworthy that among the very tall children (over the 90th percentile) there are 5 children who have had the disease for only one year, while there are

more children with long-standing disease in the lower percentiles. It is also clear that diabetic children have a tendency to be overweight. I should also like to point out another problem. In fig. 2 there are a 5-year-old boy with diabetes mellitus and marked growth retardation, and a normal boy of the same age. The short boy has all the characteristics of the syndrome of Mauriac, which are diabetes mellitus, growth retardation, hepatomegaly, cataract and petit mal. Now, at the age of 10 years, there is definite retrogression of his intellect.

Schwarz: Dr. PRADER, you have a case of Turner's syndrome in whom treatment with anabolic steroids had no effect. I should like to know whether this is your general experience. I don't think one can improve ultimate height, but in our experience the growth of these girls can be accelerated with anabolic steroids, without causing an excessive advance in bone age.

My second question is concerned with the syndrome of delayed adolescense in boys, who mature normally but late. In such patients we have used a short course of human chorionic gonadotrophin, which often seemed to trigger the onset of puberty and the pubertal spurt in height growth, thus solving psychological problems of the boys. Does Dr. PRADER have experience with this method.

Prader: In Turner's syndrome we get less effect of anabolic steroids on growth than in other short patients, using the same dose. As far as delayed adolescence is concerned, in theory no treatment is necessary, but I agree that for psychological reasons treatment is sometimes indicated. Human chorionic gonadotrophin, and sex steroids, seem to push bone age into the region where puberty will start spontaneously. Might I say something to Dr. TIDDENS? He discussed (see fig., page 220) a patient of ours with Albright's syndrome of renal acidosis, with nephrocalcinosis and rickets, who has many interesting aspects. He could not concentrate urine at all. Nevertheless, by correcting his acidosis we pushed his height above the 50th percentile. This finding proves that the inability to concentrate urine had nothing to do whatsoever with his being short, which was solely due to the acidosis.

Tiddens: I think that the concentrating ability will affect growth only if it is so severe as to cause diminished caloric intake or hypo-osmolarity. The latter point still has to be proven.

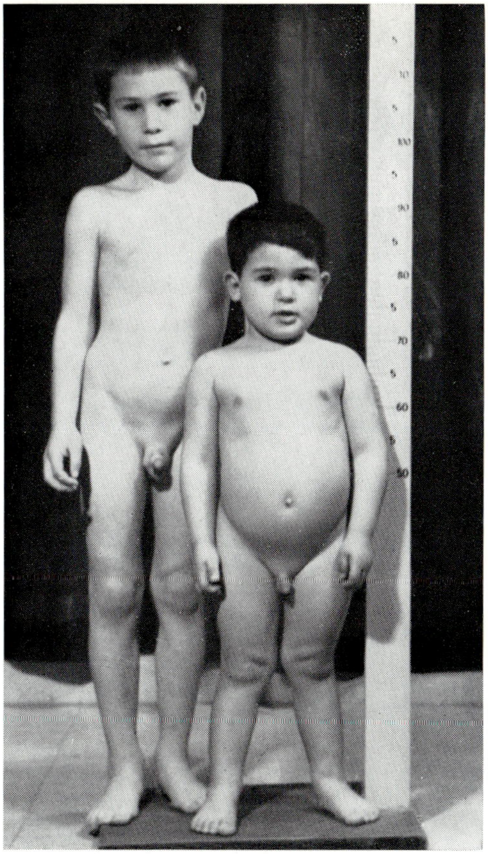

Fig. 2. The height of a five-year-old boy with Mauriac syndrome compared to a healthy boy of his age

Sobel: This growth chart (fig. 3) illustrates the findings in a patient with renal tubular acidosis and nephrocalcinosis. One can see that he was obese with retarded growth and retarded skeletal maturation. After alkali therapy was instituted there was an acceleration of growth

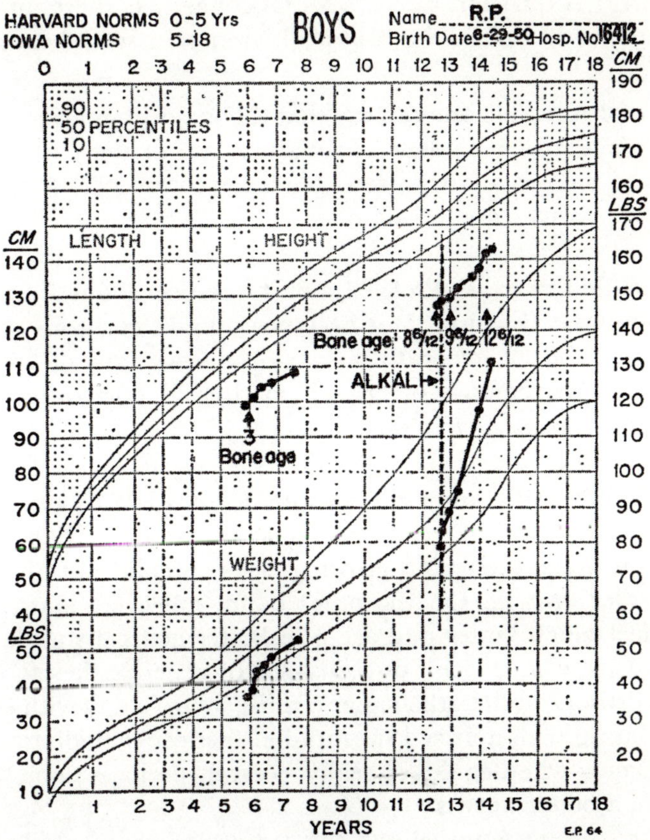

Fig. 3. Growth chart of a boy with renal acidosis. He was short and obese at 6 years of age. Progress in rate of growth and skeletal maturation was poor. The effect of therapy with alkali, began at 12 11/12, is evident in increased growth rate and advance in skeletal maturation. Reprinted with permission from Sobel, E.H., School age growth problems, in: *Biological basis of pediatric practice*, R. E. Cooke, ed., Mc Graw-Hill Book Co., In press

rate and a very marked acceleration of skeletal maturation. The boy is now in early adolescence. It seems probable that his catch-up will be so much greater in bone age than in rate of growth that he will be small as an adult. I would like to acknowledge the collaboration of Dr. CHESTER M. EDELMAN, Jr., who performed the detailed studies of renal function and acidification capacity in this child.

Van den Berg: A question to Dr. VAN GELDEREN. Is there, in different groups of mental defectives, also a difference in sexual maturation?

Van Gelderen: As a rule one can say that the majority mature normally, but there is a strong tendency to mature late in the early pre-natal groups, and there is a fairly strong tendency to precocious maturation in the groups with cerebral damage.

Otten: I would like to ask Prof. PRADER a question about the treatment of hypopituitary dwarfism. Is it necessary to give cortisone, because I think those children generally have no clinical signs of adrenal insufficiency. The response of growth to thyroid hormones might be greater if no cortisone were added.

Prader: I don't really know the answer. I don't like to give cortisone because I know they are very sensitive to cortisone. Perhaps even low doses might make them stop growing, so we should not give it if we only consider growth. On the other hand, however, many of these patients feel much better and are in a better general state of health, if they are given a little bit of cortisone. In general, therefore, we do not give cortisone at first, then after a while we try a day with cortisone, and we end up with a mixed substitution therapy including cortisone. I do not know whether this is really correct, perhaps somebody else could give a better answer.

They are insulin sensitive and this is to some extent, but not completely, corrected by giving cortisone. I feel that the lack of growth hormone is more important for insulin sensitivity than cortisone.

Sobel: In the past I was concerned that giving thyroid therapy to children with hypopituitarism might accentuate hypoglycaemia and make it necessary to give them cortisone as well despite the possibility that, even in small doses, cortisone may stop their growth entirely. Perhaps we can feel more relaxed about these problems if we are able to give somatotrophin in addition to thyroid hormone. Under these circumstances the patient may not have hypoglycaemia and it may not be necessary to give cortisone. Do you agree?

Prader: Yes, I agree with that, but I do not know the definite answer.

Wafelbakker: Dr. PRADER, I have one question asked in three different ways.

One: what is the incidence of the pathological conditions we talked about this afternoon.

Second: how big is your patient material and how large is the population which drains into your clinic.

Third: when I am a medical school officer and I see five thousand pupils per year, how often in my life can I see a Turner's syndrome, a hypopituitary dwarf etc.

Prader: I do not know the exact answer. There are 5 large paediatric departments in our country, of which the population is 5 million, so we draw on at least 1 million. It may be a little bit more. I could have brought, but did not do it because it does not mean much, the numbers of Turners or hypopituitary dwarfs. I could certainly not give a figure on delayed adolescence, because the age limits are arbitrary. Turner's syndrome, I think, will be seen in 1 of 10.000 newborns, as indicated by chromosome or buccal smear studies. And I would say that hypopituitary dwarfism has about the same incidence.

Steendijk: I am sure that there are many cases of vitamin D-resistant rickets which have not been recognized as such and which have been booked as 'intractable rickets'. I want to stress the importance of an early diagnosis, before they are 1½—2 years old, as proper treatment started at that age will often prevent the severe deformities which occur when treatment is begun at a later age. The incidence of the disease, I think, is somewhere between 1 : 10.000 and 1 : 15.000 in our country.

Prader: From table 1, from the book by WILKINS (*The Diagnosis and Treatment of Endocrine Disorders in Childhood and Adolescence*, 2nd ed., Oxford, 1957), you can see that the largest number are constitutional dwarfs, that means that they have no precise metabolic defect, no mental deficiency and no endocrine defect. Among the endocrine disturbances hypothyroidism is certainly the most frequent cause of short stature, Turner's syndrome a little less frequent and hypopituitary dwarfism perhaps even less frequent.

The relation between the various groups corresponds with what we see. We can confirm Dr. STEENDIJK's statement, because we see resistant rickets about as often as phenylketonuria. And this is very well known to be 1 in 10.000.

It was formerly believed to be 1 in 20.000, but it is a little bit more frequent. So the same frequency would be true for resistant rickets.

Table 1. *Types and incidence of stunted growth.*

		cases	%
Constitutional retarded growth and adolescent development		130	29.4
Slow growth and retarded bone age (too young for diagnosis)?		67	15.2
Primordial dwarfism	91	114	25.8
Primordial dwarfism with craniofacial anomalies ('progeroid')	23		
Hypothyroidism (dwarfism conspicuous)		53	12.0
'Syndrome of gonadal aplasia'		48	10.9
Hypopituitary or hypothalamic			
pituitary deficiency	19	30	6.7
tumours	11		
Total		442	100.0

Olthof: Several speakers have told us of the great influence of the thyroid on bone maturity. Is there any connection between the thyroid and the congenital adrenogenital syndrome?

Visser: As far as I know thyroid function in cases of congenital adrenal hyperplasia is completely normal. The acceleration of bone maturation is a pure androgen effect, and the androgens are produced by the adrenal gland.

Prader: I should like to make two points concerning Dr. VISSER's lecture. I would not agree with Dr. VISSER that the adrenogenital syndrome is so rare. We have made quite an extensive study in Switzerland, and according to our results the incidence is 1 in 5000 newborns, which makes it more frequent than for instance Turner's syndrome. The second point I wanted to make is how to control growth with this treatment. Most of us who treat these children give dosages as you have recommended but this, of course, is only the general idea of how much we should give. What we should like to do is to keep these children along their normal growth line. This is not so easy, because we do not know their genetically determined growth potential. Which channel should they follow? For many years we have made a mistake, which may please Dr. MARSHALL because we made exactly the mistake that he warned us against when he said that the height age is a bad maturity index. We tried to keep these children along the 50th percentile curve. We were sometimes successful, sometimes not. If they were below the 50th percentile, we said that we gave too much cortisone and that we inhibited growth with an overdosage, so we gave less cortisone and then bone age went off in the upper direction. We have gradually learnt that we should keep the bone age of these children along the normal line. This certainly is a better idea than the height age. And after some more experience we looked a little bit more carefully at the parents, and then we realized that some of these children have to be short. They have to move along a lower percentile, but with proper treatment their bone age now moves along the average. I think that that is the best we can do for following growth, and I think it is an important point.

Visser: I think it is very interesting that babies with congenital adrenal hyperplasia have a normal length at birth and bone age is usually also not advanced at birth. That is surprising, because the adrenal androgenic steroids are clearly effective in other ways. So we start in those babies with normal bone age, and I think with a normal length for their genetic background. And if length is at the 50th percentile at birth, this I think is their growth channel.

Laron: I think we should not disregard the influence of the androgens in the adrenogenital syndrome on the thyroid. We know that androgens decrease the circulating thyroxine binding protein and thus lower the serum PBI. I don't think we have sufficient data on this protein in the adrenogenital syndrome.

I should like to ask Dr. VISSER if he would consider the normal bone age of the newborn with the adrenogenital syndrome to be due to the increased cortisol levels during the last trimester of pregnancy; cortisol antagonizing the androgenic effect on bone.

Visser: I don't know. It is an interesting speculation of course.

Prader: Dr. SOBEL, you have studied the problem of how fast bone age will respond to androgen influence. Could it be that these babies at birth have a normal bone age, because they have not yet had the time to respond to the high androgen level with an acceleration of bone age?

Sobel: I used to think that I could answer that question, that the time-lag before the effect of androgen on skeletal maturation could become evident was the explanation for normal skeletal maturation at the time of birth in infants with congenital adrenal hyperplasia. The more recent work of BONGIOVANNI and his co-workers, on the supposedly non-androgenic progestational agents given in pregnancy, has demonstrated that bone-age can be advanced in utero (BREIBART, S., A. M. BONGIOVANNI, W. R. EBERLEIN, *New Engl. J. Med.* 268: 255, 1963).

Of course, the time phenomenon is still to be considered. When these compounds are given to women whose pregnancy is considered in jeopardy, they are probably given very much earlier in pregnancy than we might expect the androgen of foetuses with congenital adrenal hyperplasia to be produced. However, I am not sure that this interpretation is correct.

Visser: There is a very interesting hypothesis, advanced by DORFMAN in the U.S.A., that there may be steroids with anti-androgenic activity, possibly the 16-hydroxylated steroids. And there is some evidence from studies in several laboratories, that 16-hydroxylated steroids are produced in increased amounts in congenital adrenal hyperplasia. This may explain the difference with androgens given to the mother, when the 16-hydroxylated steroids may not be increased during pregnancy.

Sobel: There is still some difficulty with this explanation; how could we account for the virilization of female foetuses with congenital adrenal hyperplasia if a potent anti-androgenic compound is being produced?

CHAPTER IX

GROWTH PROMOTING AGENTS

WHAT CONSTITUTES A GROWTH PROMOTING AGENT

J. J. VAN DER WERFF TEN BOSCH

The child who is undersized in comparison with its age peers poses serious problems. The doctor faced with such a child tends to seize upon any drug that appears to hold good promises. Such promises are often explicitly given or implicitly indicated in pamphlets from pharmaceutical firms. It seems appropriate to enquire into the nature of the evidence that has been put forward to support the claims of growth promoting activity.

In the early 1930's it was found that the rate of linear growth could be raised by the administration of chorionic gonadotrophin (which stimulates secretion of testosterone by the Leydig cells of the testis) to boys with cryptorchidism or of short stature (see e.g. 11, 7, 8). It was soon discovered that testosterone preparations yielded similar results (13, 7), while recent investigations have shown that oestrogens can also stimulate growth, e.g. of tall healthy girls (18) and of stunted girls with gonadal dysgenesis (6).

It is now universally agreed that administration of a preparation of testosterone will cause an increase in the growth rate of almost any child with open epiphyses. There are two pressing reasons, however, for limiting the use of testosterone preparations as growth promoting agents. It is believed that *the minimal dose of a testosterone preparation that significantly raises the rate of linear growth* will: (1) unduly increase the rate of skeletal maturation (as happens also during normal puberty), so that an immediate gain in centimeters of stature is off-set by a postponed loss in years of potential growth, and (2) cause signs of precocious puberty (pubic and axillary hair) and of masculinization (acne, deepening of voice (4), enlargement of clitoris, male body contours through loss of subcutaneous fat and increased muscularity). It is exceedingly difficult either to substantiate or to refute these two points.

SKELETAL MATURATION (LATE EFFECT: INCREASED OR DECREASED ADULT HEIGHT?)

Quantitative assessment of an effect is easier for skeletal maturation than for 'androgenic' manifestations. Even so, some of the best studies concerning the effects of methyltestosterone have given rise to the conclusions that testosterone 'may not be a suitable agent for the promotion of growth' (17) and that it 'caused no disproportionate skeletal maturation' (3). It so happens that while androgens have been widely used in attempts to stimulate the growth rate or adult height, oestrogens have been applied in the hope of obtaining the opposite effect, a reduced rate of growth or adult stature in tall children. The conclusions from some of the best studies carried out so far, were that oestrogens 'stimulated skeletal maturation more than linear growth' (18) and that they 'stimulated linear growth and skeletal maturation proportionately' (2). There seems to be a striking resemblance between the effects of methyltestosterone and oestrogens upon growth. Both stimulate linear growth and skeletal maturation; attempts at dissociating the two effects, by careful manipulation of the dose and duration of treatment, have not yet been successful. The advent of synthetic steroids raised the hope that compounds with an inherent dissociation of these effects might be discovered. Such a find does not seem to be available yet, in spite of many a high-sounding claim. For the sake of illustration the findings of three sets of investigators who studied fluoxymesterone may be compared. By present standards all three investigations were reasonably well planned and executed. All three studies clearly showed that the drug stimulated the growth rate. One report acclaimed the drug an androgen which did not accelerate epiphyseal fusion (15), another showed the drug to be no better than methyltestosterone (12), while the third study yielded intermediate results (10).

ANDROGENICITY

In the search for steroids which might prove to be 'better' than testosterone, their androgenic potency has been a major concern. Yet no systematic studies seem to have been made to assess clinical androgenic potency. There is no information, for the growth promoting steroids now available, from which ratios can be estimated between androgenic and growth promoting potency. A dissociation between the two effects 'has not yet been proved in children. It could only be investigated by comparing a large group of children treated with testosterone to a large group of children treated with the newer anabolic steroids' (14).

THE NATURE OF ANABOLIC STEROIDS

The ill luck of pharmaceutical firms, their failure to find synthetic steroids superior to testosterone, may be the outcome of some flaws in the methods by which they hope to detect the desired steroid. The experimental model used for the primary screening of a possible effect of a new compound, is the rat. The standard reference is testosterone. Table 1 lists some of the effects of testosterone (see also page 160) in the child and in the male rat. For the growth promoting steroid that one hopes to find A is essential, whilst B and D are undesirable. The question is how such a steroid is to be found.

Table 1. *Some effects obtained after the administration of testosterone to children and to intact immature male rats.*

The child

A. Stimulation of growth in height (= skeleton)
B. Stimulation of skeletal maturation
C. Stimulation of nitrogen retention, fat loss, etc.
D. Clinical masculinization (hair, voice, acne, clitoris)

The rat

W. Diminished or unchanged growth in length (= skeleton)
X. Stimulation of nitrogen retention
Y. Stimulation of growth of levator ani muscle
Z. Stimulation of growth of ventral prostate and seminal vesicle

The present approach is to equate A and Y. Any drug that does not possess activity Y is discarded, because it is considered that if a drug does not stimulate growth of the levator ani muscle, it will not stimulate growth of the human skeleton. Note that testosterone does not stimulate the growth of the rat skeleton! The levator ani muscle is an exceptional muscle, in that (in common with the other perineal muscles) it responds to testosterone; its size is dependent on the presence of testosterone (9) and is in no other way correlated with the size (weight or length) of the animal. Current usage of the term sex characteristic justifies its application to the levator ani muscle. Or,

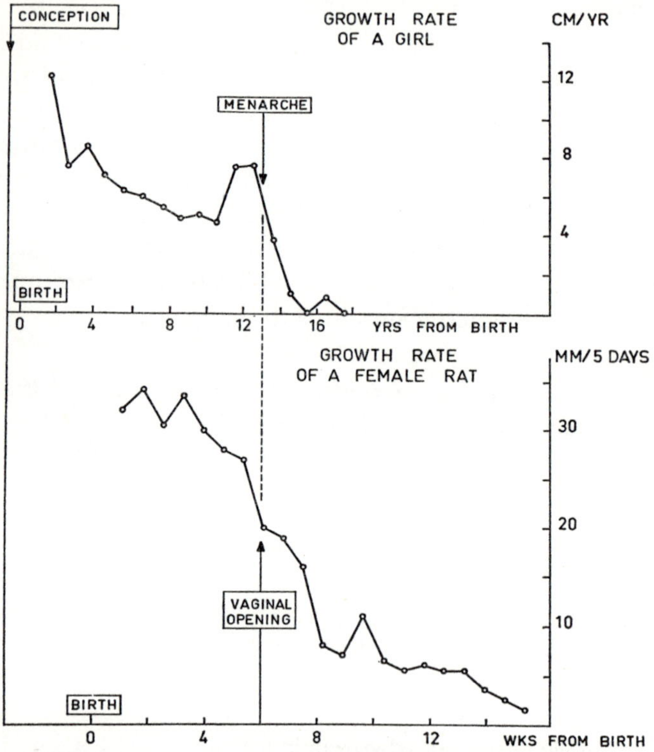

Fig. 1. To illustrate the difference in the pattern of linear growth between a girl (body height) and a female rat (length from the nose to the tip of the tail). Note the two peaks in growth velocity, around birth and during puberty, which occur in the girl. In the rat there is no evidence for an effect of puberty (vaginal opening occurs at about the time of the first ovulation) on the growth rate. The delayed peak for the rat, at 9 weeks, occurs after puberty. Age scales are arranged so that the times of conception and the times of menarche and vaginal opening are superimposed. Data from 1 (for girl) and 5 (for rat)

as Russell and Wilhelmi (16) put it: '........ in the rat, levator ani is unique even among the perineal muscles in the profound degree of atrophy which occurs after castration and in its sensitivity to androgen. On this basis, it could be classed as a component of the sexual apparatus'. The growth promoting effect of a drug upon the levator ani muscle may be denoted an androgenic effect.

The present screening methods tend to equate D and Z, although it has never been shown that the potency of drugs in terms of their effect upon the ventral prostate and the seminal vesicle of the rat is correlated with their potency on clinical criteria of masculinization.

The industrial development of a new steroid in this field depends almost entirely upon the ratio $\frac{Y}{Z}$ that is found in the primary laboratory screening test, because it is believed that this ratio will in some way be reflected in the ratio $\frac{A}{D}$. In view of the above considerations this belief seems ill-founded. It seems most likely that the purpose, the search for a non-androgenic growth promoting steroid, is defeated by the use of an androgenic parameter (levator ani muscle weight) for the detection of growth promoting potency. If there were a steroid similar to human growth hormone in its biological actions, this could never be discovered with the current tests for screening; such a steroid would be designated as non-anabolic, be discarded and left unexplored. There is a strong need for a laboratory test suitable to reveal growth promoting potency. It seems possible, but has by no means been proven, that nitrogen retaining potency is correlated with growth promoting potency, and that the screening procedure might include the study of nitrogen excretion. However, a parameter of linear growth stimulation requires the study of linear growth. In view of the great difference in growth pattern in comparison with the human (fig. 1), the rat must be considered as an unsuitable test animal for linear growth. The monkey might prove to be a rewarding subject for the testing of effects on linear growth.

REFERENCES

1. BAYER, L. M. and N. BAYLEY, *Growth Diagnosis*, 1959, Chicago.
2. BAYLEY, N., G. S. GORDAN, L. M. BAYER, M. B. GOLDBERG and A. STORMENT, Attempt to suppress excessive growth in girls by estrogen treatment: statistical evaluation, *J. clin. Endocr.* 22: 1127, 1962.
3. BAYLEY, N., G. S. GORDAN and H. LISSER, Long-term experiences with methyltestosterone as a growth stimulant in short immature boys, *Pediatr. Clin. N. Amer.* p. 819, 1957.

4. Damsté, P. H., Stem-virilisatie door het gebruik van anabole steroiden, *Ned. T. Geneesk.* 107: 891, 1963.
5. Enthoven, R., H. E. Swanson and J. J. van der Werff ten Bosch, in preparation.
6. Enthoven, R. and J. J. van der Werff ten Bosch, Lengte, skelet en gonadotrofinen bij chromatine-negatieve gonadale dysgenesie, *Maandschr. Kindergeneesk.* 32: 466, 1964.
7. Finkler, R. S., N. J. Furst and G. M. Cohn, Present status of the use of male sex hormones and chorionic gonadotropins as growth stimulating factors, *J. clin. Endocr.* 2: 603, 1942.
8. Gordon, M. B. and E. M. Fields, Effect of chorionic gonadotropic hormone and of male sex hormone on height increase and bone development, *J. clin. Endocr.* 2: 715, 1942.
9. Kochakian, Ch. D., Mechanisms of androgen actions, *Lab. Investigations* 8: 538, 1959.
10. Laron, Z., Use of fluoxymesterone in the treatment of growth retardation, *Acta paediat.* 52: 465, 1963.
11. Lurie, L. A. and J. Hertzman, Linear growth and epiphyseal closure, *J. clin. Endocr.* 1: 717, 1941.
12. Mellman, W. J., A. M. Bongiovanni, M. Garrison and D. D. Steiker, Comparison of fluoxymesterone and methyltestosterone as growth stimulants, *Pediatrics* 28: 525, 1961.
13. Moricard, P. and P. R. Bize, Premières observations de développement du pénis provoqué chez l'enfant par l'injection d'acétate et de propionate de testostérone, *Bull. Soc. de pédiat. Paris* 35: 26, 1937.
14. Prader, A., *Acta endocr.* (*Kbh.*) suppl. 63: 106, 1962.
15. Reilly, W. A. and G. S. Gordan, Dissociation of growth-stimulating and skeleton-maturing actions of the synthetic androgen, fluoxymesterone, *J. Pediat.* 59: 188, 1961.
16. Russell, J. A. and A. E. Wilhelmi, Growth (hormonal regulation) *Ann. Rev. Physiol.* 20: 43, 1958.
17. Sobel, E. H., C. S. Raymond, K. V. Quinn and N. B. Talbot, The use of methyltestosterone to stimulate growth: relative influence on skeletal maturation and linear growth, *J. clin. Endocr.* 16: 241, 1956.
18. Whitelaw, M. J., T. N. Foster and W. H. Graham, Estradiol valerate: its effects on anabolism and skeletal age in the prepubertal girl, *J. clin. Endocr.* 23: 1125, 1963.

EFFECTS OF HUMAN GROWTH HORMONE AND TESTOSTERONE ON PROTEIN METABOLISM IN MAN

A. HAAK

Administration of growth hormone to the rat causes accumulation of water and protein, and loss of fat (4, 6, 7, 15, 20).

Similar effects can be observed in humans upon the administration

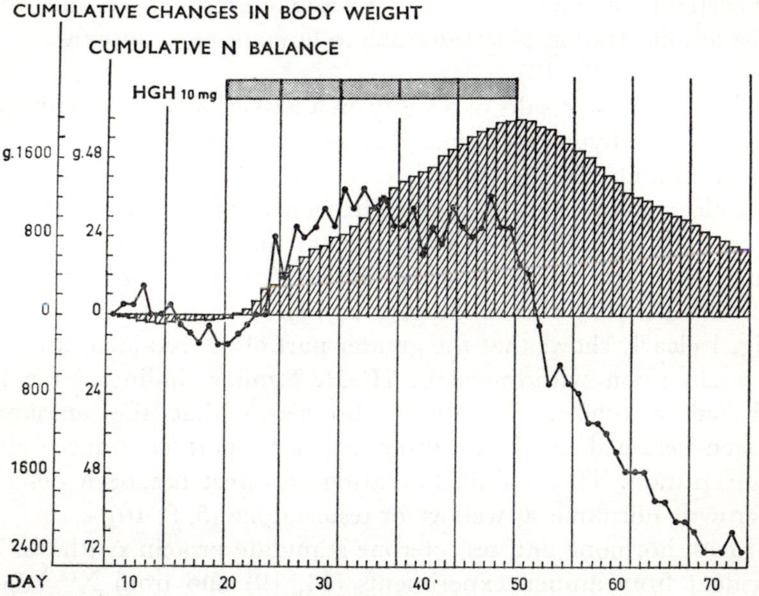

Fig. 1. Effect of human growth hormone on the cumulative nitrogen balance and on the cumulative changes in bodyweight, in a male patient suffering from panhypopituitarism

of human growth hormone (HGH). A metabolic study of a 53-year-old male with panhypopituitarism may serve to illustrate the effects of HGH. The growth hormone administered was prepared by the Raben-method and kindly supplied by N.V. Organon (Netherlands).

Fig. 1 contains curves showing the cumulative nitrogen balance and the cumulative changes in body weight. The scales are matched so, that changes in weight would result in identical changes in nitrogen balance, if the latter changes were due exclusively to losses or gains in muscle protoplasm. The first effect of HGH is a gain in weight surpassing the change in nitrogen retention, so that it would seem that water is retained in excess of the amount needed for tissue growth. An opposite effect may be seen when HGH-administration is stopped: at first there is excess weight loss, presumably due to excessive loss of water. During HGH-administration about 60 g nitrogen was retained, most of which was excreted again subsequently. At the end of the study the body had gained about 20 g nitrogen, although it had lost 2400 g in total weight. The composition of the body had obviously changed, almost certainly by the loss of fat during and after HGH-administration.

The administration of testosterone to humans also causes accumulation of protein (12, 13).

Fig. 2 shows the results of a study on a 34-year-old male with hypogonadotropic hypogonadism. Testosterone propionate in daily doses of 25 and 12.5 mg caused retention of nitrogen and potassium, and a clear rise in body weight. Nitrogen retention averaged 68 mg per kg body weight per day. A normal male, treated in the same manner, retained nitrogen at the rate of 27 mg per kg body weight, which confirmed earlier findings (12, 13).

Fig. 1 clearly shows that the greater part of the retained nitrogen is lost again upon withdrawal of HGH. Similar findings have been published by others. This study also shows that the amount of nitrogen retained tends to grow smaller upon continued HGH-administration. This so-called wearing-off effect has been described for growth hormone as well as for testosterone (5, 8, 10).

Growth hormone and testosterone stimulate protein synthesis. This is evident from animal experiments (14, 19) and from N^{15} labelled glycine studies in man (8, 9). The latter studies have also shown that the two hormones produce an increase of the amino acid pool which remained unchanged when nitrogen retention decreased. The results along with data obtained on acromegalics, suggest that continued stimulation by nitrogen-retaining hormones leads to a state of equilibrium between protein synthesis and protein catabolism. However, the daily amounts of protein synthesized and broken down are now greater than before treatment.

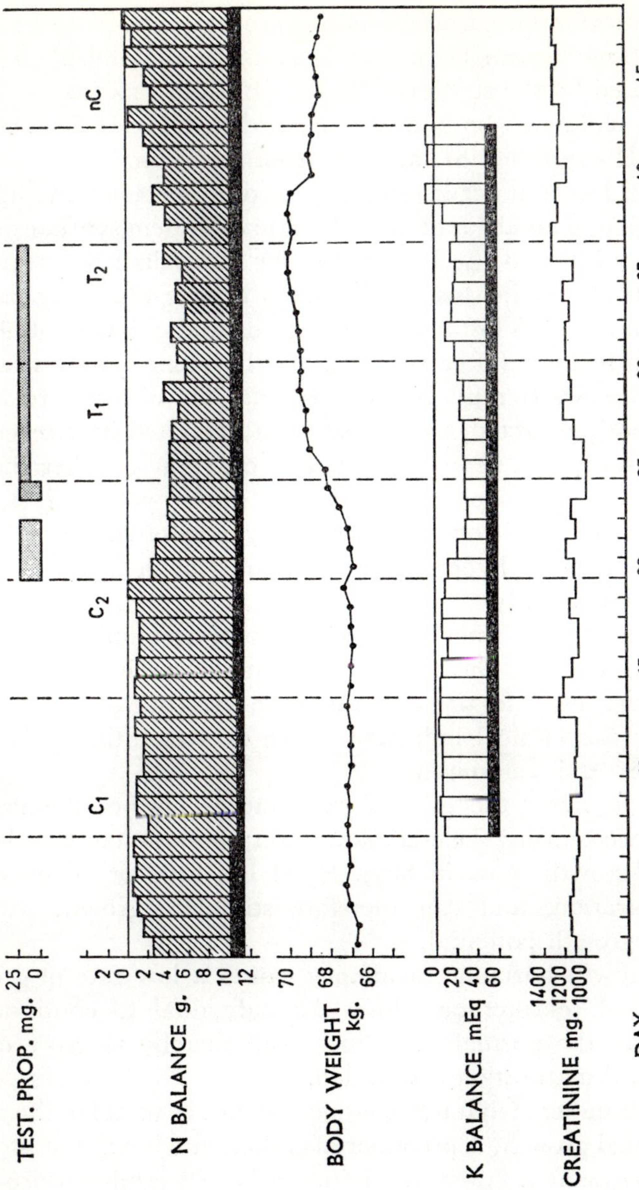

Fig. 2. Effect of testosterone propionate on the nitrogen and potassium balance, body weight and excretion of creatinine in the urine of a male patient suffering from hypogonadotropic hypogonadism

It seems possible that the equilibrium is reached much later when the opportunities for protein accumulation are higher, as in the growing child, when growth hormone induces irreversible anatomical changes. This is indicated by the studies of RABEN (18) and PRADER (16) who found that in children who had been treated with HGH for a couple of years, HGH continued to cause nitrogen retention.

The protein loss that occurs after a period of hormone administration may be due to an abrupt fall in the rate of protein synthesis while catabolism continues at the higher rate for some time before a new equilibrium is attained. Most investigators believe that only part of the retained nitrogen is lost subsequently, but studies have not always been sufficiently long (after stopping the hormone administration) to justify this view. It must be assumed that the nitrogen retained, and subsequently excreted, must have been deposited in a reversible condition, possibly as a depot protein. The question whether the organism possesses such depots has not been settled yet (1, 2, 3, 11). It seems possible that nitrogen utilised for hypertrophy may be labile, while nitrogen used for hyperplasia (as during growth of a child) may be retained permanently.

Growth in stature is associated with protein accumulation.

It is understandable, therefore, that hormones such as HGH and testosterone are used to try and raise the growth rate in stunted children. For this clinical indication there exist essential differences between HGH and testosterone.

1. Testosterone raises the growth rate but diminishes the growth potential by accelerating skeletal maturation; this also happens during the pubertal growth spurt in boys. HGH has little or no effect on skeletal maturation, and can therefore stimulate growth without affecting the growth potential.

2. Lack of growth hormone in infancy causes a low rate of growth whereas lack of testosterone allows the individual to continue his growth beyond the normal time limit, and thereby to grow taller, because skeletal maturation is retarded.

These points indicate that testosterone may not be useful in the treatment of retarded growth. A prepubertal child treated with testosterone will usually grow at a faster rate initially, but its adult stature may remain below that which it would have reached without treatment.

HGH-administration causes accelerated growth in children who are stunted because of growth hormone deficiency. RABEN (18) has described 3 cases of pituitary dwarfism who have reached a normal adult height following treatment with HGH for 4—7 years, at doses of 2—5 mg three times per week. One patient grew from 125 cm to a height of 165 cm in 5½ years' time. Although antibodies for growth-hormone were demonstrable after 5 years of treatment, HGH appeared to remain effective over the last 6 months of treatment. PRADER and TOUBER (16) have published 3 cases who failed to gain in height, and who had already high HGH-antibody titres in the serum during the first month of treatment.

The effect of the HGH on protein metabolism is less in normal children than in children with deficient endogenous growth hormone (16). This implies that the use of growth hormone in cases of growth retardation not caused by a growth hormone deficiency is questionable (17).

REFERENCES

1. ALBRIGHT, F., Does 'deposit protein' exist? *Conference on Metabolic Aspects of Convalescence, including Bone and Wound Healing*, 5th Meeting, p. 25, Josia Macy, Jr. Foundation, New York, 1943.
2. ALLISON, J. B., Interpretation of nitrogen balance data, *Fed. Proc.* 10: 676, 1951.
3. ALLISON, J. B. and W. H. FITZPATRICK, *Dietary Proteins in Health and Disease*, Charles C. Thomas, Springfield, Ill., U. S. A., 1960.
4. BODO, R. C. DE and N. ALTSZULER, The metabolic effects of growth hormone and their physiological significance, in: *Vitam. and Horm.* 15: 205, 1957, Ac. Press, New York.
5. FINKEL, M. J., Human growth hormone, *Amer. J. Med.* 32: 588, 1962.
6. GREENBAUM, A. L., Growth hormone and fat metabolism, in: *Hypophyseal Growth Hormone. Nature and Actions*, p. 330, Mc. Graw-Hill, New York, 1955.
7. GREENBAUM, A. L. and P. MCLEAN, The influence of pituitary growth hormone in the catabolism of fat, *Biochem. J.* 54: 413, 1953.
8. HAAK, A., *Studies over de werking van humaan groeihormoon en testosteron op de eiwitstofwisseling van de mens*, J. J. Groen & Zoon, Leiden, 1963.
9. HAAK, A., A. A. H. KASSENAAR and A. QUERIDO, Studies of protein metabolism in humans with the aid of N^{15} labelled glycine, in: *Protein Metabolism. An International Symposium*, p. 150, Springer-Verlag, Heidelberg, 1962.
10. HENEMAN, PH. H., A. P. FORBES, M. MOLDAWER, E. F. DEMPORY and E. L. CARROL, Effects of human growth hormone in man, *J. clin. Invest.* 39: 1223, 1960.
11. HOLT, L. E., E. HALAC and C. N. KAJDI, The concept of protein stores and its implications in diet, *J.A.M.A.* 181: 696, 1962.

12. KENYON, A. T., I. SANDIFORD, A. H. BRYAN, K. KNOWLTON and F. C. KOCH, The effects of testosterone propionate on nitrogen, electrolyte, water and energy metabolism in eunuchoidism, *Endocrinology* 23: 135, 1938.
13. KENYON, A. F., K. KNOWLTON, J. SANDIFORD, F. E. KOCH and G. LOTUIN, A comparative study of the metabolic effects of testosterone proprionate in normal men and women and in eunuchoidism, *Endocrinology* 26: 25, 1940.
14. KORNER, A., The effect of growth hormone on protein synthesis, in: *Protein Metabolism. An International Symposium*, p. 8, Springer-Verlag, Heidelberg, 1962.
15. LEE, M. O. and G. B. AYRES, The composition of weight loss and the nitrogen partition of tissue in rats after hypophysectomy, *Endocrinology* 20: 489, 1936.
16. PRADER, A., Specific human growth hormone (H.G.H.). Antibodies in patients treated previously with H.G.H., *Proceedings of the second International Congress of Endocrinology*, p. 993, Excerpta Medica Foundation, London, 1964.
17. RABEN, M. S., Growth hormone, 2. Clinical use of human growth hormone, *New Engl. J. Med.* 266: 82, 1962.
18. RABEN, M. S., Effect of human growth hormone on dwarfed children, *Proceedings of the second International Congress of Endocrinology*, p. 989, Excerpta Medica Foundation, London, 1964.
19. WILSON, J. D., Regulation of protein synthesis by androgens and estrogens, in: *Protein Metabolism. An International Symposium*, p. 26, Springer-Verlag, Heidelberg, 1962.
20. YOUNG, F. G., Growth and diabetes in normal animals, treated with pituitary (anterior lobe) diabetogenic extract, *Biochem. J.* 39: 515, 1945.

THE USE OF ANABOLIC STEROIDS IN THE TREATMENT OF GROWTH RETARDATION

ZVI LARON

Besides its androgenic activity, testosterone possesses 'protein anabolic' properties, i.e. nitrogen retention and increased protein synthesis (12), leading to an increase in body weight, resulting from increase in muscle mass and water retention. Testosterone has been found to stimulate growth in animals and man (22). It has not yet been established whether the androgenic and anabolic properties of testosterone can be dissociated (10) and whether the androgenic and anabolic activity play separate roles in the growth promoting action.

The method generally used to determine the androgenic activity is to measure the degree of restitution of the weight of the seminal vesicles in castrated male rats. The anabolic activity is measured by the degree of restitution of the levator ani muscle in the same animal (4). This is called the myotropic effect. The myotropic and androgenic activity of a drug are then related to those produced by testosterone under similar experimental conditions, and the quotient obtained by dividing the relative myotropic activity of the substance tested, by its relative androgenic activity is called the therapeutic ratio or index.

In the search for a steroid which has primarily anabolic and no androgenic activity many steroids, most of them derivatives of testosterone, have been synthesized in recent years. Some of the mostly used anabolic steroids are shown in fig. 1. According to the rat therapeutic ratio many of them are much less androgenic and far more anabolic than testosterone. However, the rat therapeutic ratio is not an exact index in man and all anabolic steroids have been shown to be more androgenic than expected. At present no anabolic steroid free from androgenic activity has become available.

During recent years the use of anabolic steroids in many fields of medicine, including pediatrics has increased. Several reviews have critically analyzed the pediatric use of these drugs (5, 7, 17). One of the possible indications for the use of anabolic steroids is treatment of growth retardation. Before discussing their growth promoting properties, it is necessary to discuss the possible undesirable effects of anabolic steroids, since their appearance is one of the main limiting factors for the prolonged use of these drugs.

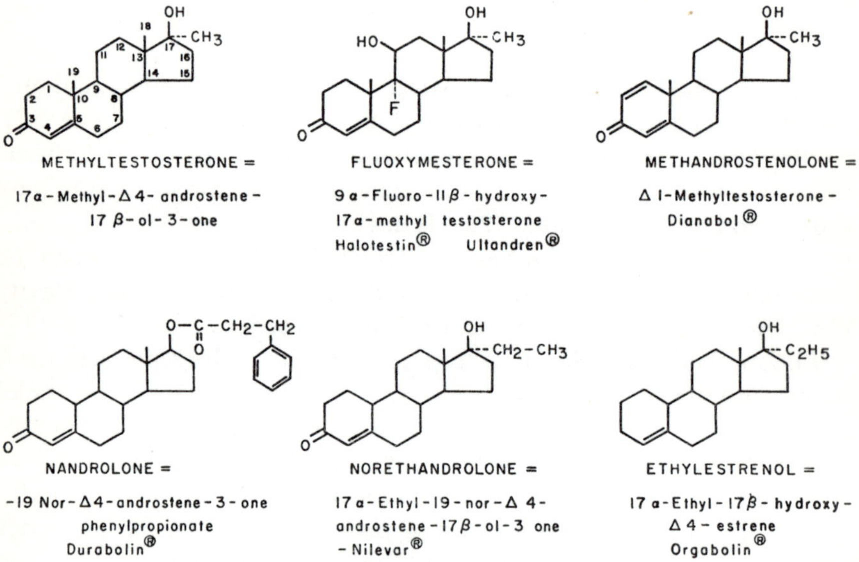

Fig. 1. The chemical structure, nomenclature and generic names of several anabolic steroids as compared to methyltestosterone

Virilization is by far the most frequent undesirable effect. In boys the earliest sign is an increased frequency of erections. The penis or clitoris enlarges (fig. 2), the voice deepens and pubic hair may appear. These changes are reversible only if arrested in their earliest stages. As acceleration of skeletal maturation parallels the virilizing signs, it is at least to some extent an androgenic effect.

Because of the wide variations in individual sensitivity to anabolic steroids, it is impossible to establish a generally valid scheme of non-virilizing doses for these steroids. We have found that for fluoxymesterone (Halotestin, Ultandren) 0.2 mg/kg/day given for three months, or 0.1 mg/kg/day for six months usually are the maximal non-virilizing doses (13, 15). These figures show that doubling of the time of administration reduced the safety limits to half. In accordance with others (21) we have found that methandrostenolone (Dianabol) 0.04 mg/kg/day for 3 to 4 months is non-virilizing in most of the cases. It has been reported that nandrolone propionate (Durabolin) 0.1 mg/kg/month is non-virilizing (3) and that ethylestrenol (Orgabolin) in a dose of 0.1 mg/kg/day causes only minimal virilizing effects in some patients treated for several months (25). More prolonged use of any of these drugs will enhance the androgenic effect. For this reason and the finding that after discontinuation of the drug (13, 15) the growth rate remains at a higher than the pretreatment level for some time, we feel that an intermittent therapy scheme is to be preferred.

Feminization. With what we now consider to be virilizing doses of methandrostenolone, 0.08 mg/kg/day or more, several prepubertal boys have developed gynaecomastia (14) (fig. 3) accompanied by increased oestrogen excretion (16), probably due to conversion of the anabolic steroid in the liver. No such changes have been obtained with fluoxymesterone, but methyltestosterone is known to cause breast enlargement (2).

Other effects of large doses of anabolic steroids, such as should never be used in the paediatric age group, are: liver damage by the C-17 alpha alkylated anabolic steroids such as fluoxymesterone, methandrostenolone and norethandrolone (1, 18, 27). Gonadal hypotrophy (19) and amenorrhea (6) can be caused by suppression of gonadotrophins; lowered urinary 17-ketosteroid and 17-hydroxycorticosteroids by suppression of ACTH secretion (9, 29). Serum PBI concentration can also be lowered by reduction of the serum thyroxine binding capacity (20).

All the undesirable effects except the androgenic effect, seem to be reversible (slow regression taking weeks or months) if the drug is discontinued immediately upon recognition of the undesirable effect.

In considering treatment of growth retardation with anabolic steroids several questions arise: a. which kind of growth retardation is prove to respond to such treatment; b. which is the optimal age at which treatment should be initiated; c. will treatment be of temporary benefit only or can it improve final stature; d. should the sex of the child influence the scheme of treatment; e. can one outline a scheme of treatment which will promote growth without causing undesirable side effects? Partial answers to these questions, and the importance to get full answers, may be illustrated by a few cases. They are taken from our experience with several hundreds of children treated with anabolic steroids during the last six years. The patients were carefully examined before, during and after treatment at intervals of at least 3 months, and bone age determinations were made at most of these

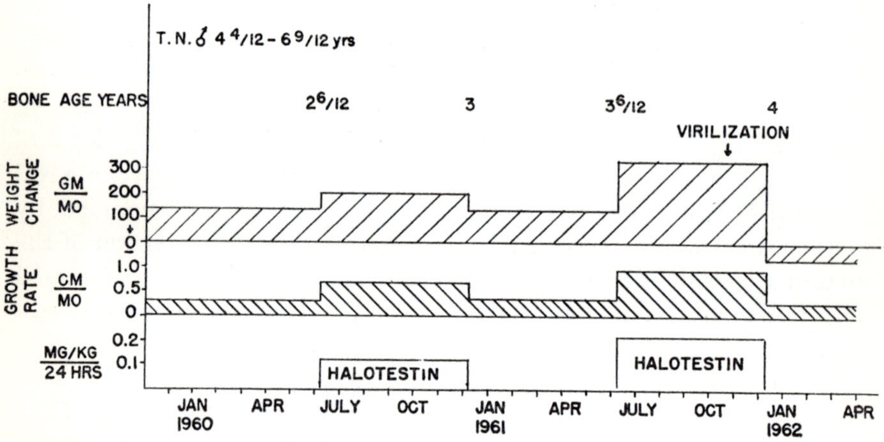

Fig. 4. Mean body weight changes, mean growth rates and skeletal maturation in a prepuberal boy with growth retardation treated with fluoxymesterone (Halotestin ® — Upjohn). From 15

examinations. The anabolic steroids employed were fluoxymesterone (Halotestin ® — Upjohn), methandrostenolone (Dianabol ® — Ciba) and 7α-17-dimethyltestosterone (Myagen ® — Upjohn). In the vast majority of cases the steroids were administered for three months, followed by periods of at least three months without treatment. In a small number of children the treatment period was extended to six months.

Figure 4 illustrates that the administration of Halotestin 0.1 mg/kg/day to a 5-year-old boy accelerated his growth rate in height and body weight. Doubling the dose increased the response but virilizing signs appeared.

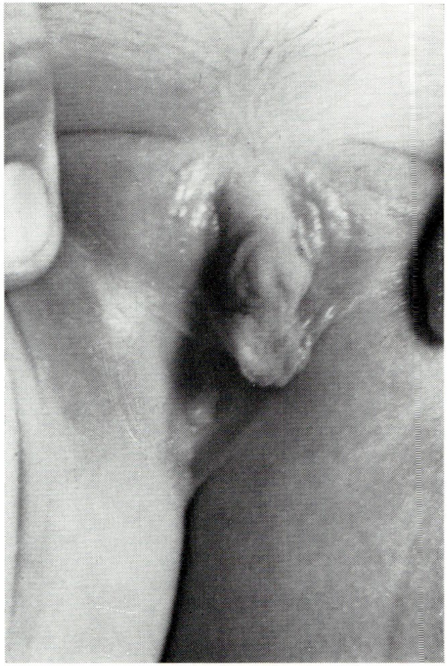

Fig. 2. Enlargement of the clitoris in a $5^1/_2$ year old girl with growth retardation treated with methandrostenolone (Dianabol^R-Ciba, 0.08 mg/day)

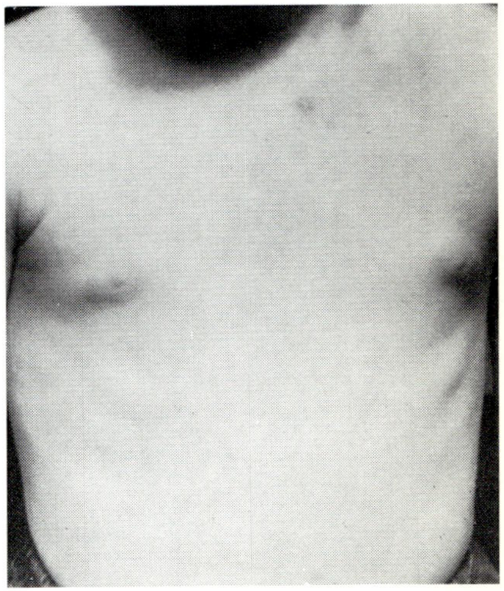

Fig. 3. Breast enlargement in a 5 year old boy induced by methandrostenolone (Dianabol-Ciba). The gynecomastia regresses several months after discontinuation of the therapy

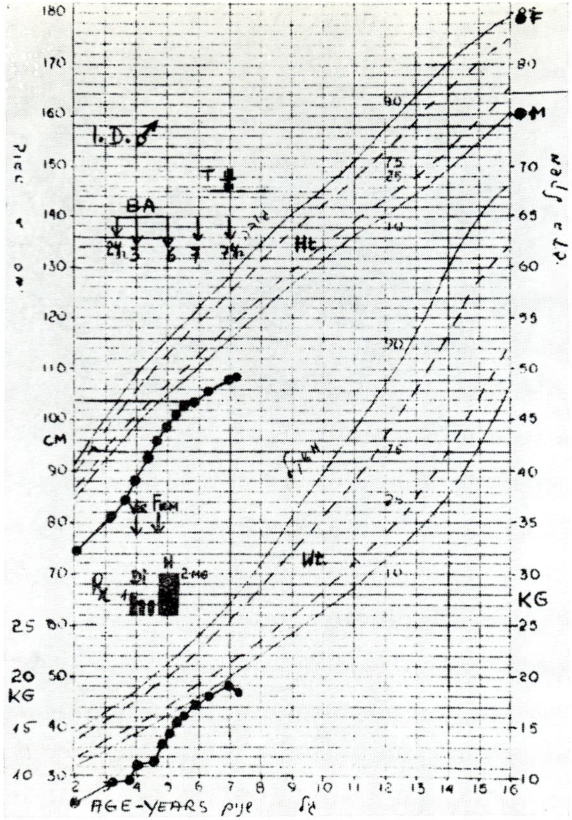

Fig. 6. Growth chart of boy with Bloom's syndrome treated with methandrostenolone (Dianabol) and fluoxymesterone (Halotestin). F represents the height of the patient's father, M that of the mother, BA = bone age

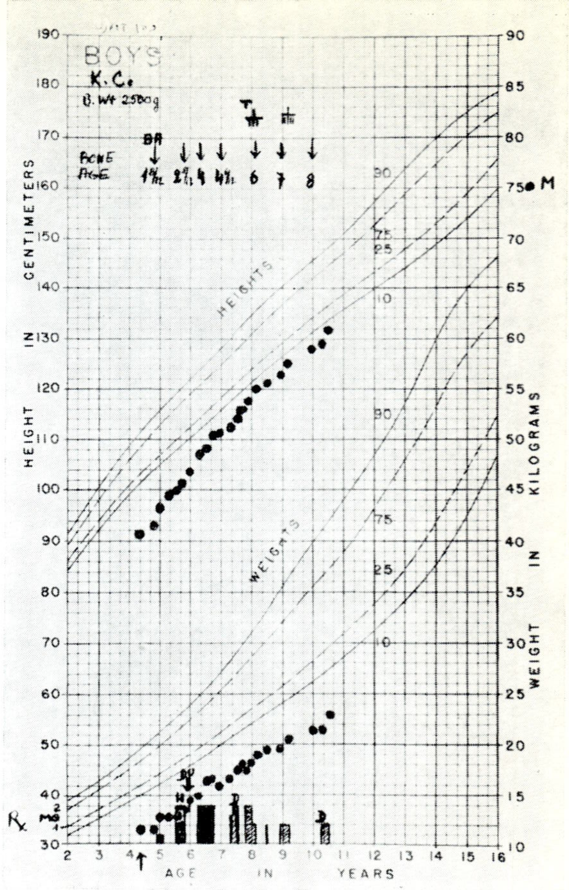

Fig. 7. Growth chart of a boy with nondefined growth retardation and pseudoepiphysis treated with fluoxymesterone (Halotestin) and methandrostenolone (Dianabol). M represents the height of the patient's mother, BA = bone age

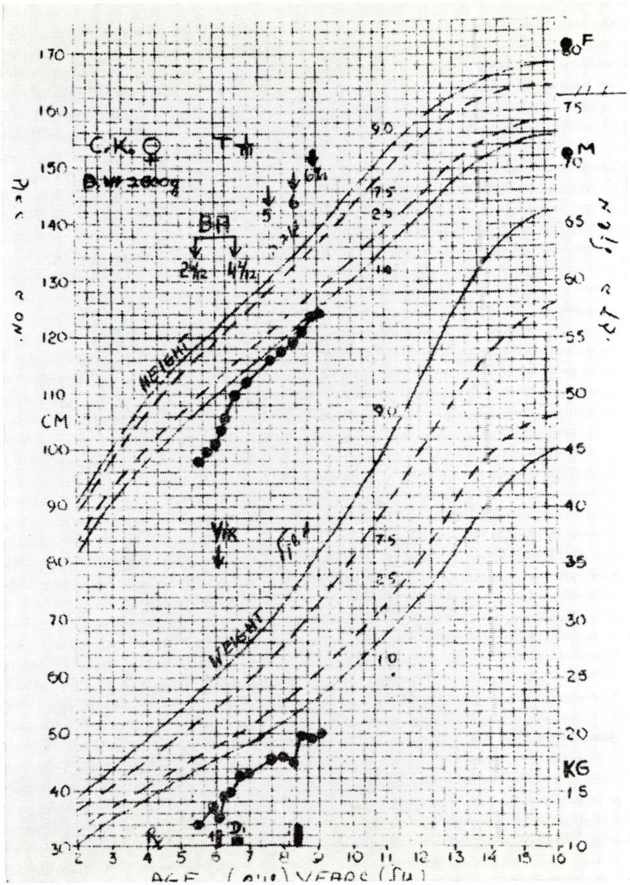

Fig. 8. Growth chart of a girl with nondefined growth retardation treated with methandrostenolone (Dianabol). F = height of patient's father and M = mother, BA = bone age

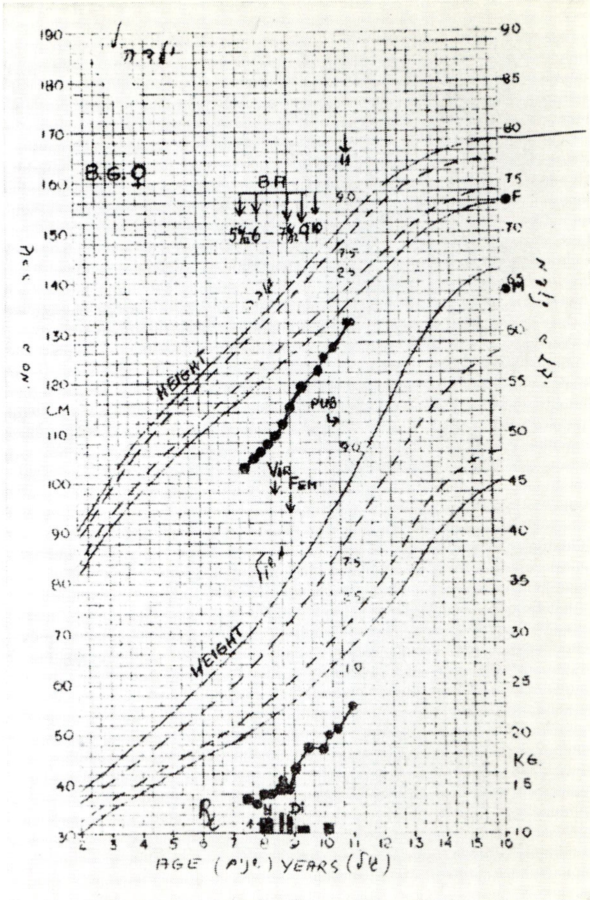

Fig. 9. Growth chart of a Yemenite girl with growth retardation treated with fluoxymesterone (Halotestin) and methandrostenolone (Dianabol). F = height of patient's father and M = mother, BA = bone age

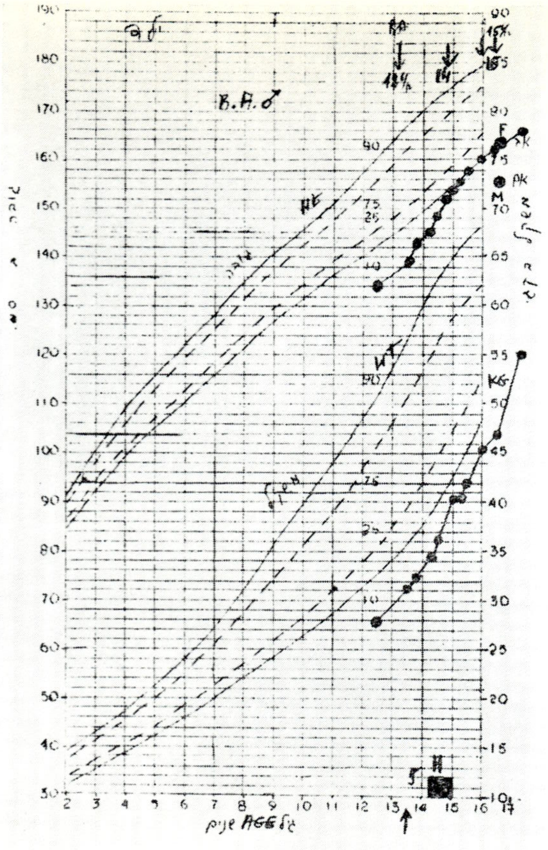

Fig. 10

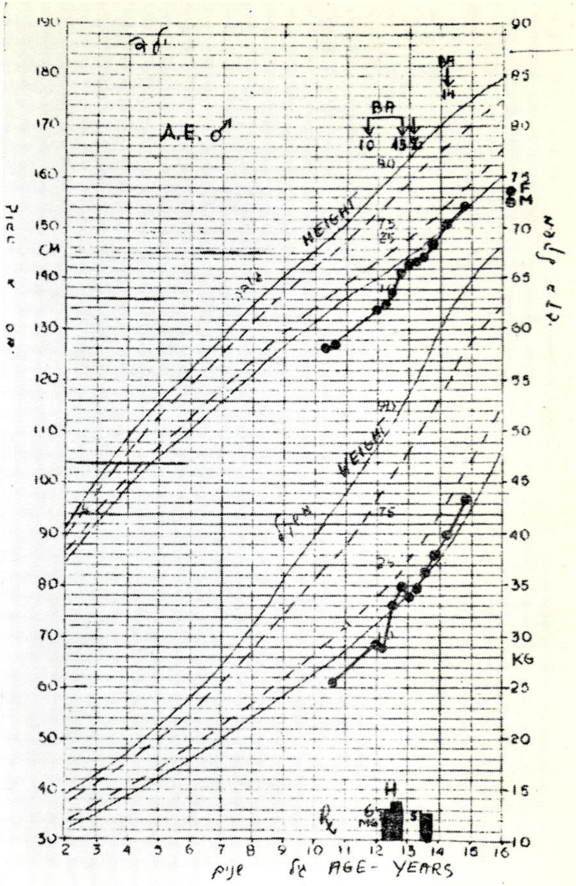

Fig. 11

Fig. 10 and 11. Growth charts of two boys with growth retardation associated with delayed puberty, treated with fluoxymesterone (Halotestin). F = height of patient's father and M = mother, BA = bone age

Figure 5 shows the results of intermittent treatment with Dianabol in a boy of 9 6/12 years with growth retardation. It is clear that after discontinuation of treatment the growth rate in height remains above the pretreatment level for a few months. In contrast, body weight gain stops abruptly after discontinuation of therapy, and actual weight loss may occur. We interpret this as release of accumulated water.

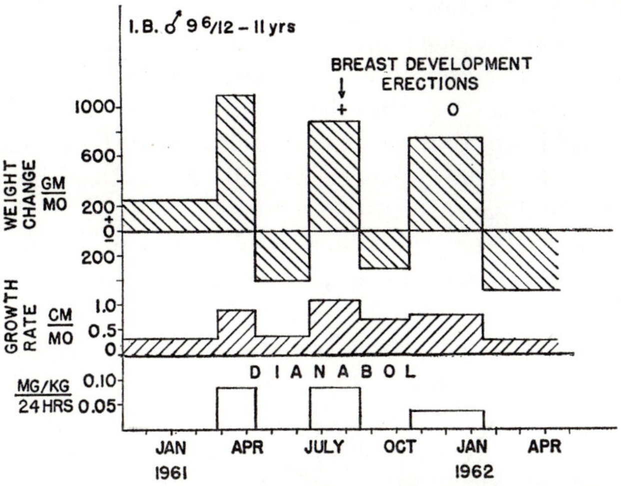

Fig. 5. Mean body weight and mean growth changes in a prepuberal boy with growth retardation treated with methandrostenolone (Dianabol ® — Ciba). From 16

We shall now look at several growth charts of children with growth retardation, to illustrate the long term effect of anabolic steroids therapy.

Figure 6 represents the growth of a boy with Bloom's syndrome (11) who was started on anabolic therapy at the age of 2 8/12 years. It may be seen that there was little if any bone age retardation and that bone maturation was accelerated by the treatment. During treatment there was also a spurt in growth, but after discontinuation of treatment the growth rate decreased and his present height is at about the same percentile as before treatment, whereas his bone age is now advanced for his age. In conclusion: no success and possibly a loss of final height.

The next chart (fig. 7) shows the growth spurt of a boy who besides growth retardation had a systolic heart murmur and a 'pseudoepiphysis' of the second metacarpal bone (26). Though his bone age was 3 years retarded, no endocrine disturbance could be detected. Intermittent treatment with either fluoxymesterone or methandrostenolone caused a marked growth spurt which brought the child to the 3rd percentile. Whenever treatment was interrupted the growth rate decreased. During the first 2 years of treatment bone age advanced quickly, but for the last two years, with smaller doses and longer intervals between treatment, bone age advanced parallel with chronological age. Since the bone age is now still two years behind, therapy can be continued, I hope, until normal puberty. Not having found evidence for an endocrine disorder, we think that without treatment this boy would have continued to grow slowly but for a longer period of time. Anabolic therapy has successfully normalized his growth at the critical school age.

Figure 8 illustrates the growth chart of a girl with undefined growth retardation accompanied by a retardation in skeletal age of three years, at the beginning of the study. Two courses of methandrostenolone improved the growth rate markedly, while the bone age advanced almost two years within one year. Thereafter growth continued along the 3rd percentile and bone age advanced in a parallel fashion. As bone maturity is still retarded, we are attempting to improve the growth rate further.

The next figure (fig. 9) illustrates the growth pattern of a Yemenite girl who at the beginning of the study had a 2 year retardation in skeletal age. Intermittent therapy with fluoxymesterone and methandrostenolone improved her growth rate and she approached the 3rd percentile. However, at this stage bone age is equal to chronological age and continuation of treatment could impair final height by advancing bone age faster than linear growth. Eight months after the last course of anabolic therapy the growth rate had not decreased, probably because of beginning puberty. But will she continue to grow along this percentile? It should be noted that her mother (M) is very short (136 cm).

The following two graphs (fig. 10, 11) illustrate two boys with delayed puberty, growth retardation and retardation in skeletal age. Institution of treatment with fluoxymesterone stimulated both the growth rate and bone maturation. After 1 or 2 courses of treatment puberty had advanced to such an extent that growth continued along the improved channel on endogenous stimulation alone. It has been stated that advancement of the bone age to about 13 to 14 years stimulates by some unknown mechanism the secretion of the gonadotrophins (24). If it is true that acceleration of bone age to pubertal age leads to an earlier onset of puberty (19), it can be argued that growth retardation associated with delayed puberty should be treated with either anabolic steroids or testosterone itself.

COMMENTS

The degree of response of children to the various anabolic steroids varies in an unpredictable manner. As shown in the case with Bloom's syndrome, anabolic steroids should not be given to children with growth retardation when bone age is not retarded. It has been repeatedly shown that children with primordial or constitutional dwarfism, chondrodysplasia, and gonadal dysgenesis do not respond adequately to anabolic steroids (8, 9, 13, 15, 19, 28) and impairment to the already reduced final stature can be expected. It has also been shown that anabolic steroids have little if any growth promoting effect in premature babies (23). Therefore therapy with anabolic steroids should only be attempted in children with bone age retardation of one year or more. As it is very difficult, at least in the first periods of treatment, to prevent that skeletal maturation is accelerated more than the growth in height, only children with a marked retardation in skeletal maturation will be able to benefit from prolonged treatment. As the growth rate will continue at an increased rate for some time after discontinuation of the treatment, we feel that intermittent therapy should be used.

We think that therapy should be initiated, if possible, before school age to minimize unfavourable effects, including psychological ones, of the short stature on the school performance. A second important age group is the growth retardation associated with delayed puberty. Advancement of bone age to pubertal age may indirectly advance the onset of spontaneous puberty. In this age group treatment has marked beneficial effects from the psychological point of view.

We feel that the sex of the child should not influence our decision on treatment, as we attempt to stop therapy at the first sign of undesirable effects. In boys older than 13 years, signs of virilization are not considered an indication to discontinue therapy. In this age group virilizing doses could be used.

Currently anabolic steroids are being used in attempts to counteract the growth inhibiting effects of corticosteroids (see p. 329).

IN CONCLUSION

Anabolic steroids are a useful asset in the treatment of growth retardation, if children are carefully selected and their bone age is retarded.

Considering the necessity of repeated thorough medical examinations, body measurements and accurate bone age assessment at regular intervals, before, during and after therapy, and the difficulty in assessing achievement and indication for further therapy, we feel that treatment with anabolic steroids should only be administered by specialized clinics.

REFERENCES

1. ARIAS, I. M., in ref. 7, p. 434.
2. BAYLEY, N., G. S. GORDAN and H. LISSER, *Pediat. Clin. North Amer.* Nov. 1957, p. 819.
3. BIERICH, J. R., B. BECKER and L. BORNER, *Xth International Congress of Pediatrics*, Sept. 1962, Lisbon.
4. CAMERINO, B. and G. SALA, *Progress in Drug Research* 2: 71, 1960.
5. Editorial, *Brit. Med. J.* 1: 1035, 1963.
6. EVANS, R. G., *Acta Allergol.* 17: 220, 1962.
7. GROSS, F., Ed., *Protein metabolism — Influence of growth hormone, anabolic steroids and nutrition in health and disease*, Springer Verlag, Berlin-Göttingen-Heidelberg, 1962.
8. HUBBLE, D. and D. R. MACMILLAN, *Arch. Dis. Childh.* 37: 518, 1962.
9. JAMES, V. H. T., J. LANDON and V. WYNN, *J. Endocrin.* 25: 211, 1962.
10. JOSS, E. E., K. A. ZUPPINGER and E. H. SOBEL, *Endocrinology* 72: 123, 1963.
11. KATZENELLENBOGEN, I. and Z. LARON, *Arch. Derm.* 82: 609, 1960.
12. KOCHAKIAN, C. D., *Vitam. and Horm.* 4: 255, 1946.
13. LARON, Z., *Acta Endocrin.* (*Kbh.*) 36: 541, 1961.
14. LARON, Z., *J. clin. Endocrin.* 22: 450, 1962.
15. LARON, Z., *Acta Paediat.* (*Uppsala*) 52: 465, 1963.
16. LARON, Z., in ref. 7, p. 398.
17. LARON, Z. and S. GITTER, *Clin. Paediat.* 2: 594, 1964.
18. MARQUARDT, G. H., C. I. FISHER, P. LEVY and R. M. DOWBEN, *J. Amer. Med. Ass.* 175: 851, 1961.
19. PRADER, A. and R. ILLIG, in ref. 7, p. 383.

20. Rosenberg, I. N., C. S. Ahn and M. L. Mitchell, *J. clin Endocrin.* 22: 612, 1962.
21. Scharer, K., H. Habich and A. Prader, *Helv. med. Acta* 27: 530, 1960.
22. Sobel, E. H., in: L. I. Gardner, *Adrenal function in infants and children*, p. 137, Grune and Stratton, Inc., New York, 1956.
23. Todd, R. M., *Xth International Congress of Pediatrics*, Sept. 1962, Abstr. no. 321, Lisbon.
24. Tonutti, E., *11 Symposion der Deutschen Gesellschaft für Endokrinologie*, Springer Verlag, in the press.
25. Visser, H. K. A. and W. Croughs, see page 290.
26. Wagner, R., *J. Diss. Child.* 91: 6, 1956.
27. Werner, M., A. Hitz, F. Gloor and H. Tholen, *Klin. Wschr.* 39: 1006, 1961.
28. Whitelaw, M. J., S. F. Thomas, W. H. Graham and T. N. Foster, *Amer. J. Obstet. Gynec.* 84: 501, 1962.
29. Wynn, V., J. Landon and V. H. T. James, *J. Endocrin.* 25: 199, 1962.

EFFECTS OF ANDROGENS AND ANABOLIC STEROIDS ON GROWTH RATE AND HEIGHT

H. K. A. VISSER* and WIM CROUGHS

INTRODUCTION

There is not much known about the production of androgenic hormones by the gonads and the adrenal glands during infancy and childhood. It is probable that small amounts of these substances are produced. Accurate data of production rate studies are not available so far but 17-ketosteroids(17-KS) can be estimated in the urine of children. It is however not before puberty that a considerable rise in the urinary excretion of 17-KS can be observed and it is generally accepted that an increased production of androgenic substances by the gonads (in boys) and the adrenal glands (in girls as well as boys) is responsible for the development of several signs of puberty. Up to now there is no evidence that the production of adrenocortical steroids is different in males and females. **

Androgens promote growth and skeletal maturation and produce secondary male sex characteristics. During puberty a typical increase in growth velocity is seen in boys and girls, followed by a decline in growth rate until after a few years epiphyseal fusion occurs and adult height is reached (39, 43). The pubertal growth spurt in males can easily be explained by the increased production of testosterone by the gonads. The cause of the female adolescent spurt is not well understood. Adrenal androgens may be responsible and it is possible that the ovaries produce small amounts of testosterone when puberty starts. An increased secretion of growth hormone cannot be ruled out. The role of estrogenic hormones in these processes is not clear, but there is

* Supported in part by a PHS returning research fellow grant (RF-41) from the Public Health Service, National Institutes of Health, Bethesda, Md., U.S.A., and a grant from the Netherlands Organization for the Advancement of Pure Research (Z.W.O.).

** There is now (1966) evidence for different production of △y-androstenedione by the adrenal glands in adult men and women.

evidence that these substances also stimulate growth in girls and promote epiphyseal fusion (44).

Some 'experiments of nature', diseases with an increased or decreased production of hormones from the gonads and adrenal glands give a unique opportunity to study the effects of these hormones on growth and development and in this paper we will shortly summarize what can be learned from these observations.

Androgens, and in particular anabolic steroids (anabolic steroids are in fact androgens), are now widely used in the treatment of children with growth disorders. We think it is possible to use the term 'anabolic' for those substances, which have a growth-promoting effect and a low androgenic activity when given in small doses. Treatment with these substances generally results in an accelerated growth rate, but at the same time skeletal maturation becomes advanced. It has been very difficult so far to evaluate the results of treatment with anabolic steroids in regard to its effect on ultimate height (9, 20, 30). We have limited experience with the anabolic steroid ethylestrenol (Orgabolin) and the results of treatment of some children with retarded growth will be reported in this paper. We have tried to evaluate the effect on ultimate height by plotting the growth rate not only against chronological age but also against bone age, and we believe that in this way a better insight can be obtained in what anabolic steroids do to ultimate adult height.

EFFECTS OF ANDROGENS ON GROWHTH RATE AND HEIGHT IN NORMAL CHILDREN AND CHILDREN WITH PREMATURE ADRENARCHE, CONGENITAL ADRENAL HYPERPLASIA AND PRECOCIOUS PUBERTY

The onset of puberty is more correlated with bone age than with chronological age*. Puberty normally appears in girls when bone age has reached about 11 years, and in boys when bone age is about 13 years. As long as chronological age and bone age are the same, puberty of course will also start at the chronological age of 11 and 13 years

* An accurate correlation between the sequence of events at puberty and bone age has not been made so far. We use 'onset' of puberty here as beginning of height spurt, which correlates generally with the appearance of pubic hair and elevation of breast and papilla in girls, and which in boys may start a year after the appearance of pubic hair.

respectively. In early and late maturers there is a dissociation of chronological age and bone age when puberty starts. This is illustrated in figs. 1 and 2.

Fig. 1 demonstrates the growth curves for a normal boy. Length in cm and growth velocity in cm per year were plotted against chronological age (continuous lines), and against bone age (dotted lines). In

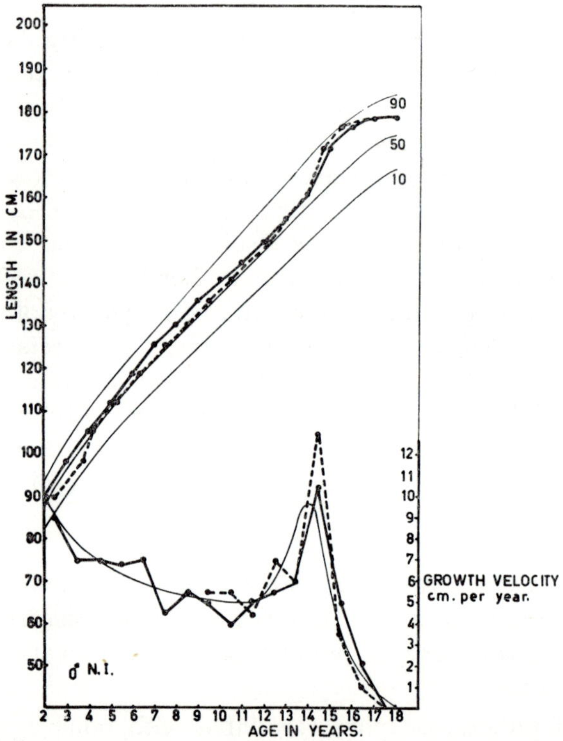

Fig. 1. Growth curves and growth velocity curves of a normal boy; plotted against chronological age (•—•) and skeletal age (•----•). See text. Data from 3

this chart and all following charts the 10, 50 and 90 percentiles for length are those for Dutch children of De Wijn and De Haas (48). The standard curves for growth velocity (cm per year) were constructed using data from the growth velocity curves of Bayer and Bayley (3) for North-American children and of Prader, Tanner and Von Harnack (31) for West-European children. Predicted mature height

(PMH) was calculated using the radiographic atlas of Greulich and Pyle (13) (for estimation of bone age) and the tables of Bayley and Pinneau (5). Using the atlas of Greulich and Pyle skeletal maturation before puberty advances generally one year per chronological year, and the same is true during puberty. The standards for bone age in this atlas are not mean values from a group of children, but represent

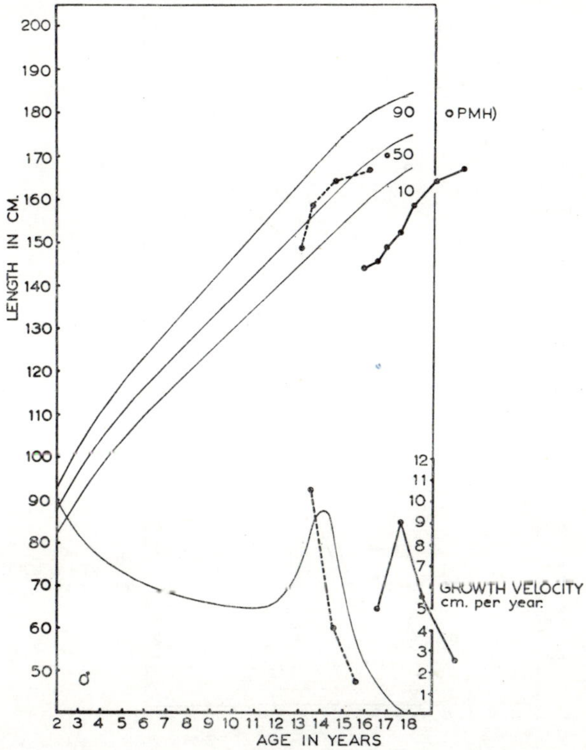

Fig. 2. Growth curves and growth velocity curves of a late maturing boy; plotted against chronological age (•—•) and skeletal age (•----•). See text. Data from VAN DER WERFF TEN BOSCH, J. J. (personal communication)

X-rays of a median child in a group. Calculating the data of 8 normal children from Bayer and Bayley (3), skeletal age advanced with 2 3/12 year (average value) in a period of 2 chronological years of maximal growth during puberty. Fig. 1 represents one of these children. It can be seen that annual increments in height for skeletal age as well as for chronological age are about the same. There are individual differences, and increments in height for chronological and skeletal age may show discrepancies when they are studied for short intervals.

Fig. 2 demonstrates the growth curves, plotted in the same way,

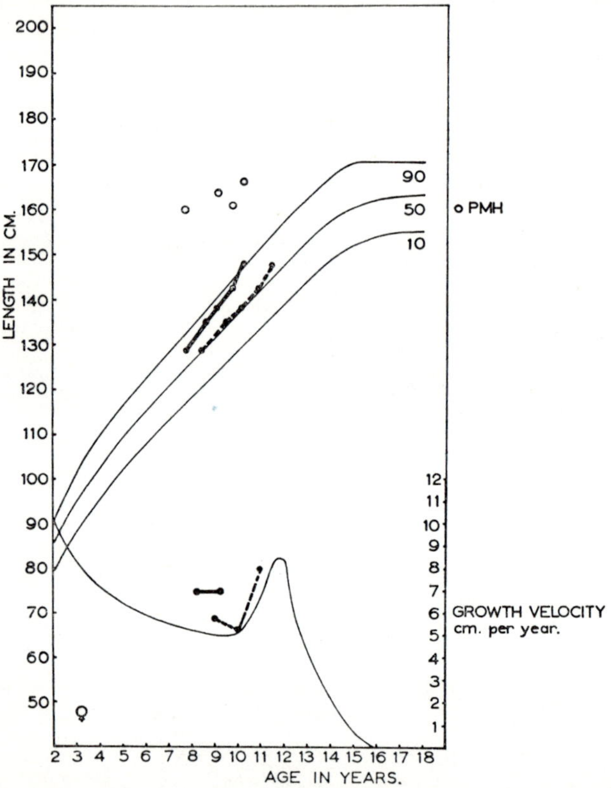

Fig. 3. Growth curves and growth velocity curves of a girl with premature adrenarche; plotted against chronological age (•—•) and skeletal age (•-----•). See text. PMH = predicted mature height

for a 'late maturer'. The dissociation of chronological and skeletal age at the time of puberty can be clearly seen.

Fig. 3 shows the growth curves of a girl with premature adrenarche. At the age of 4 years pubic hair appeared and the clitoris became enlarged. Bone age was advanced for chronological age, but increases of skeletal maturation and height were at the same rate and predicted adult height did not decrease. No symptoms of increased production of estrogens were observed. Urinary excretion of 17-KS was slightly high for age. This syndrome has been called premature adrenarche and is explained by an early maturation of the adrenal glands which produce more androgenic substances than normally before puberty (12, 47). There is some evidence for an increased excretion of dehydroepiandrosterone, an androgenic steroid produced by the adrenal glands, in this condition (50). Premature adrenarche can be 'idiopathic', as precocious puberty, but may also be the result of an intracranial lesion (24).

In children with precocious puberty growth is much faster than normal and these children are very tall during childhood, particularly when the symptoms develop at an early age. Bone age however increases faster and epiphyseal closure occurs at an age before normal adult height is reached. As a result those patients are mostly short adults, even dwarfs, and this 'experiment of nature' is a most important example of the effect of androgens on linear growth and bone maturation: growth is accelerated at the expense of a decrease in adult stature. Fig. 4 illustrates this in a girl with precocious puberty at a very early age. This patient, from Bayer and Bayley (3), had her first period at the age of 7 months! Her ultimate height was 142 cm. The growth curves demonstrate that this 'loss' in height has occurred before her bone age was 11 years. Growth velocity in cm per year of bone age was less than normal during this period. However, the pubertal growth spurt plotted against bone age is almost normal (see fig. 1). It is very likely that an increased production of androgens promotes bone maturation excessively when bone age is less than about 11 years, and the more as bone age is younger; the same amount of androgens is a normal growth stimulant when bone development shows a bone age of 11 years and more, and then growth velocity per years of bone age is the same as during normal puberty. It seems to make no difference what the chronological age is during this period. This is again an example of the correlation between bone age, rather than chronological age, and what we would like to call biological age: the onset of puberty. Growth velocity in fig. 4 plotted against chronological age shows that this patient had a growth spurt around her second year of life; the growth curve since her 5th year remarkably has the same slope as the final part of the normal growth velocity curve between 12 and 16 years (standard curve).

It seems to us that congenital adrenal hyperplasia takes an intermediate position between premature adrenarche and precocious puberty. Growth and bone maturation advance more than in patients

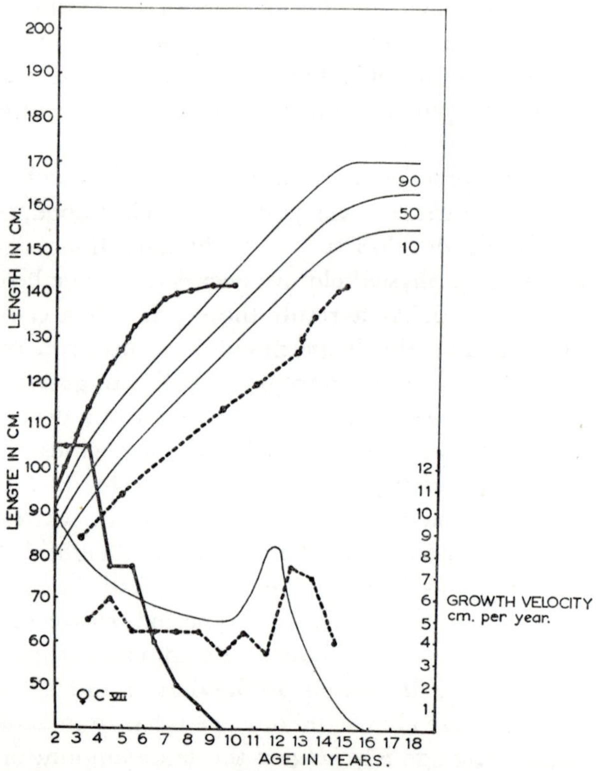

Fig. 4. Growth curves and growth velocity curves of a girl with precocious puberty at a very early age; plotted against chronological age (•—•) and skeletal age (•----•). See text. Data from 3

with premature adrenarche. There is some 'loss of height' with decreased adult stature. This is however mostly not as excessive as in patients with precocious puberty. The effects of androgens on growth and height in patients with congenital adrenal hyperplasia are discussed in chapter VIII, p. 248.

In these syndromes with increased production of androgens an eventual decrease in adult stature is probably dependent on the chemical nature (and biological activity) and the amount of androgenic substances.

The differences in ultimate adult height between patients with premature adrenarche and congenital adrenal hyperplasia might depend primarily upon the differences in amount of adrenal androgens produced. In patients with premature adrenarche excretions of 17-KS are somewhat increased (1—2 times normal) and ultimate height is not influenced, while in congenital adrenal hyperplasia urinary 17-KS excretion is 5—10 times normal and ultimate height is mostly decreased (12). Moreover in the last condition the increased production of androgens starts much earlier than in premature adrenarche. In precocious puberty gonadal androgens are also involved and in this condition ultimate height is even more decreased, particularly when the symptoms start at an early age. Urinary excretion of 17-KS in precocious puberty is generally not increased above values normal for adolescence or adulthood. In a 3-year-old boy with precocious puberty an increased production of testosterone has been reported (25).

GROWTH RATE AND HEIGHT IN CHILDREN WITH INSUFFICIENT FUNCTION OF THE GONADS AND ADRENAL GLANDS (TURNER'S SYNDROME, ADDISON'S DISEASE ETC.)

In patients with gonadal dysgenesis or Turner's syndrome the production of gonadal androgens and estrogens must be very low or absent. There is also some evidence for a subnormal production of adrenal androgens in this condition (21). Several investigators, as VAN DER WERFF TEN BOSCH (41, 42) and ACHESON and ZAMPA (1) have pointed out that skeletal maturation is normal until the age of puberty, but then bone development becomes retarded.

There are only a very few observations in the literature on growth in children who had no functioning gonads as a result of traumata, X-ray castration and operation, or in boys with anorchia for unknown reason. BAYER and BAYLEY (3) describe a girl who underwent X-ray castration at the age of 13 years for a Ewing tumour of the fourth lumbar vertebra. At that time however her pubertal growth spurt was almost finished. After X-ray treatment bone maturation became retarded and epiphyseal fusion did not occur. Prader (29) has made a unique observation on a pair of male identical twins. One of the boys had undescended testicles from birth on and at operation free ends of the spermatic cord were found. Growth curves in both boys were identical until puberty started in the normal boy. At least in this case gonadal androgens had no influence on statural growth during childhood.

From these and other observations it may be concluded that epiphyseal fusion is dependent on the presence of functioning gonads. It is not clear if the growth spurt during puberty is completely dependent on gonadal hormones. It might be considered that in the absence of functioning gonads the adrenal androgens may cause a small acceleration of growth over a long period. In any case ultimate adult height is not decreased when the gonads are absent. In patients castrated before puberty ultimate adult height may even become some centimeters larger as a result of the delayed epiphyseal fusion.

Children with Turner's syndrome are different in this respect and in fact do not represent 'normal' children without gonads. These children react differently upon growth hormone and anabolic steroids compared with normal children. Prader (28, 30) and others (7, 14, 45) have suggested that there is a tissue-insensitivity for the growth stimulating effect of these anabolic compounds.

We are not aware of longterm studies on growth in children with Addison's disease. It is not known that adrenal androgens have a role in statural growth during childhood. Blodgett et al. (8) have observed that substitution therapy with cortisone may have prompted some acceleration of growth in children with Addison's disease.

EFFECTS OF ANDROGENS AND ANABOLIC STEROIDS ON GROWTH RATE AND HEIGHT IN THE TREATMENT OF CHILDREN WITH RETARDED GROWTH

All anabolic steroids available at this time are in fact androgens. The best anabolic steroid to use for the treatment of children with retarded growth is that compound which has the lowest possible 'androgenic' effects (virilizing symptoms and stimulation of bone maturation) and the highest possible 'anabolic' effects (stimulation of protein synthesis and thus of growth).

Testosterone, isolated in 1935 (10), has highly androgenic activities. It seems to stimulate bone maturation excessively when administered to children with a bone age of less than about 11 years. When given for a short period an acceleration of linear growth is observed together with a faster acceleration of bone age. After the withdrawal of testo-

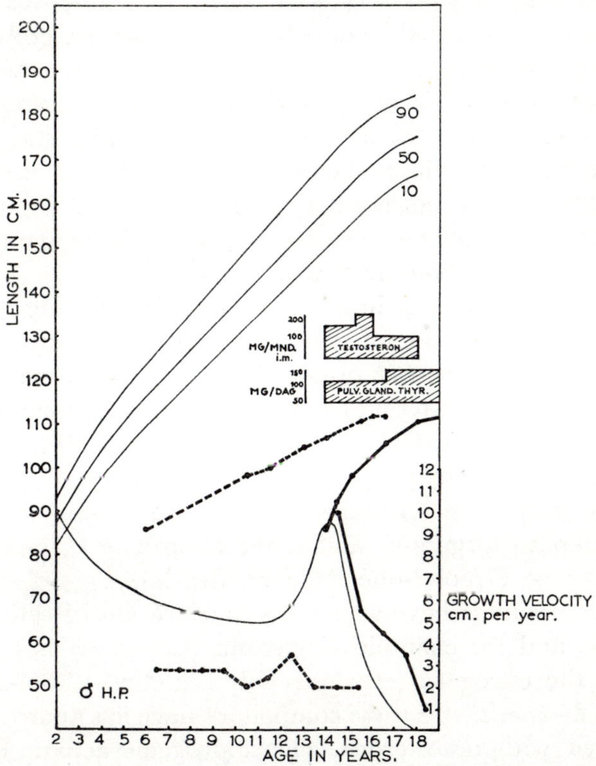

Fig. 5. Growth curves and growth velocity curves of a boy with idiopathic pituitary insufficiency, during treatment with testosterone. Curves plotted against chronological age (•—•) and skeletal age (•----•). See text

sterone, this acceleration of height and bone maturation often continues for some period of time, and bone maturation again faster than linear growth! These effects, after treatment has been discontinued, have been overlooked in the past. A long period of observation in these patients is necessary. Improvement of growth with testosterone, achieved at the cost of decreased adult height has been reported a.o. by WILKINS (46), SOBEL et al. (38), PRADER and ILLIG (30), and others.

An example of these effects of testosterone is shown in fig. 5. This is a patient with pituitary insufficiency. Retardation of growth started at the early age of six months. At the age of 14 years his bone age was 6 years. He was treated with testosterone over a period of 4 years and it can be seen that his growth velocity during this time was normal for chronological age. Plotted against bone age however, growth velocity was much below normal. In this period of 4 years bone age increased more than 9 years! It is interesting that when plotted against bone age the growth spurt was not observed. The early start of growth retardation in this patient makes it likely that a severe and early deficiency of growth hormone must have existed. In our opinion testosterone should not be given to boys before bone age has reached the development of about 13 years.

Several anabolic steroids have been synthetized during recent years. Some of them are testosterone derivatives as methyltestosterone (17α-methyl-Δ_4-androsterone-17β-ol-3-one), fluoxymesterone (9α-fluoro-11β-ol-17α-methyltestosterone) and methandrostenolone (Δ_1-methyl-testosterone, Dianabol, CIBA). Others are called 19-nortestosterone compounds (these compounds have no side chain at C_{19}), as nandrolone-phenylpropionate (19-nor-Δ_4-androsterone-3-one-phenylpropionate, Durabolin, Organon) and norethandrolone (17α-ethyl-19-nor-Δ_4-androsterone-17β-ol-3-one, Nilevar, Searle).

Newer compounds have structures that are not directly related to testosterone and for example Orgabolin (Organon) has a structure related to the estrogens (ethylestrenol, 17α-ethyl-17β-ol-Δ_4-estrene).

In animal experiments these compounds have less androgenic activity compared with testosterone. The androgenic activity is evaluated by measuring the degree of restitution of the weight of the seminal vesicles. The anabolic effect is called the myotropic effect and is based on the measurement of the degree of restitution of the specifically sensitive levator ani muscle of the castrated male rat (11, 27).

It should be emphasized that up to now there are no satisfactory results from animal experiments in regard to the effects of the anabolic compounds on bone maturation compared with growth. The pharmaceutical industries, supplying us with an increasing number of anabolic drugs, so far have given no exact information on the effects of these drugs on bone maturation in animals, and these effects have in fact to be studied on the growing child. The so-called therapeutic ratio of a drug, the ratio of androgenic over myotropic activities in the castrated male rat in comparison with the activities of testosterone, cannot be considered the ideal criterion for a drug for clinical treatment of children with retarded growth.

Fluoxymesterone has been used by several investigators in the treatment of children with growth retardation (16, 18, 19, 32, 23). REILLY and GORDAN (32) have reported that on a dose of 5 mg orally per day, growth in height increased more than bone age, in other words predicted adult height increased. This has not been confirmed by the other investigators and SOBEL (37) has criticized the observations of REILLY and GORDAN. LARON (18) recommended a dose of 0.1 mg/kg/day if used continuously for six months, and 0.2 mg/kg/day if used for three months only.

Methandrostenolone (Dianabol, CIBA) has been studied by PRADER and ILLIG (30), LARON (19) and BAYER and BAYLEY (4). In a dose of 0.04 mg/kg/ day PRADER and ILLIG (30) did not observe virilizing effects. However, bone maturation increased usually more than growth in length. BAYER and BAYLEY (4) report no decrease in predicted adult height (PMH) using 0.02—0.03 mg/kg/day.

Nandrolone-phenylpropionate (Durabolin, Organon) was studied by BIERICH (6) and PRADER and ILLIG (30). The last authors report no virilizing effects in a dose of 1 mg/kg/month, but bone maturation increased again in most cases more than height.

Ethylestrenol (Orgabolin, Organon) in a dose of 0.1 mg/kg/day did not increase bone maturation more than linear growth (7). Our experience with this anabolic steroid is limited and will now be reported.

Twelve children with various types of growth retardation have been treated with ethylestrenol for periods ranging from 6 months to 2 6/12 years. All, except one of the children were boys, and chronological ages were 10—14 years. Some typical examples representing this group are illustrated in the next charts.

Fig. 6 shows the effects of treatment with testosterone and ethylestrenol on growth and bone maturation in a boy with 'constitutional delay of growth and adolescence' and retarded bone age. Testosterone was given in a dose of 10 mg intramuscularly per week during 8 months. There was an acceleration of growth, but after treatment was discontinued bone age increased 20 months during the following 9 months, while height increased only 4 cm. As a result PMH declined considerably. Ethylestrenol 0.1—0.2 mg/kg/day orally was then given,

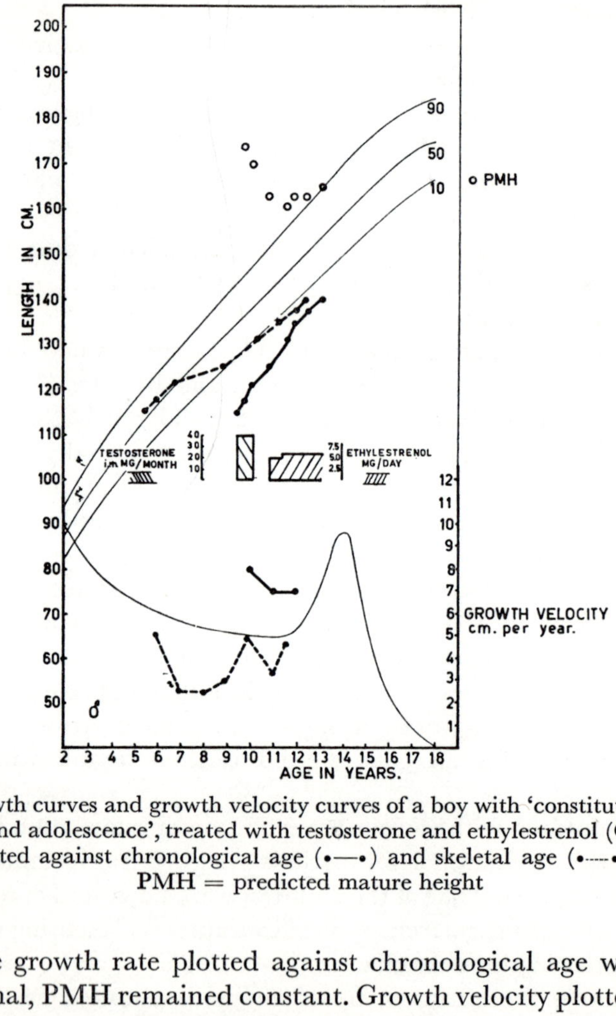

Fig. 6. Growth curves and growth velocity curves of a boy with 'constitutional delay in growth and adolescence', treated with testosterone and ethylestrenol (Orgabolin). Curves plotted against chronological age (•—•) and skeletal age (•-----•). See text. PMH = predicted mature height

and while growth rate plotted against chronological age was higher than normal, PMH remained constant. Growth velocity plotted against bone age shows the 'loss in height' during the testosterone period; on ethylestrenol the growth rate was more or less normal for bone age.

These children, mostly boys, with 'constitutional delay of growth and adolescence' have retarded bone age and on this basis one can predict when puberty will start. It may be that estimations of serum growth hormone or androgens will in the future enable us to classify these children as endocrine patients, but by current criteria they are endocrinologically normal. Usually predicted adult height is not below the 10th percentile, but in these children predictions are difficult to make. Using the tables of Bayley and Pinneau (5) a retardation of bone age of more than 2 years will result in an overestimated PMH. Is bone age advanced by more than 2 years, then PMH will be underestimated (see TANNER, 39). Psychologically these children may be handicapped for a long period, and we have seen several of them with psychological problems at school and at home. The boy illustrated in fig. 6 had problems at school, was difficult to handle at home and had enuresis nocturna. There was a remarkable improvement in this situation during treatment.

Another example of this group is shown in fig. 7. This patient had always been small for his age, but his growth velocity, plotted against chronological age, was normal. Since the age of 9 6/12 years he has been treated for diabetes mellitus with insulin and a regular diet. At 10 8/12 years his height age was 8 6/12 years and bone age 6 6/12 years. There were serious psychological problems at home and at school, and it became difficult to control his diabetes. He was treated with ethylestrenol for 1 6/12 years (0.1—0.2 mg/kg/day). Meanwhile psychiatric treatment of the boy and his family was undertaken (Dr. SANDERS-WOUDSTRA, Dept. Child Psychiatry, State University, Groningen). There was remarkable improvement in the general condition of the boy. He gained 14.5 cm and 10 kg during 1 6/12 years and he grew more muscular. Diabetes was controlled more easily and his school results improved dramatically. At 13 years his bone age was also 13 years, and there were signs of puberty. During therapy predicted adult height fell from 186 cm to 176 cm. This loss in height is also evident from the curve for velocity per year of bone age.

Treatment with ethylestrenol in this type of patients may move the onset of puberty to an earlier age without a significant change in adult stature. Puberty, indicated by the first period in girls (menarche) has moved along the age axis to an earlier age during the last century. Since ± 1850 a difference of 4½ year has been observed in several West-European countries. Children are much taller at earlier ages, but ultimate adult height is not as different as it has been calculated (26). Better nutrition and disappearance of chronic infections have been regarded as important causes for this 'secular trend'.

It is highly interesting that in these children with retarded growth and adolescence, who represent the general pattern of growth one

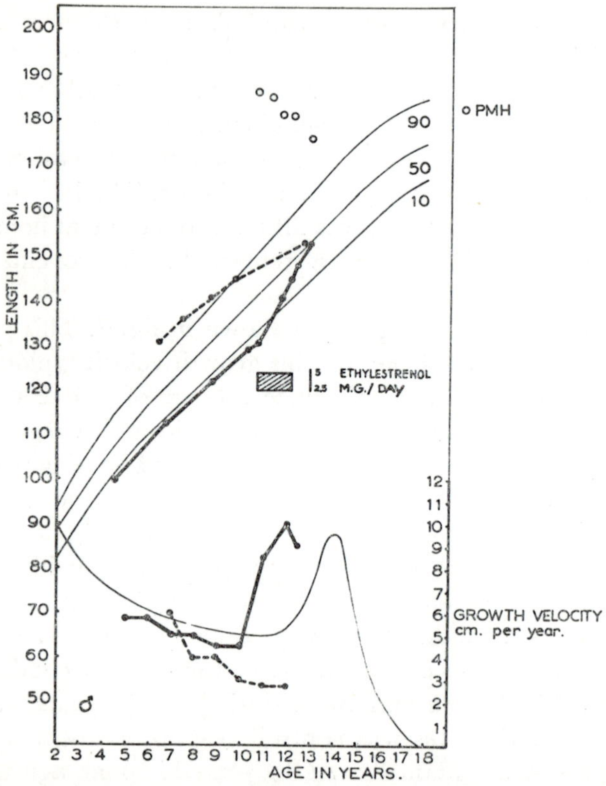

Fig. 7. Growth curves and growth velocity curves of a boy with 'constitutional delay in growth and adolescence' and diabetes mellitus, treated with ethylestrenol (Orgabolin). Curves plotted against chronological age (•—•) and skeletal age (•----•). See text. PMH = predicted mature height

hundred years ago, anabolic steroids can move the onset of puberty to an earlier age. We believe that treatment of these children with anabolic steroids is indicated when it is not desirable to wait until natural puberty starts, e.g. when there are psychological problems.

Testosterone and anabolic steroids have a stimulating effect on

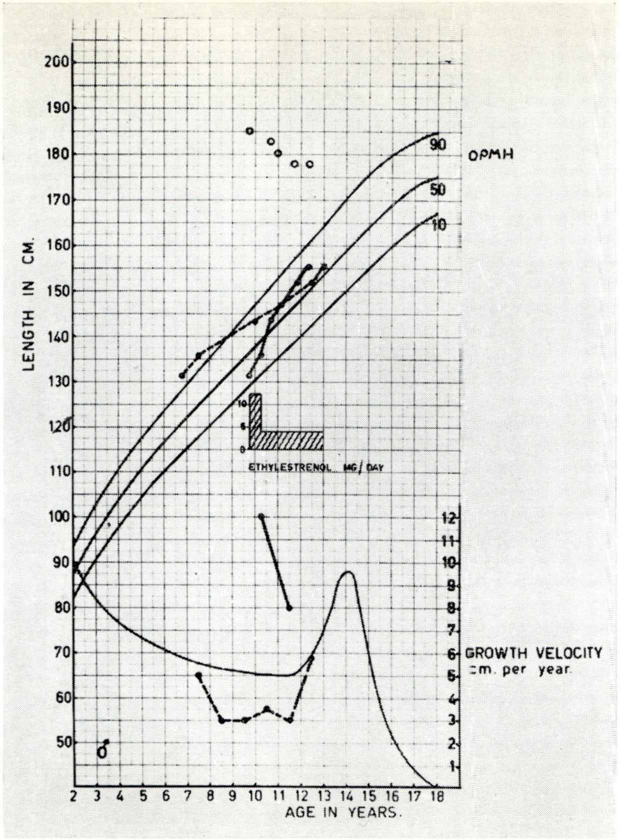

Fig. 8. Growth curves and growth velocity curves of a boy with 'constitutional delay in growth and adolescence' and aplastic anaemia, treated with ethylestrenol (Orgabolin). Curves plotted against chronological age (●——●) and skeletal age (●·······●). See text. PMH = predicted mature height

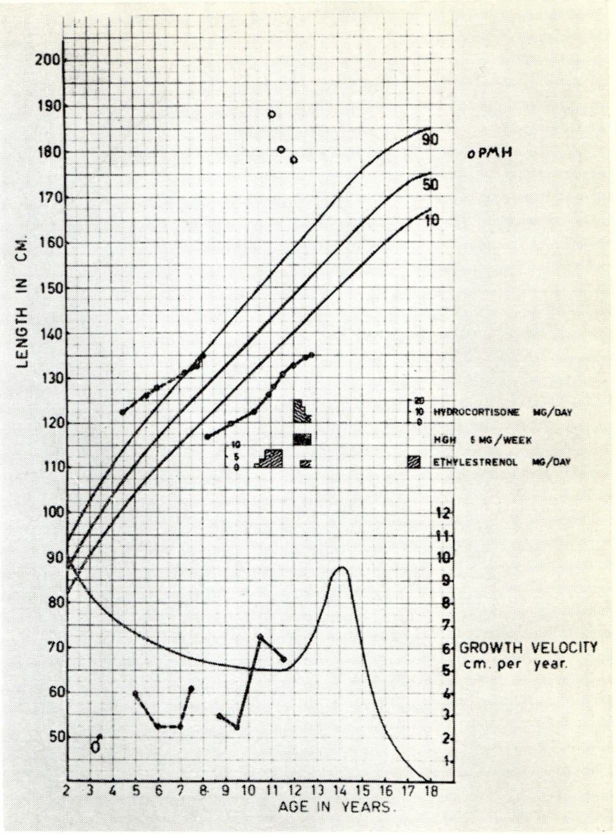

Fig. 9. Growth curves and growth velocity curves of a boy with idiopathic pituitary insufficiency, treated with ethylestrenol (Orgabolin). Curves plotted against chronological age (●——●) and skeletal age (●·······●). See text. PMH = predicted mature height

erythropoiesis, and have been used successfully in the treatment of some types of congenital or acquired aplastic anaemia, sometimes in combination with corticosteroids (34, 35). Fig. 8 illustrates growth of a boy with aplastic anaemia, treated for more than 2 6/12 years with ethylestrenol. At the age of 9 10/12 years his height was just above the 10th percentile, his bone age was 6 9/12 years. During ethylestrenol treatment the haemoglobin concentration rose in a few months' time from 6.5 to 12—13 g/100 ml. Blood transfusions were no longer needed. Leucocytopenia and thrombocytopenia were much less influenced. Over a period of 2 years his height increased 20 cm, weight 11.6 kg. Growth velocity plotted against bone age shows a loss in height between 8 and 12 years, and a normal growth velocity between 12 and 13 years. Consequently PMH decreased somewhat but stays now at 178 cm. These patients have to be followed carefully to see what PMH predictions actually mean in those cases.

As long as human growth hormone is not available in sufficient amounts, children with hypopituitarism can be treated with androgenic steroids. Results of treatment of such patients with testosterone have been reported by Van der Werff ten Bosch (42) and with anabolic steroids by Prader (28) and Prader and Illig (30). In our opinion treatment with testosterone should be avoided as long as bone age is less than about 13 years. Treatment with anabolic steroids should be preferred under those conditions and will advance bone maturation less, in comparison with height, than testosterone. When bone age has become about 13 years, testosterone can be used in male patients. We have treated 3 boys with idiopathic hypopituitarism with ethylestrenol. Fig. 9 shows the results in one patient. On a dose of 0.1—0.2 mg/kg/day for 14 months, height increased by 8.5 cm. However bone age increased 2 6/12 years, and both the growth velocity per year of bone age, and PMH, indicate a 'loss in height' during this period. In the two other boys similar effects were observed. Stimulation of growth cannot always be expected in children with pituitary insufficiency. In some patients operated for craniopharyngeoma minimal effects of anabolic steroids have been observed by Prader (30) and the theory has been advanced that anabolic steroids are not effective in the absence of growth hormone (11, 30, 36).

Anabolic steroids have had little if any growth stimulating effect in children with so-called primordial dwarfism (14, 16, 30). This is an ill-defined group of small children, including 'low birth weight dwarfism', children with congenital anomalities and other types.

We like to emphasize that at this moment no definite conclusions can be made on the use and the indications of anabolic steroids in the treatment of children with retarded growth. Virilizing symptoms of anabolic steroids are enlargement of penis and clitoris, erections, appearance of pubic hair, and deepening of the voice. These symptoms are clearly time and dose dependent. Deepening of the voice is a very undesirable virilizing symptom in girls and further work has to be done on the possible reversibility of this effect (33).

In higher doses the production of pituitary gonadotropins may become suppressed, but PRADER and ILLIG have reported that such steroid-induced gonadal atrophy, even of several months' duration, is completely reversible (30).

Increased serum levels of bilirubin, transaminase and lactic dehydrogenase have been described, indicating liver damage (2, 22). Anabolic steroids may cause gynaecomastia in boys (17). Methandrostenolone, given to adults in a dose of 0.2 mg/kg/day interfered with the production or release of ACTH and the metabolism of hydrocortisone (15, 49). Recently VERMEULEN has found that ethylestrenol inhibits the metabolism of hydrocortisone in the liver (40).

We have observed minimal virilizing symptoms in some patients when ethylestrenol was given over a period of several months in a dose of 0.1 mg/kg/day. In a dose of 0.2 mg/kg/day virilizing symptoms were more pronounced. Serum bilirubine and transaminase levels were always normal.

REFERENCES

1. ACHESON, R. M. and G. ZAMPA, Skeletal maturation in ovarian dysgenesis and Turner's syndrome, *Lancet* I: 917, 1961.
2. ARIAS, I. M., The effects of anabolic steroids on liver function, *Ciba symp. on Protein Metabolism*, Springer Verlag, Berlin, Germany, p. 131, 1963.
3. BAYER, L. M. and N. BAYLEY, *Growth diagnosis*, The University of Chicago Press, Chicago, Ill., U.S.A., 1949.
4. BAYER, L. M. and N. BAYLEY, Growth pattern shifts in healthy children: spontaneous and induced, *J. Pediat.* 62: 631, 1963.
5. BAYLEY, N. and S. R. PINNEAU, Tables for predicting adult height from skeletal age, revised for use with the Greulich-Pyle hand standards, *J. Pediat.* 40: 423, 1952.

6. BIERICH, J. R., Effects and side-effects of the therapy with anabolic steroids in children, *Het Hormoon* XXV: 55, 1961.
7. BIERICH, J. R.. L. FISCHER and B. BECKER, Clinical and pathogenetic differences in constitutional growth disturbances and their response to anabolic steroids, *Abstracts Xe Intern. Congress Ped.*, p. 280. Lisbon, 1962.
8. BLODGETT, F. M., L. BURGIN, D. IEZZONI, D. GRIBETZ and B. N. TALBOT, Effects of prolonged cortisone therapy on the statural growth, skeletal maturation and metabolic status of children, *New Engl. J. Med.* 254: 636, 1956.
9. BONGIOVANNI, A. M., Anabolic drugs to promote growth, *Pediatrics* 27: 519, 1961.
10. DAVID, K., E. DINGEMANSE, J. FREUD and E. LAQUEUR, Über Kristallinisches mannliches Hormon aus Hoden (Testosteron), wirksamer als aus Harn oder aus Cholesterin bereitetes Androsteron, *Ztschr. f. Physiol. Chem.* 233: 218, 1935.
11. DESAULLES, P. A. and C. KRAEHENBUHL, Differentiation of action of various anabolic steroids, *Ciba symp. on Protein Metabolism*, Springer Verlag, Berlin, Germany, p. 170, 1963.
12. FERRIER, P., T. H. SHEPARD II and E. K. SMITH, Growth disturbances and values for hormone excretion in various forms of precocious sexual development, *Pediatrics* 28: 258, 1961.
13. GREULICH, W. W. and S. I. PYLE, *Radiographic atlas of skeletal development of the hand and wrist*, Stanford University Press, Calif., U.S.A., 1959.
14. HUBBLE, D. and D. R. MACMILLAN, A study of growth promotion in children, *Arch. Dis. Childh.* 37: 518, 1962.
15. JAMES, V. H. T., J. LANDON and V. WYNN, Effect of an anabolic steroid (methandienone) on metabolism of cortisol in the human, *J. Endocrinol.* 25: 21, 1962.
16. LARON, Z., Effectiveness of fluoxymesterone on linear growth and weight in children with growth retardation and underweight, *Acta Endocrinol.* 36: 541, 1961.
17. LARON, Z., Breast development induced by methandrostenolone (Dianabol), *J. Clin. Endocrinol. and Metab.* 22: 450, 1962.
18. LARON, Z., Use of fluoxymesterone in the treatment of growth retardation, *Acta Paediat.* 52: 465, 1963.
19. LARON, Z., Discussion on use of anabolic agents in disorders of growth, *Ciba symp. on Protein Metabolism*, Springer Verlag, Berlin, Germany, p. 398, 1963.
20. LARON, Z. and S. GITTER, Anabolic steroids: their clinical use and specific dangers in pediatrics, *Clin. Pediatrics* 2: 594, 1963.
21. LIPSETT, M. B., Decreased adrenal androgen biosynthesis in patients with gonadal dysgenesis, *J. Clin. Endocrinol. and Metab.* 22: 119, 1962.
22. MARQUARDT, G. H., C. I. FISHER, P. LEVY and R. M. DOWBEN, Effect of anabolic steroids on liver function tests and creatine excretion, *J. Amer. Med. Ass.* 175: 85, 1961.
23. MELLMAN, W. J., A. M. BONGIOVANNI, M. GARRISON and D. D. STEIKER, Comparison of fluoxymesterone and methyltesterone as growth stimulants, *Pediatrics* 28: 525, 1961.
24. MIGEON, C. J., Comment on study of eight cases of isolated precocious pilosity or 'premature pubarche', *The Yearbook of Pediatrics*, 1962—1963, Yearbook Med. Publ., Chicago, p. 354.
25. NEW, M., P. PITT and R. E. PETERSON, Testosterone production in a 3-year-old male with isosexual precocity, *J. Pediat.* 63: 703, 1963 (abstract Society for Pediatric Research, 33rd Annual Meeting, 1963).
26. OPPERS, V. M., *Analyse van de acceleratie van de menselijke lengtegroei door bepaling van het tijdstip van de groeifasen*, Proefschrift, Amsterdam, 1963.

27. Overbeek, G. A., A. Delver and J. de Visser, Pharmacological comparisons of anabolic steroids (ethylestrenol, nandrolone esters), *Het Hormoon* XXV: 43, 1961.
28. Prader, A., The influence of anabolic steroids on growth, *Het Hormoon* XXV: 53, 1961.
29. Prader, A., Personal communication.
30. Prader, A. and R. Illig, Use of anabolic agents in disorders of growth, *Ciba symp. on Protein Metabolism*, Springer Verlag, Berlin, Germany, p. 383, 1963.
31. Prader, A., J. M. Tanner and G. A. von Harnack, Catch-up growth following illness or starvation, *J. Pediat.* 62: 646, 1963.
32. Reilly, W. A. and G. S. Gordan, Dissociation of growth-stimulating and skeleton-maturing actions of the synthetic androgen, fluoxymesterone, *J. Pediat.* 159: 188, 1961.
33. Shadidi, N. T., Personal communication, 1964.
34. Shadidi, N. T. and L. K. Diamond, Testosterone-induced remission in aplastic anemia, *Am. J. Dis. Child.* 98: 293, 1959.
35. Shadidi, N. T. and L. K. Diamond, Testosterone-induced remission in aplastic anemia of both acquired and congenital types, *New Engl. J. Med.* 264: 953, 1961.
36. Simpson, M. E., C. W. Asling and H. M. Evans, Some endocrine influences on skeletal growth and differentiation, *Yale J. Biol. Med.* 23: 1, 1950.
37. Sobel, E. H., Comment on ref. 32, *The Yearbook of Pediatrics*, 1962—1963, Yearbook Med. Publ., Chicago, U.S.A., p. 355.
38. Sobel, E. H., C. S. Raymond, K. B. Quinn and N. B. Talbot, Use of methyltestosterone to stimulate growth: relative influence on skeletal maturation and linear growth, *J. Clin. Endocrinol. and Metab.* 16: 241, 1956.
39. Tanner, J. M., *Growth at adolescence*, 2nd ed., Blackwell Scientific Publ., Oxford, England, 1962.
40. Vermeulen, A., Influence des stéroides anabolisants sur l'axe hypophyso-surrénalin chez l'homme, *Societa Italiana di' Endocrinologica, X Congresso Nationale*, Paria.
41. Werff ten Bosch, J. J. van der, *Normale en abnormale geslachtsrijping*, Universitaire Pers Leiden, The Netherlands, 1959.
42. Idem, Hypophysaire dwerggroei, *N. T. v. G.* 106: 1282, 1961.
43. Werff ten Bosch, J. J. van der and R. Enthoven, De normale lengtegroei, *N. T. v. G.* 108: 1174, 1964.
44. Werff ten Bosch, J. J. van der and R. Enthoven, The healthy tall child and its adult stature in the press.
45. Whitelaw, M. J., S. F. Thomas, W. H. Graham and T. N. Foster, Growth response in gonadal dysgenesis to the anabolic nonethrandrolone, *Am. J. Obstet. Gynaec.* 84: 501, 1962.
46. Wilkins, L., Dwarfism, in: *Current Therapy*, ed. H. F. Conn, W. B. Saunders, Phil., U.S.A., 1956.
47. Wilkins, L., *The diagnosis and treatment of endocrine disorders in childhood and adolescence*, C. Thomas Publ. Springfield, Ill., U.S.A., 1957.
48. De Wijn, J. F. and J. H. de Haas, *Groeidiagrammen van 1—25 jarigen in Nederland*, Nederlands Instituut voor Praeventieve Geneeskunde, Leiden, The Netherlands, 1960.

49. Wyn, V., J. Landon and V. H. T. James, Effect of an anabolic steroid (methandienone) on pituitary-adrenal function in the human, *J. Endocrinol.* 25: 199, 1962.
50. Zurbrügg, R. P. and L. I. Gardner, Urinary C 19 steroids in two girls with precocious sexual hair, *J. Clin. Endocrinol. and Metab.* 23: 704, 1963.

EFFECTS OF ANDROGENS ON THE GROWTH OF RATS*

EDNA H. SOBEL

The search for an agent appropriate for treating children with short stature must consider its effect on skeletal maturation as well as on linear growth, since an increase in mature stature is to be expected only if an increase in rate of linear growth is not offset by a greater acceleration of skeletal maturation (8, 10, 13, 14, 15). Children with virilizing disorders are giants in infancy but, if untreated, dwarfed adults. Another example of this situation is shown in figure 1. This little boy, a patient at the Children's Cancer Research Foundation in Boston, had true sexual precocity. At the age of 3 years his height-age was 6 years and his bone-age was 12 years. The risk of short stature in adult life as a consequence of androgen therapy is, I believe, real although of lesser degree than one can anticipate for a patient with sexual precocity.

Many years of carefully planned studies are required to determine whether any of the modified androgens, hopefully designated as anabolic agents by their manufacturers, are indeed able to increase the adult stature of children (10). Dr. VAN DER WERFF TEN BOSCH (see p. 269) has discussed the fallacy of attempts to equate increase in the weight of the levator ani muscle of castrated male rats with 'anabolic' potency of a synthetic steroid (3, 7; 11). This effect must indeed be considered an indication of androgenic potency, for androgens promote growth of the levator ani even in animals on a protein-free diet while other muscles, such as the diaphragm, fail to grow (9). The end-point used for androgenic action in the screening tests of the pharmaceutical houses, increase in weight of the seminal vesicle of the castrated rat, also provides evidence of androgenic potency. So the ratio of these

* Funds for this project were supplied by the Public Health Service, National Institutes of Health (NIH HD 01204).

two actions in male rats cannot provide the information needed for selecting compounds that might be useful in the treatment of short stature in childhood. We need to know whether a compound is able to increase rate of linear growth without advancing skeletal maturation or virilizing the child. Experiments in animals, using these same criteria, might be of some advantage in selecting drugs to be used in children. Most investigators have been unable to demonstrate an effect of androgens on the epiphyseal cartilage of rodents. However, in 1941 SILBERBERG and SILBERBERG described histologic evidence of accelerated atrophy and disintegration of epiphyseal cartilage of growing mice treated with testosterone propionate (12). Accelerated skeletal maturation of newborn mice treated with several androgenic compounds has been reported recently (4). Our own first efforts with testosterone propionate in nursing rats yielded negative results, but we then found that it advanced the skeletal maturation of older rats, treated from the 28th to the 70th day of life (6); figure 2 shows this effect.

Having achieved this encouraging result, we went on to do more detailed studies, using pair-fed weanling female litter-mate rats. The experimental design, method of evaluating skeletal maturation, and other technical details have been described (5, 6). Testosterone propionate was injected subcutaneously on alternate days in 0.1 ml of sesame oil; control animals received only sesame oil. The doses used were 0.25, 1.0, 2.5 or 6.0 mg/kg/day, given from the 28th until the 70th day, when the animals were killed. The results are shown in figure 3, where they are represented as differences between the treated animal and its control litter-mate. Skeletal maturation is expressed as difference in number of maturity points between treated and control litter-mates; maturity points are derived from the number of epiphyseal fusions. Open circles indicate differences significantly different from zero, at $p = 0.05$ or 0.01. The *body weight* of the treated animals was progressively and significantly increased at all doses greater than 0.25 mg/kg/day; there was no further increase in weight above the dose of 2.5 mg/kg/day (figure 3, E). The length of the *tibia* and of the *radius* was significantly longer in the animals given 1.0 mg/kg/day; there was no effect from either smaller or larger doses (figure 3, A and B). The lengths of the 3rd metatarsal and 3rd metacarpal bones

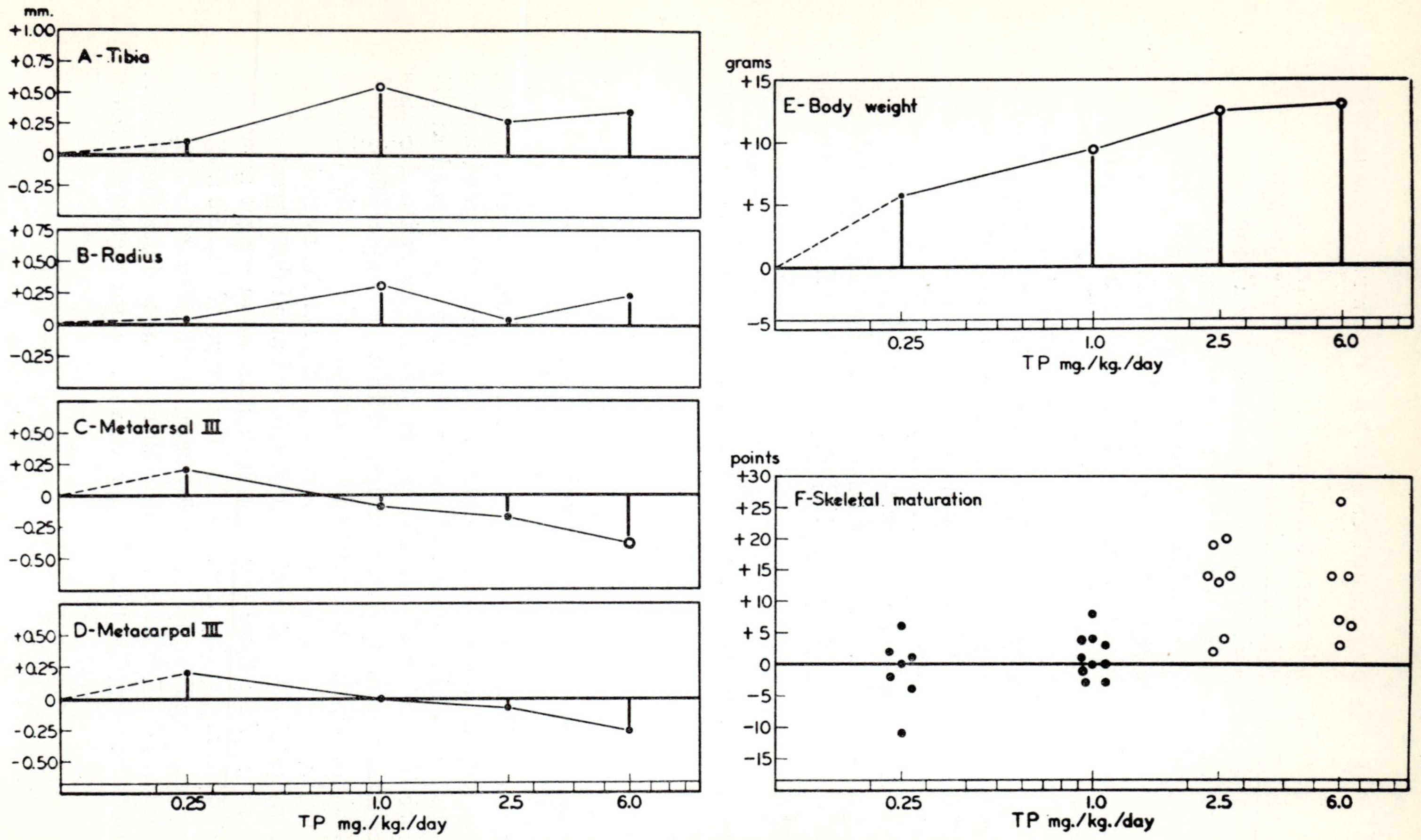

Fig. 3. Effect of testosterone propionate on body weight, length of individual bones and skeletal maturation of female rats at age 70 days. Results are represented as differences between treated animals and their control litter-mates. Open circles represent differences significantly different from zero (at $p = 0.05$ or 0.01)

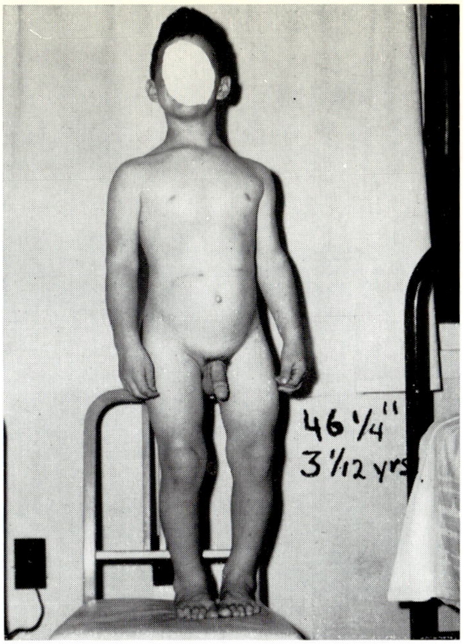

Fig. 1. Photograph of patient with true sexual precocity. At age $3^1/_{12}$ height-age was 6 years and bone-age 12 years. Patient of the Children's Cancer Research Foundation, Boston

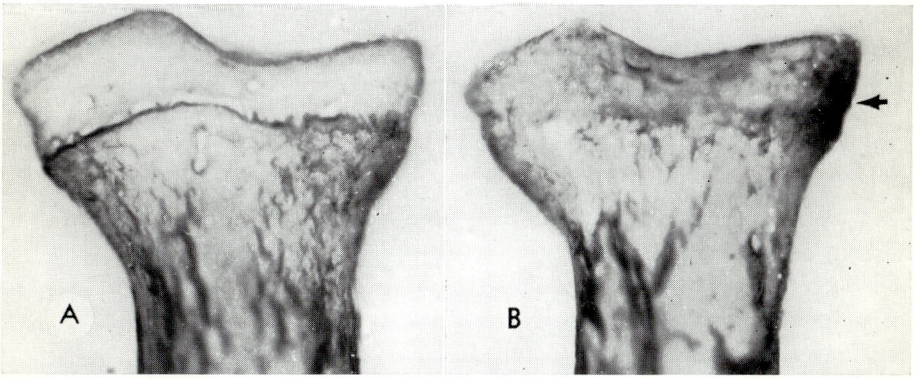

Fig. 2. Photographs of proximal epiphysis of radius; intact bones cleared and stained with Alizarin Red S. Female rats, 70 days old. A. Untreated animal, B. Litter-mate given 2.5 mg/kg/day testosterone propionate from 28 days. Reprinted with permission from reference 6, fig. 1

suggested an increase in the animals receiving low doses and a decrease with the larger doses; there was a significant decrease in the length of the *3rd metatarsal* in the animals treated with 6.0 mg/kg/day (figure 3, C and D). Skeletal maturation was significantly advanced by either 2.5 or 6.0 mg/kg/day (figure 3, F).

As Dr. VAN DER SLUYS VEER explained (see p. 52), rats can grow at the knee and wrist after growth at the elbow and ankle has ceased. The radius and tibia each have two epiphyses, one of which, (proximal radius and distal tibia) fuses at 65 to 100 days, while the other remains open much longer (2). The growth characteristics of the tubular bones of the paws are different: the 3rd metacarpal completes its growth at about 70 days (1) and epiphyseal fusion is complete approximately 20 to 30 days later (5). Growth of the 3rd metatarsal follows a similar pattern, with obliteration of the epiphysis at 90 to 110 days (5). We interpreted these results, which have been published in detail (6), as indicating that 1.0 mg/kg/day stimulated rate of growth without increasing rate of skeletal maturation in the 6 weeks of treatment; we do not know what would have happened had treatment been continued. The decreased length of the 3rd metatarsal with the largest dose given indicated that any stimulus to growth was negated by accelerated maturation of its single epiphysis.

One might think we had demonstrated that an appropriate dose of testosterone propionate had been found, that its effects on growth and skeletal maturation can be separated. I would like to emphasize that we did not interpret the findings in this way. The conditions of our studies permitted only the conclusion that the system could be used for evaluation of potentially useful drugs in terms of the criteria that are relevant to their use in patients. We already knew that testosterone is not good for the child and wanted to find out whether it also is not good for the rat. We have tested some compounds that seem more promising for the rat than testosterone, but cannot possibly say that they will therefore be suitable for children. An interesting aspect of our experiments is an acromegalic appearance in the treated rats. Perhaps the mechanism of enhanced growth includes increased production of somatotrophin. The experimental design, with all its limitations, offers the possibility of investigating several aspects of mammalian growth.

REFERENCES

1. Becks, H., C. W. Asling, D. A. Collins, M. E. Simpson and H. E. Evans, Changes with increasing age in the ossification of the third metacarpal of the female rat, *Anat. Rec.* 100: 577, 1948.
2. Dawson, A. B., The age order of epiphyseal union in the long bones of the albino rat, *Anat. Rec.* 31: 1, 1925.
3. Eisenberg, E. and G. S. Gordan, The levator ani muscle of the rat as an index of myotrophic activity of steroidal hormones, *J. Pharmacol. Exp. Ther.* 99: 38, 1950.
4. Howard, E., Steroids and bone maturation in infant mice: relative activities of dehydroepiandrosterone and testosterone, *Endocrinology* 70: 131, 1962.
5. Joss, E. E., E. H. Sobel and K. A. Zuppinger, Skeletal maturation in rats with special reference to order and time of epiphyseal closure, *Endocrinology* 72: 117, 1963.
6. Joss, E. E., K. A. Zuppinger and E. H. Sobel, Effect of testosterone propionate and methyl testosterone on growth and skeletal maturation in rats, *Endocrinology* 72: 123, 1963.
7. Kochakian, C. D., Mechanisms of androgen actions, *Lab. Invest.* 8: 538, 1959.
8. Laron, Z., see p. 281.
9. Nimni, M. E. and E. Geiger, Non-suitability of levator ani method as an index of anabolic effect of steroids, *Proc. Soc. Exp. Biol. Med.* 94: 606, 1957.
10. Prader, A., The influence of anabolic steroids on growth, *Acta Endocrin.*, Suppl. 63: 78, 1962.
11. Russell, J. A. and A. E. Wilhelmi, Growth (hormonal regulation), *Ann. Rev. Physiol.* 20: 43, 1958.
12. Silberberg, M. and R. Silberberg, Response of cartilage and bone of growing mice to testosterone propionate, *Arch. Pathol.* 32: 85, 1941.
13. Sobel, E. H., C. S. Raymond, K. V. Quinn and N. B. Talbot, The use of methyltestosterone to stimulate growth; relative influence on skeletal maturation and linear growth, *J. Clin. Endocrin.* 16: 241, 1956.
14. Van der Werff ten Bosch, J. J., see p. 269.
15. Visser, H. K. A., see p. 290.

DISCUSSION

Marshall: The rate of growth in the normal child is constantly decreasing, with the exception of the period of the adolescent spurt. We don't know what controls this pattern of growth. I should like to hear Prof. PRADER's opinion as to whether the decreasing rate of growth under treatment with human growth hormone might reflect the fact that whatever mechanism controls the normal growth curve is still functioning in those children whose rate of growth has declined during treatment with growth hormone.

Prader: I cannot give you the exact answer, but I would like to point out that in patients who develop high titers of antibodies, there is no growth response at all, right from the beginning. Patients who show a progressive decline in their response, sometimes develop antibodies. We favour the hypothetical explanation, that this represents insufficient catch-up. If you study a hypothyroid patient who is put on thyroid treatment you see the same thing. First, for a short period, you can see a tremendous acceleration of growth, and then growth slows down. Now, the amount of catch-up is dose-dependent, and it may be that our dose is then too low.

Stoelinga: Dr. HAAK showed that during administration of human growth hormone weight is gained, and that after stopping this hormone the weight goes down. In fact, however, the weight gain stopped already during treatment. Dr. HAAK said that the weight loss is possibly caused by mobilization of fat. Prof. PRADER, have you in your long-term experiments seen a loss of fat tissue in these children, or does this occur only in adults.

Prader: I am sorry to say that we have not adequately studied this problem. We did not measure skin folds. The patients looked as if they lost fat. Since they gain muscle weight, the weight alone does not mean anything.

Thomson: I should like to ask Dr. VAN DER WERFF TEN BOSCH why adolescence is so often associated with acne, and with infectious lesions. This may seem a trivial problem but it causes a great deal of misery, and is difficult to treat.

A question to Dr. HAAK. I understood from what he said that in some cases the administration of growth hormone resulted in the retention of large quantities of nitrogen. This was equated to the nitrogen content of muscle tissue, and it was implied that the increase of body weight was attributable to increase of muscle. In one of the diagrams, the increase of weight was nearly 3 kg. Surely such a gain, occurring over a relatively short period of time, could not possibly be due to muscle? Muscle is meat, and I do not think it anatomically possible that such subjects could lay down 3 kg of new meat.

Van der Werff ten Bosch: All I know about acne is that their occurrence requires the presence of functioning sebaceous glands and that the latter condition is testosterone-dependent (see: HAMILTON, J. B., *J. Clin. Endocr.* 1: 570, 1941; RONY, H. R. and S. J. ZAKON, *Arch. Derm. Syph.* 48: 601, 1943).

Acne can be produced by testosterone and it is logical to assume that in normal boys they are produced by testosterone. Why they disappear again at later ages, is a different question, that I cannot answer. Establishment of a new hormonal dynamic state? (see also the Annotation, *Lancet* 2: 26, 1964, and: ANDREWS, G. C., *Medical Clinics of North America* 49: 737, 1965).

Laron: I think that we have evidence that corticosteroids have some effect on acne. This may be a permissive action and does not imply that testosterone is not needed to produce acne.

Haak: STRAUSS and PUCHI (*Proc. of the Snd. Int. Congr. of End.* 1964, p. 407) have developed a technique for the measurement of androgenicity of drugs that is based on the production of sebum from the sebaceous glands of the forehead. Dr. THOMSON, all the calculations of the workers who have studied the nitrogen balance, are based on the assumptions of ALBRIGHT and REIFENSTEIN (*J. Clin. Endocr.* 5: 367, 1945) The water content of muscle is approximately 80 %. I don't know where the retained nitrogen is going in the body. I should like to ask Dr. PRADER whether it is correct that during the treatment with human growth hormone the muscular apparatus develops.

Prader: That is my clinical impression, but I can not prove it. Creatine excretion usually goes down in patients who receive growth hormone. This is something very interesting. It depends how high creatine excretion is before the treatment. The higher it is, the more it comes down. However, the patients were on their own diet, rigidly constant, but individual. And I don't know how much creatine was in each patient's diet.

Haak: Where is the retained nitrogen deposited during the growth caused by administered growth hormone? We have looked at acromegalic patients. Acromegaly is a complicated disease, for instance by hypogonadism. We have never observed excessive muscular strength in acromegalic patients. I do not know whether muscles can indeed increase in size under the influence of growth hormone.

Sobel: I would like to ask Prof. PRADER about his procedure for performing insulin tolerance tests in children suspected of having hypopituitarism. Have you ever encountered any difficulty when giving 4 units/m^2 intravenously to the patient? What precaution do you advise?

Prader: I know that a problem is involved here. We give the full dosage, because otherwise we cannot compare the results. And we have glucose ready, formerly we had adrenalin, now we have glucagon ready. We have seen patients become unconscious, and twice we have had a convulsion, in which cases glucose is given intravenously. The doctor who performs the test always remains on the spot to do whatever is necessary.

Querido: I would like to ask Dr. PRADER whether he carries out growth hormone determinations in the blood of the patients before he starts treatment. The diagnosis of hypopituitary dwarfism is so difficult, we feel, that now the determination is available, it would be nice to check it in that way.

Prader: There is so much progress in this field that one is always behind. First we did not determine growth hormone. Then we did it by the Read method and were happy about it, and then we realized that the method is bad. Then Dr. TOUBER assayed the growth hormone level of some of our patients radio-immunologically and found zero values. Now we know that this does not mean anything, because you should do the assay after having given insulin, so finally my answer is we have not done what could according to our present knowledge have been done. But I think that the nitrogen retention effect is a standardized metabolic test for growth hormone. I think this test has offered us some diagnostic help. If you get a high increase in nitrogen retention, it supports the diagnosis hypopituitary dwarfism or pituitary insufficiency, and a low increase in nitrogen retention argues against these diagnoses.

Laron: When studying the metabolic effects of growth hormone, the most striking finding is the extremely fast increase in free fatty acids in the blood. I wonder if the nitrogen retention could also be detected early enough, if adequate technical facilities were available.

Another finding which is interesting and cannot be explained, is the calciuria in patients treated with growth hormone. I would like to ask whether anybody would like to suggest a working theory of the action of growth hormone or the androgens, with the metabolic data available at present.

Prader: In our hands there has been about the same hypercalciuria in hypopituitary as in control patients that were given growth hormone. So, in contrast to the nitrogen retaining effect, we could not find a difference between these two groups of patients and controls, and as far as I know others have had the same experience. I also think that there is no difference between hypopituitary patients and controls, in the increase of free fatty acids, when growth hormone is given. Isn't that correct?

Laron: Generally speaking there seem to be certain patients who respond differently as to the free fatty acid mobilization. We have some data on that; but interpretation is difficult because the resting level of free fatty acids, are different and the question always arises as to how one should express the data.

Sobel: I should like to go back to the question of insulin tolerance tests in patients suspected of hypopituitarism, because I think the test is really risky without all the precautions Prof. PRADER mentioned. We often are able to demonstrate an impairment in insulin tolerance by giving 2 units/m^2 intravenously, and sometimes with as little as 1 unit/m^2. I realize that this precaution might require the performance of a second test in a suspected patient who responds with an adequate rise in blood sugar at the end of 90 minutes. However, I wonder if it might not be wiser to do this than to run the risk of severe and prolonged hypoglycaemia if one does not have a supply of glucagon and a physician who can sit with and take adequate care of the patient throughout the test. On one occasion I saw hypoglycemic coma persist for several hours despite every therapeutic effort in a well-equipped children's hospital. Fortunately, the patient eventually made a satisfactory recovery.

Prader: I fully agree with you, Dr. SOBEL.

Querido: Some strong opinions on anabolic steroids that I had, and which I wanted to express after the earlier papers that have been presented, have been more or less weakened by the beautiful presentation of Dr. SOBEL. She has actually succeeded, in a very confused field, to pin-point precisely what we are looking for. The confusion in the field shows how difficult it is to get away from the bias created in the past. I think the bias is introduced by this word anabolic, just as it is introduced by applying the term catabolic to cortisone. Anabolic and catabolic are words that are related to metabolic events in an overall organism or in a tissue, but they need to be defined. Cortisone is catabolic in a number of tissues in the sense that it decreases the amount of tissue, but anabolic in other tissues like the liver and the intestinal tract. So in using the term anabolic one implies that from the fact that certain steroids cause nitrogen retention, it follows that every pool of protein metabolism, and every reaction in the body, should be in an anabolic condition. I think this absolutely confusing, and the only terminology we like to use is based on the pharmacological results, that is that we infer that most of the compounds that have been tested on the levator ani muscle can cause nitrogen retention, as has been shown in experiments. Therefore you just have to do away with all terminology, and use the term nitrogen retaining steroids.

The second confusing term is: side-effects. Side-effects are no side-effects. They are inherent to the natural action of testosterone. They are just part of the pattern of the reaction to testosterone. This does not mean that we cannot obtain compounds that are devoid of certain actions of testosterone, because the pattern of action of testosterone in an organism is brought about by the affinity of certain tissues to this preparation. But theoretically it seems possible to make steroids in the laboratory that are devoid of an action on some tissues, while maintaining the effects on other tissues. So the term side-effects should be dismissed. One can say that a compound is nitrogen retaining, and has an affinity for certain tissues. Dr. SOBEL came just the other way around. She did away with all of the original story and she said, and I think this is the only right way, that we can probably make pharmacological agents that have certain properties; so she went to look for the pharmacological end-points which correspond with those she wants to study in a child. Of course she stated extremely cautiously that the end-points she was studying in the rat, are not necessarily the end-points properly comparable to those that she is concerned with in a child.

To give you an idea of how confused the situation is, I shall recount some work by KASSENAAR, in this department. He has shown very clearly and elegantly, that by varying the time of injection and the dose of testosterone, one can obtain any androgenic-anabolic ratio that one desires. It is possible thus to design an experiment from which testosterone appears to be a beautiful anabolic agent. There is for us only one conclusion, to be scientifically honest, to do away with all words that imply something and have no real meaning, but to realize that we are looking for a steroid which has a certain action in the human which may not even be based on one of the natural actions of testosterone. Most of the compounds are selected for an effect on nitrogen retention, and are therefore, if you want to talk about these steroids in a general term, nitrogen retaining steroids. However, nitrogen retention and the promotion of growth that one desires in a child, are not necessarily related. Again I want to congratulate Dr. SOBEL on her experiments because, as far as I can see, they are the best attempt at pin-pointing the problem, even though they may not lead to the finding of the compound for children.

Prader: I think these statements were necessary to clarify the situation. Could I ask you more specifically, Prof. QUERIDO, do you think that there is no real advantage in using the so-called anabolic steroids, that one can just as well use testosterone, provided one uses the right dose; was not that your conclusion?

Querido: No, I don't think so. I could visualize the possibility that you want to induce nitrogen retention. I think that there are, at the moment, a few compounds which can induce nitrogen retention in doses with an androgenic activity which is less than the androgenicity of testosterone doses required for a similar amount of nitrogen to be retained. I think that there may be two, Dianabol and probably Bolasterone. It is certainly true that for nitrogen retention there seem to be synthetic compounds that are less androgenic in the conventional terminology. But I don't think that in the growth promotion field compounds have been formulated and synthesized, of which there is proof that their growth promoting action in the human is better than the growth promoting action of testosterone, on an equal biological level of androgenic activity. Which does not mean that very carefully designed experiments, like those discussed by VISSER and LARON, should not be conducted.

Van der Werff ten Bosch: May I stress the point, that as long as the screening methods in the pharmaceutical laboratories are based on a test which will screen for androgenicity, in other words, as long as they test for effects on the levator ani muscle, and then only continue to study the substances that have an effect on this muscle, there is a good chance that they are throwing away all those substances that we want to have, the substances that are not androgenic at all. The first screening is: are they androgenic or not; and then the secondary screening is: can we by any other test find that they are not androgenic.

This seems to be an enormous waste of time and possibly a waste of substances that could be useful.

Laron: I would like to add to the very useful remarks by Prof. QUERIDO. We should remember that the androgens are protein anabolic and fat catabolic; without using the word protein anabolic, we do not really make this clear. I also agree that the term side-effect is not accurate and I would ask Prof. QUERIDO to agree to use the terms 'desirable effects' and 'undesirable effects'. Concerning the use of testosterone and the less androgenic so-called anabolic drugs in children, I would like to state that under well-controlled conditions and in well-chosen children these drugs are useful. There is no favourable evidence for the use of testosterone in prepubertal children. On the other hand, we have pharmacological evidence that in a growth promoting dose testosterone is more androgenic in children than the newer compounds. We also have some evidence that there are certain conditions or certain ways of treatment in which these anabolic compounds, given for a certain length of time, increase the growth rate without causing virilization.

Querido: I think that words as desirable and undesirable are wrong. We know that nature has developed testosterone. We call such effects of testosterone which counteract the changes caused by orchidectomy, the androgenic effects. We can now make compounds more or less at will, with actions that we choose, and this is the point I think that Dr. SOBEL stressed. She said: I want to have a compound that does this, and I am looking for the pharmacological end-point that could define this compound. Dr. VAN DER WERFF TEN BOSCH has said, in the past we have thrown away a number of compounds because we have been testing on the wrong end-point. Now, of course it is much simpler to do an assay on a levator ani, which gives an answer in 1 or 2 weeks, than to do the more involved experiments such as Dr. SOBEL has carried out. Still, only experiments of the latter type can answer our problems.

Sobel: I think that Dr. LARON asked whether there is any circumstance under which one might use some of the modified androgens successfully in a short child. Is that the question?

Laron: Not exactly. I just asked what would be your personal choice between testosterone and the newer synthetic anabolic compounds, if it is decided that a child should get some treatment.

Sobel: It is a good question, but it is difficult to answer. I have been very reluctant to treat children with short stature just in order to make them larger than nature had perhaps planned them to be. I do not know what is 'normal' height; there is a great deal of variation in height among people who appear to be perfectly normal. I do think that perhaps I have been too conservative in avoiding treatment with androgens. It is certainly possible, for example, that in some normal older boys with retarded adolescence, there may be a psychologic advantage without too great a therapeutic disadvantage in treating them very cautiously. I have been interested and delighted to see the careful work done by others in human beings, although I myself have been unwilling to do it for some years. On the basis of such work it may be possible to define a drug that can be used in essentially healthy short children. I am still not inclined to use these drugs in patients without a very good indication. Aplastic anemia is a good indication; severe short stature which may lead to a very severe handicap in adult life, is a good indication if one cannot find the ideal therapy for the patient. Ideal therapy might be: treatment of renal tubular acidosis, discovery and correction of a disorder in nutrition or in intestinal function. Ideal therapy would include giving somatotrophin to a pituitary dwarf. Such treatment, specific for the patient's disease, would be very much better than use of a growth-stimulating modified androgen, even one without some of the major disadvantages of testosterone. On the whole I think I will continue to be perhaps a little bit more conservative than I should be and will not use such compounds for most short patients, especially when their shortness is of only moderate degree.

Visser: I would like to add to Prof. Querido's statement, concerning two promising drugs. We have now treated a group of patients with Orgabolin and we have found that over short periods there were no indications that the growth velocity per year of bone age was less than the growth velocity per chronological year. Prof. Querido, do you use the terms glucocorticoids and mineralocorticoids? If you give cortisone in a somewhat high dose, it has salt-retaining activity. If you treat a patient with cortisone you might get osteoporosis, you may get short stature. Do you call these effects side-effects?

Querido: I don't call them side-effects. There is much confusion on this in the litterature and in the minds of many people. If you think that a greater activity per mg makes a compound a better drug, it is essential also to look in more detail at the spectrum of biological activities, for instance at the glucocorticoid activity.

Prader: I would like to ask the speakers for their opinion as to whether we alter final (adult) height by giving these steroids. There is no doubt that we increase the height at the moment we give it, but what about the final height?

Visser: I have seen no case, so far, in whom final height was increased. The general pattern is that you move puberty forward. This is a very interesting phenomenon. You get a growth spurt, and you should not give it for too long a time because as bone age advances, natural puberty will start when the bone age is about 12 years.

Prader: Dr. Laron, you stated that this therapy should not be given if bone age is normal or advanced, compared to chronological age. This statement shows that you are afraid of the effect of these steroids, but I don't think there is any scientific basis for that statement.

Laron: I would like to answer your question first. We have no evidence whatsoever that final height is not decreased when more prolonged therapy is given. If we treat a patient for growth retardation, we have to assume that therapy will have to be given for a prolonged period of time, with the exception of cases of delayed adolescence, where treatment for 3 or 6 months results in signs of puberty. Summing up our experience of several years, we find that usually at the beginning of treatment the bone age tends to increase far more than height and therefore if we do not start with a retarded bone age, we cannot be certain that we are not rendering the patient a bad service. We hope that by treating a patient who has a retarded bone age we do not damage the final height. But if we treat patients whose bone age is equal to chronological age with the present drugs, we are prone to ultimately advance the bone age more than we accelerate his linear growth.

Sobel: I really think it is not very important whether one reduces adult height by two or three centimeters in treating a boy with late adolescence. This small difference is probably not at all significant. My conservatism is much more related to treatment of the really short child where there is a possibility that, with treatment, he will be even shorter as an adult. I don't think it matters a great deal for a person who is going to end up, as far as one can tell, within the average range of stature for any population on this planet. Whether such a person ends up two or three centimeters taller or shorter than he would have been without treatment could not be considered of real consequence.

CHAPTER X

GROWTH INHIBITING AGENTS

EFFECTS OF CORTICOSTEROID AND COMBINED CORTICOSTEROID-ANABOLIC THERAPY ON BODY HEIGHT

Z. LARON

In view of the effects that cortisone and its analogues exert on the structure and growth of bones in experimental animals (see p. 63, ref. 9), it is not surprising that the increased endogenous secretion of cortisol in Cushing's syndrome causes impairment of the growth of children with this disease (15, 8). The wide use of cortisone or its more potent derivatives in clinical practice, has yielded ample evidence of the growth suppressing effect of such steroids. Nevertheless, it is astonishing that in comparison to the number of papers written on the use of corticosteroids in diseases of the paediatric age, the number of reports dealing with the adverse effect on growth is very limited. The first to draw attention to this problem were Blodgett et al. (1) who, in 1956, reviewed allergic children — suffering from asthma and eczema — given corticosteroids for pharmacological reasons, and children suffering from pituitary insufficiency, adrenal insufficiency and the adrenogenital syndrome, given corticosteroids as replacement therapy. These authors found that in children normal from an endocrine point of view, doses of cortisone of over 50 mg/m² body surface/day are usually required to reduce the rate of growth, whereas in patients suffering from pituitary insufficiency a dose averaging 20 mg/m²/day of cortisone already reduced the growth rate. Data on asthmatic children requiring prolonged therapy (12, 4, 6) showed that a dose of prednisolone exceeding 6 mg/m²/day induced reduction of the linear growth rate, whereas asthmatic children receiving 50—70 mg cortisone per m²/day grew satisfactorily. It therefore appeared as if the new synthetic steroids (prednisone, methylprednisolone, triamcinolone and fluoprednisolone) were more active than cortisone with regard to linear growth inhibition. Retardation in skull growth by high doses of corticosteroids has also been reported (2). Even excessive use of 1 % hydrocortisone ointment has been found to retard the growth of an infant (7).

When the dose of cortisone which impairs the growth rate is reduced or the treatment is stopped, growth is resumed at a rate faster than before treatment (7) (fig. 1), with the exception of children with pituitary insufficiency, who lack the stimuli for this rebound phenomenon which has been called 'catch-up growth' (13). The child with an adrenal tumour, or the child receiving only one course of corticosteroids such as in many cases of rheumatic fever or nephrotic syn-

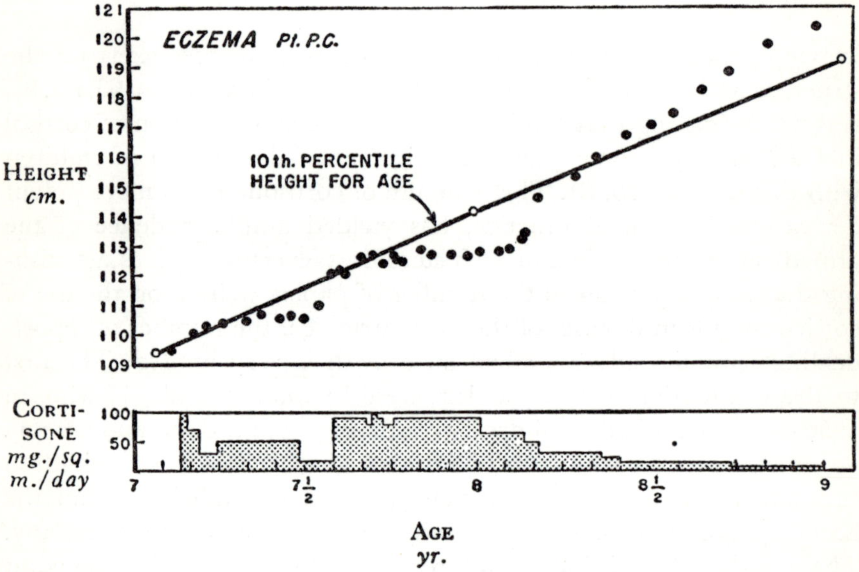

Fig. 1. Growth during various doses of cortisone in a patient with eczema (from 1)

drome, will catch up their previous growth; what is the fate of the child who requires prolonged and repeated treatment with corticosteroids or the child with adrenogenital syndrome requiring continuous therapy? SOBEL stated that 'very small amounts of cortisone, barely adequate to prevent progressive virilism, have a deleterious effect on growth' (14).

One asset favouring the 'catch-up' is the finding that corticosteroids retard skeletal maturation simultaneously with the growth retardation (1).

A good recovery in height would require that the catch-up in height is not less than that in skeletal age; increased growth hormone secretion for a longer period of time could play a role here. However, there is not enough data available to answer the question what actually happens to the ratio: 'height' catch-up/'skeletal maturation' catch-up, when corticosteroid therapy is given intermittently.

Theoretically the use of steroids which have a growth promoting property, in order to counteract the growth depressing action of corticosteroids, seems justified. However the question arises whether counteraction of some undesired effect of the corticosteroids will not also interfere with some of the desired effects such as antiinflammatory of antiallergic actions (11). Experience with children on this subject is so far very limited and difficult to interpret. A small number of children with asthma (3, 6) receiving combined therapy were reported to grow at a normal rate without signs of virilization, in spite of the fact that the anabolic steroids were administered in what we consider 'virilizing' doses. It may well be that the corticosteroids antagonized the virilizing properties of the anabolic steroids, without affecting their growth-promoting effect, thereby increasing the non-virilizing dose of the anabolic steroids.

I should like to demonstrate two cases who receive combined corticosteroid-anabolic therapy. The first patient is a 12 6/12-year-old boy referred to us because of growth retardation. From the age of two years he has been suffering from asthma and he has since been receiving various corticosteroids with short interruptions. His height at 4 years was close to the 10th percentile. During the last year before admission he received 4 mg Triamcinolone a day. On his first visit to us his height fell below the 10th percentile (fig. 2). There were no signs of sexual development and his bone age was 8 6/12 years (fig. 3). X-rays of the bones revealed osteoporosis. It was not possible to interrupt the corticosteroid therapy but we reduced the dose to 2 mg Triamcinolone per day, which was the minimal dose which prevented severe asthmatic attacks. As the child did not grow even on this lower dose Fluoxymesterone (Halotestin-Upjohn) 5 mg per day was added and growth was resumed (fig. 2).

The second patient is a girl with adrenogenital syndrome of the salt losing type who requires for her well-being doses of corticosteroids that impair her growth in height as well as bone maturation (fig. 4).

It is very difficult to adjust the corticosteroid dose in such a manner that ACTH secretion is sufficiently suppressed to prevent virilization, that cortisol requirements are met and that body growth is not impaired.

Sometimes small amounts of corticosteroids hardly sufficient to check virilization will interfere with normal growth. One of the main difficulties in simple adrenal insufficiency or adrenogenital syndrome

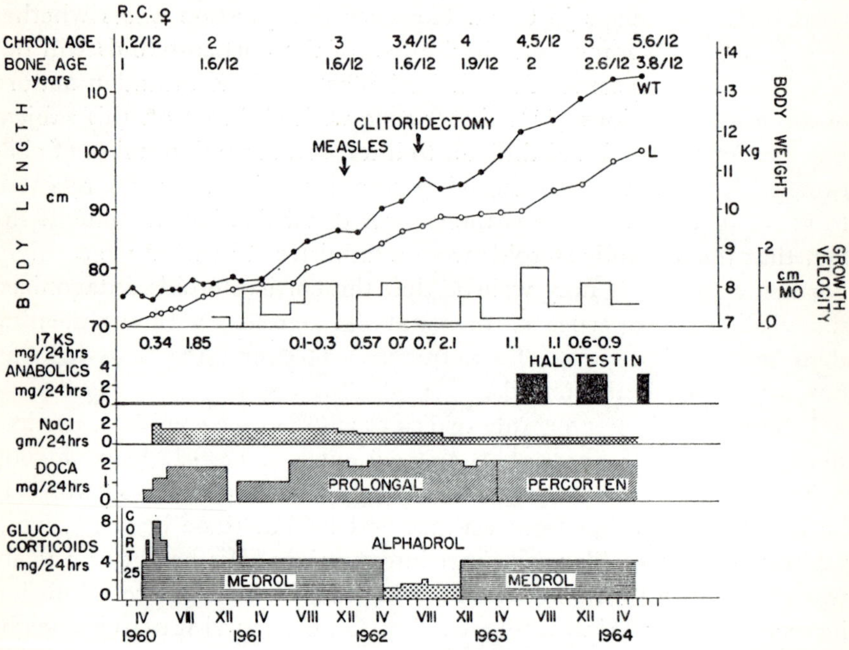

Fig. 4. Developmental chart of a patient with adrenogenital syndrome demonstrating the relationship between growth and various treatment regimens. Halotestin = Fluoxymesterone — Upjohn. DOCA = Prolongal = crystalline suspension Zori; Percorten M = DOCA trimethyl acetate — Ciba; CORT = Cortisone; Medrol = 6α-methylprednisolone — Upjohn. Alphadrol = 6α-fluoro prednisolone — Upjohn

is the lack of an endogenous stress mechanism and the necessity, therefore, to increase the exogenous corticosteroid dose at times of stress such as extensive exercise, illness etc. The desire to be on the safe side usually leads to the use of excessive doses. Another point is the increase in the physiological requirement with advancing age, body weight and height.

We therefore proceeded in the above case with the following trial:

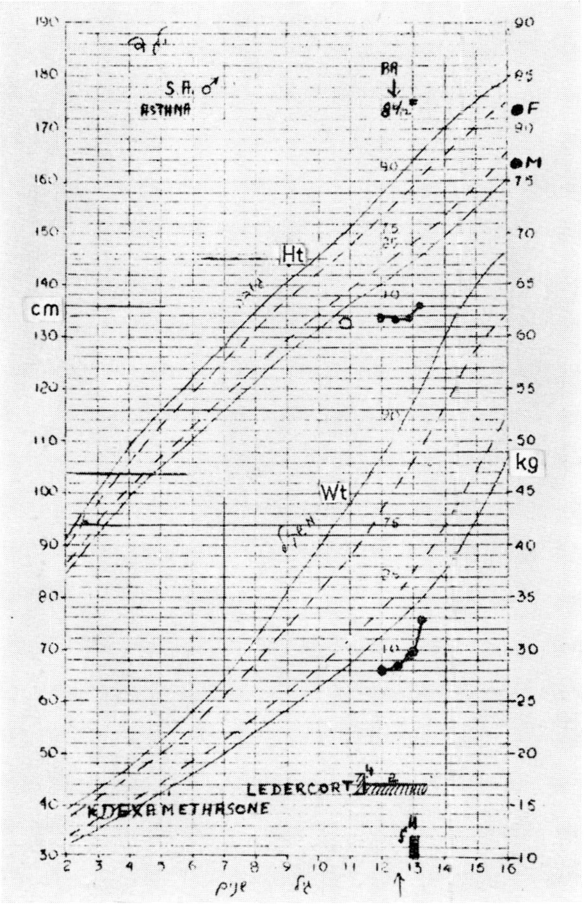

Fig. 2. Body height and weight of an asthmatic boy during treatment with corticosteroids alone or in combination with Fluoxymesterone (H = Halotestin - Upjohn) 5 mg per day

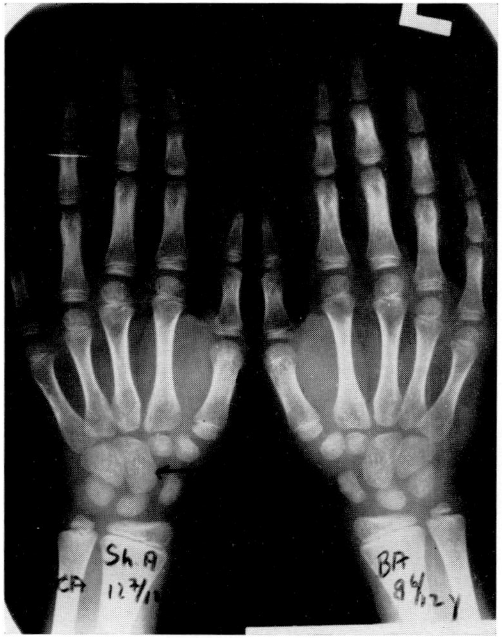

Fig. 3. Radiograph of hands and wrists of patient from fig. 2. CA = chronological age; BA = bone age

to administer corticosteroids at a minimal adequate dose as judged by the urinary 17-ketosteroids, electrolyte balance and clinical well-being, adding an anabolic steroid to overcome the retardation in growth. Such a scheme should enable control over the exogenous anabolic supply, whereas release of the endogenous androgen is more difficult to regulate.

Institution of combined therapy of 6-methyl prednisolone (Medrol-Upjohn) and Fluoxymesterone (Halotestin-Upjohn) has improved the growth rate and actual height but has also advanced the bone age (20 months advancement in 12 months). We intend to repeat this study with smaller doses. Our own experience and that of others, as far as we know, is still insufficient to indicate the proper dose relationships which could make the anabolic steroids a useful adjuvant to corticosteroid therapy, without superimposing the undesirable effects of the two drugs. The value of anabolic steroids in counteracting the corticosteroid-induced osteoporosis or in preventing its occurrence, has not yet been proven. Human growth hormone would probably be a better choice than the anabolic steroids (10): it is a pity that the amounts available are limited. If corticosteroids suppress growth and their administration cannot be interrupted to permit 'catch-up' growth, the use of anabolic steroids should be critically considered.

ACKNOWLEDGEMENT

This study was supported in part by a grant from the Upjohn Co., Kalamazoo, Michigan, U.S.A.

REFERENCES

1. Blodgett, F. M., L. Burgin, D. Iezzoni, D. Gribetz and N. B. Talbot, *New Eng. J. Med.* 254: 636, 1956.
2. Drescher, A. N. and N. B. Talbot, *New Eng. J. Med.* 257: 1280, 1957.
3. Evans, R. G., *Acta Allergol.* 17: 220, 1962.
4. Falliers, C. J., J. Szentivanyi, McBridge and S. C. Bukantz, *J. Allergy* 32: 420, 1961.
5. Falliers, C. J., J. Szentivanyi, L. S. Tan and S. C. Bukantz, *Abstr. 230 Xth International Congress of Paediatrics*, Lisbon, Sept. 1962.
6. Falliers, C. J., L. S. Tan, J. Szentivanyi, J. R. Jorgensen and S. C. Bukantz, *Sur. J. Dis. Child* 105: 127, 1963.
7. Fanconi, G., *Helvet. Paediat. Acta* 17: 267, 1962.

8. Grob, M., A. Prader and H. V. Zollinger, *Helvet. Paediat. Acta* 8: 202, 1953.
9. Laron, Z., see p. 63.
10. Laron, Z., B. Z. Arie and S. Kende, *Endocrinology* 72: 470, 1963.
11. Laron, Z. and S. Gitter, *Clinical Pediatrics* 2: 594, 1963.
12. Van Metre, T. E., Jr., W. A. Nierman and L. J. Rosen, *J. Allergy* 31: 531, 1960.
13. Prader, A., J. M. Tanner and G. A. von Harnack, *J. Pediat.* 62: 676, 1963.
14. Sobel, E. H., in: *Adrenal function in infants and children*, Report of the 13th M & R Pediatric Research Conference, p. 76, 1955.
15. Talbot, N. B. and E. H. Sobel, in: C. Z. Levine, *Advances in Pediatrics* 2: 238, 1964.

EFFECTS OF OESTROGENS AND PROGESTATIONAL AGENTS ON THE GROWTH OF CHILDREN

J. J. VAN DER WERFF TEN BOSCH

INTRODUCTION

The factors responsible for the attainment of a certain height at any particular age, may be said to exert their effect through influencing the *rate of linear growth* and/or through influencing the *rate of skeletal maturation*, which determines the length of the growth period. Thus the tall stature of an adult may have been brought about by an abnormally high rate of growth during infancy (genetic tallness, see p. 241), by an abnormally long length of the growth period (hypogonadotrophic hypogonadism, see p. 242), or by a combination of these two factors (true gigantism, see p. 242). Conversely, short adult stature may be the result of an abnormally low growth rate during infancy (e.g. in genetically short people), or of an abnormally short length of the growth period (due to premature ossification of the epiphyses, as in sexual precocity). Further, a slow rate of growth may be compensated for by extension of the growth period (as in 'slow maturers', short healthy children with late onset of puberty, and in some conditions of stunted growth, see fig. 1), whilst a fast rate of growth may be compensated for by shortening of the growth period (as in obese tall girls, see p. 246).

It is difficult, in all these instances, to assess the degrees of abnormality, and the degrees of success of the compensating mechanisms. This difficulty stems from the inherent inability to obtain more than a rough estimate of the potential adult height of an individual, particularly in tall (p. 245) and in short children, when the prediction tables of Bayley and Pinneau (4) are used. A more fractionated estimation of bone age (11, 12), the incorporation of parental size (2), and longitudinal studies of large groups of untreated tall and short children (e.g. by the pooling of data from different study centres), may contribute to the establishment of a more reliable method for predicting the potential adult height of children with abnormal stature.

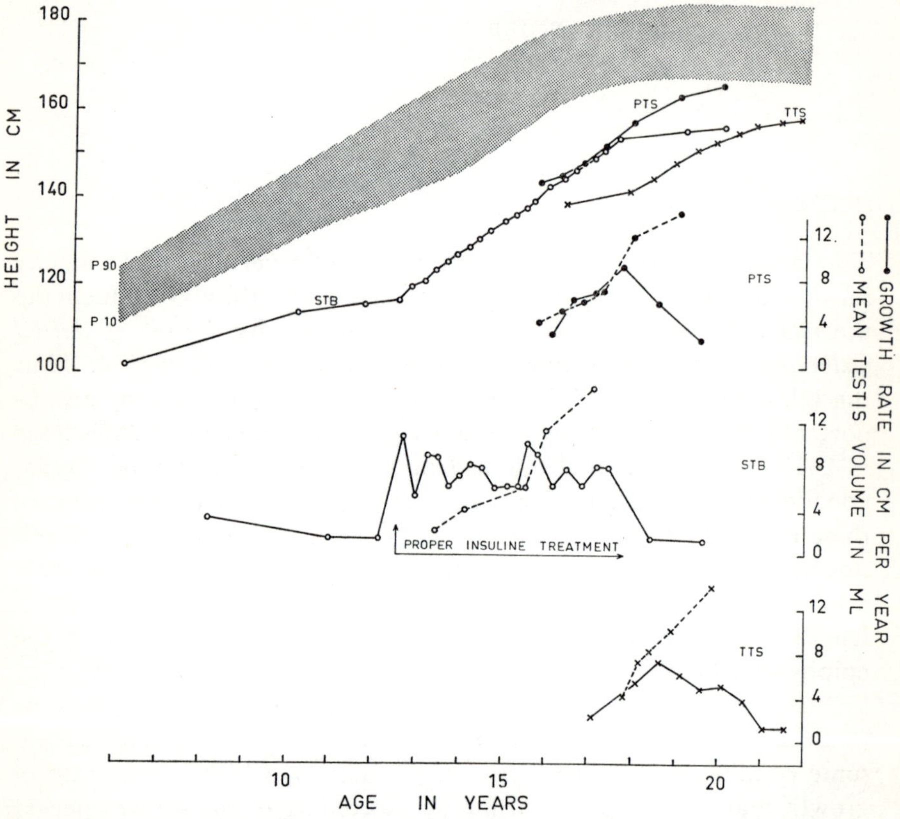

Fig. 1. Growth and testis size of three stunted boys, two with isolated growth disturbance (PTS and TTS) and one with diabetes mellitus (STB). Note the progress and effect on height, of puberty, which occurred relatively late. Percentiles from 14

OESTROGEN TO TALL GIRLS

The rationale behind the advocated treatment of tall children with sex hormones is quite obvious. In natural experiments, large amounts of sex hormones cause the 'pubertal' acceleration in growth and the concomitant acceleration in skeletal maturation, to take place at a very early age. The results of such natural experiments (the various forms of sexual precocity), are an initial marked increase in stature, followed by termination of growth at an age when other children often have not yet started to come in puberty, so that the giant child becomes a stunted adult, as a result of early ossification of the epiphyseal cartilages. These effects also occur both in children with an androgen-producing tumour, and in children with an oestrogen-producing tumour. There is no doubt that exactly the same processes can be brought about artificially, in healthy children, by exogenous androgen or oestrogen. For historical reasons androgens appear seldom to have been applied to this purpose, whereas oestrogens have been given to numerous children.

Fig. 2 summarizes in a schematic way the considerations upon which the treatment of tall children with oestrogens is based. If by such treatment the onset, and the end, of the 'pubertal' spurt in height were hastened by two years, then the contribution of two years of growth at the prepubertal rate of say 5 cm per year (totalling 10 cm) would be detracted from the potential adult height. From the age of eight years A would grow a further 36 cm, and B only 26 cm. In fact, however, a situation arises that is sketched on the right side of the figure. The spurt induced at an earlier age contributes more to adult height than the normal, later spurt would have done (C versus A). Instead of a loss of 10 cm (B), a loss of only 5 cm (C) occurs. It is well known (see fig. 1 on p. 241), that in sexual precocity the pubertal spurt reaches higher values for the growth rate (as in fig. 2, C), and that moreover, the spurt is of longer duration (not indicated in fig. 2) than during normal puberty. It is not certain whether these differences are solely due to the difference, between the two conditions, in bone age at the onset of the spurt, or whether the blood level of sex steroids is also involved. These facts have also emerged from a study in which early and late maturing normal girls were compared (9). Table 1 shows the average increment in height from 7 to 17 years in these two groups of girls. The difference is 4.7 cm. When the spurt started, the late maturers had grown 10 cm more, from the age of 7 years, than the early maturers. This is due to the fact that (over this age span) the late maturers had had 4 years of prepubertal growth, against 2 years in the early maturers. However, from the onset of the pubertal spurt, the early maturers gained more in stature than the late maturers, a difference of 5.3 cm. Thus the loss incurred by the earlier onset of

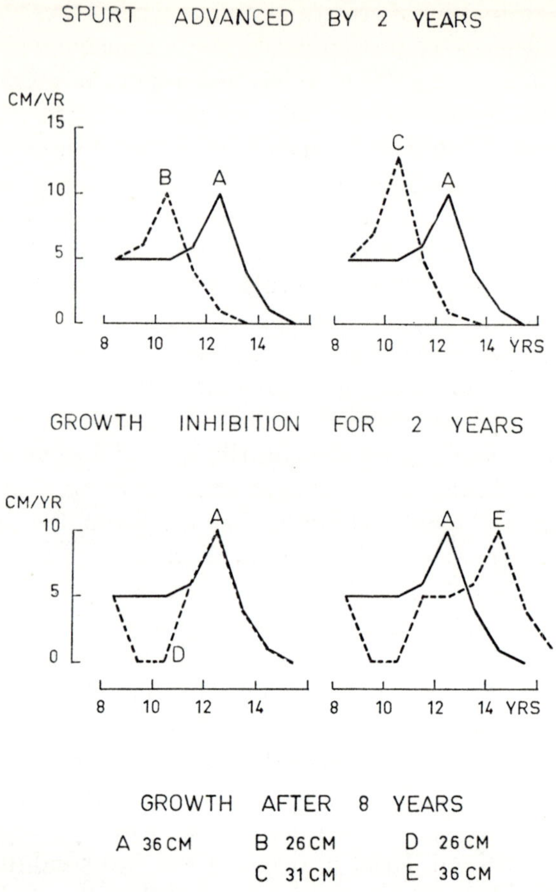

Fig. 2. Diagram to illustrate hypothetical effects on the growth rate pattern, caused by advancement of the sex steroid growth spurt (from the normal endogenous pubertal spurt A to the spurt induced by exogenous sex steroids, B or C), or by temporary complete inhibition of growth e.g. by corticosteroids (from A to D or E). Maximal effects of the two procedures would be obtained in the absence of compensating mechanisms (B and D), but it seems probable that some compensation will always take place (peak of higher magnitude in C because the skeleton is less mature at onset of peak; delay of onset of peak in E through the unknown mechanism that strives to integrate general body growth with skeletal and sexual maturation)

Table 1. *Differences in the growth in height before and during puberty between early and late maturing girls (data from 9).*

		Early girls	Late girls	Difference
Age at menarche (yrs.-months)		10-0—11-11	13-0—15-5	
Approximate average age at onset of pubertal spurt (yrs.)		9	11	+ 2
Increment in height (cm)	7 yrs. till onset of spurt	12.6	22.6	+ 10.0
	onset of spurt till 17 yrs.	27.8	22.5	— 5.3
	7—17 yrs.	40.4	45.1	+ 4.7

Table 2. *Height and bone age, at onset and after one year and two (or nearly two) years of treatment with oestrogen, of two tall girls (data from 13). Note the high rate of growth and of skeletal maturation.*

Case	Age (yrs.-months)	Height (cm)	Growth rate (cm/yr.)	Bone age (yrs.-months)	Skeletal maturation rate (yrs./yr.)
W.C.	8—7	143.8		8—6	
			13.3		2.5
	9—7	157.2		11—0	
			5.0		2.7
	10—5	161.3		13—3	
N.C.	9—6	141.3		9—6	
			13.0		2.5
	10—6	154.3		12—0	
			5.7		1.5
	11—6	160.0		13—6	

puberty, was partially compensated by the greater gain during that earlier growth spurt.

Views concerning the effect of therapeutic doses of oestrogens on growth vary. Some workers believe that such doses depress the growth rate, others believe that they accelerate skeletal maturation. In fact, oestrogens appear able to stimulate both the rate of linear growth and the rate of skeletal maturation (table 2). The question that remains is whether it may be possible, by the selection of an optimal preparation, an optimal dose and an optimal age of treatment, to accelerate skeletal maturation more than linear growth. The natural experiments referred to above, indicate that this must be possible. The 'limiting' factor for practical utilisation of this possibility is the optimal age for commencement of treatment. Table 3 shows the differences between predicted and actual adult height observed in two studies of tall girls treated with oestrogen. These differences are very similar to

Table 3. *The differences between predicted and observed adult heights of tall children treated with oestrogens (A from 3; B from 13). For comparison with tall children who have not received steroid therapy, see table 2 on p. 245.*

Source	Case	Duration of treatment (months)	Bone age for height prediction (yrs.)	Adult height (cm)		
				Observed	Predicted	Difference
A						
	DA	13	12.3	172.7	176.5	3.8
	TC	16	14.0	169.7	171.7	2.0
	LA	17	14.5	174.2	176.0	1.8
	RJ	21	10.9	176.0	178.3	2.3
	NG	23	12.0	175.3	180.3	5.0
	GG	29	10.9	174.8	173.7	— 1.1
	KL	38	11.8	182.4	176.0	— 6.4
B	JA	12	12	179.1	188.4	9.3
	EF	12	11	178.8	180.1	1.3
	VS	18	10	175.3	180.5	5.2
	WC	22	8½	166.4	177.6	11.2
	LC	24	11	173.4	178.0	4.6
	KH	24	11	167.0	170.7	3.7
	NC	28	9½	165.1	167.4	2.3

those observed in untreated tall girls (table 2 on p. 245), and the apparent effect of treatment may well be due to the error involved in predicting the adult height of tall girls (see p. 245). It would seem that convincing effects of oestrogen treatment of tall girls are to be expected only, when such treatment is started at an age well below 10 years. The choice then lies between: 1. a tall young girl, made temporarily a yet taller girl with precocious pseudo-puberty, and: 2. a tall girl who comes in puberty in the normal age range, but who will be a taller adult than 1. We do not advocate such treatment.

PUBERTY-SUPPRESSING DRUGS TO CHILDREN WITH TRUE SEXUAL PRECOCITY

In children with sexual precocity, the endogenous sex steroids induce the precocious appearance of external signs of sexual maturity (pubic and axillary hair, breast development), the menstrual periods and the pubertal spurt in body growth and skeletal maturation. In precocious pseudo-puberty it is possible to prevent such development by removal of the gonad tumour or, in congenital adrenal hyperplasia, by suppressing the secretion of sex steroids through corticosteroid administration (see p. 253). In true sexual precocity the pituitary secretes gonadotrophins in amounts that are abnormally high for the age of the patient. It seems logical to try and suppress true sexual precocity by drugs that may inhibit the secretion of gonadotrophic hormones. It is obvious, that such drugs should not possess the undesirable activities of androgens or oestrogens that the treatment attempts to suppress. The aims of such treatment are: to prevent the (further) appearance of external signs of puberty, to prevent or stop menstrual bleedings, to slow down growth and to slow down skeletal maturation.

With a progestational drug it has been possible to achieve some of these aims, i.e. to stop menstrual bleedings and the further development of breasts, but it seems difficult to influence the skeleton (8, 7, 10). There are at least three possible reasons for this difficulty: 1. the drugs may be ineffective with respect to the skeleton; 2. the methods used to ascertain effects may be too crude; 3. the patients to which the drugs have been given may been have too far advanced.

The drugs could be ineffective by failing to suppress the pituitary gland (the effects on uterus and breast might be due to direct actions of the progestational drugs on these structures), or by exerting a stimulating effect upon the bone which compensates for the fall in endogenous androgen or oestrogen output.

The skeletal effects are studied by measuring linear growth and by assessing skeletal maturation. Both these parameters are usually satisfactory only when employed in a long-term study, so as to overcome disturbing factors such as the errors involved in measurements and assessments, and the 'spontaneous' variations in growth and skeletal maturation associated with the seasons and with the quick changes characteristic of puberty. It is desirable to know the natural history of the growth pattern of untreated cases. Some data on three girls depicted in fig. 3, may exemplify these points. All three are cases of constitutional or cryptogenic (see 5) true sexual precocity. Patient LDN has not been given any hormone treatment. Her growth curve covers the age span from 3.5 years to adulthood. At 12 years she had reached her adult height of 157 cm. It can be seen that at 3.5 years her bone age was 10.2 years, and her growth rate was already on the decline. The pubertal spurt in height had obviously followed the perinatal spurt very closely. Menarche occurred at 5.25 years, after the peak in height growth. The rate of skeletal maturation, at first greatly exceeding that of one bone age year per chronological year, decreased once the bone age had passed the level of 13 years. The pattern just described seems to be fairly representative for girls of this kind, apart from differences in the age at which precocious puberty begins. This is illustrated by the curves for the second untreated girl, SDN, which seem to be following the same pattern 2—3 years later.

The task for the experimenter, is to demonstrate whether it is possible to alter this pattern. More specifically: to see if the growth rate which is already declining, can be depressed further. Note that it seems highly unlikely that even an effect of total sex hormone 'withdrawal' — suppression of its production — would result in either a very quick or a very marked change in the growth rate. On the one hand, it is to be expected that there will be a latent phase before the skeletal response to a lack of further stimulation by sex steroids becomes apparent in a difference in the growth rate. On the other hand, the difference in the growth rate between a normal prepubertal child and a normal child in the middle of its steroid-induced pubertal spurt, is often less than 50—100 % when the growth rate is measured over

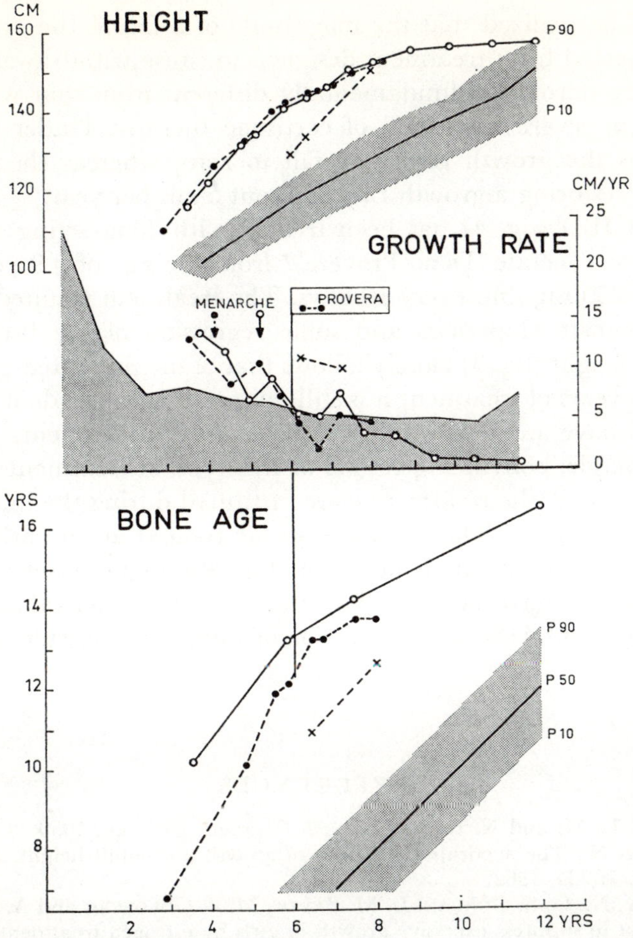

Fig. 3. Growth and skeletal maturation of three girls with cryptogenic true sexual precocity. Percentiles for height, see 14; bone age method, see 11 and 12. For comparison the height curve (drawn line) and the growth rate curve (shaded area) of a normal average girl are also shown (from 1).
Patient IBD (•-----•) has now been treated with medroxyprogesterone acetate, Depoprovera, for more than two years (this patient is being studied in collaboration with Dr. H. Janse, Department of Paediatrics, Leiden University Hospital).
o—o = patient LDN; ×-----× = patient SDN

periods of a year (e.g. 5 versus 7 cm per year, a difference of 40 %). It should be realized that the magnitude of a fall in the growth rate to be expected from treatment designed to cause withdrawal of endogenous sex steroids, is fundamentally different from that which may result from severe starvation of cortisone therapy. Under the latter conditions the growth rate may fall to zero, whereas the former is aimed at restoring a growth rate of about 5 cm per year.

Patient IBD (fig. 4) has been treated with long-acting medroxyprogesterone acetate (Depo-Provera)* from the age of 5.9 years, with a dose of 250 mg i.m. every 10 days. The treatment resulted in cessation of menstrual periods and some regression of the breasts. Her curve for height (fig. 3) closely follows that of the untreated girl LDN. After two years of treatment it is still not possible to decide if the treatment will have an effect on the adult height of the patient.

In principle, convincing results of this type of treatment might be expected only if the treatment were instituted during the initial phase of sexual precocity. The few cases so far treated at an early age, do not seem to warrant high hopes of thus obtaining better results, inasmuch as they have failed to show that the rate of skeletal maturation can be lowered by the administration of medroxyprogesterone acetate (7, 10).

REFERENCES

1. Bayer, L. M. and N. Bayley, *Growth Diagnosis*, Chicago, 1959.
2. Bayley, N., The accurate prediction of growth and adult height, *Mod. Probl. Paediat.* 7: 234, 1962.
3. Bayley, N., G. S. Gordan, L. M. Bayer, M. B. Goldberg and A. Storment, Attempt to suppress excessive growth in girls by estrogen treatment: statistical evaluation, *J. clin. Endocr.* 22: 1127, 1962.
4. Bayley, N. and S. R. Pinneau, see 6.
5. Donovan, B. T. and J. J. van der Werff ten Bosch, *Physiology of Puberty*, London, 1965.
6. Greulich, W. W. and S. I. Pyle, *Radiographic atlas of skeletal development of the hand and wrist*, 2nd ed., Stanford, 1959.
7. Hahn, H. B., A. B. Hayles and A. Albert, Medroxyprogesterone and constitutional precocious puberty, *Mayo Clinic Proceedings* 39: 182, 1964.
8. Kupperman, H. S. and J. A. Epstein, Medroxyprogesterone acetate in the treatment of constitutional sexual precocity, *J. clin. Endocr.* 22: 456, 1962.

* This drug has been kindly supplied by Upjohn-Nederland.

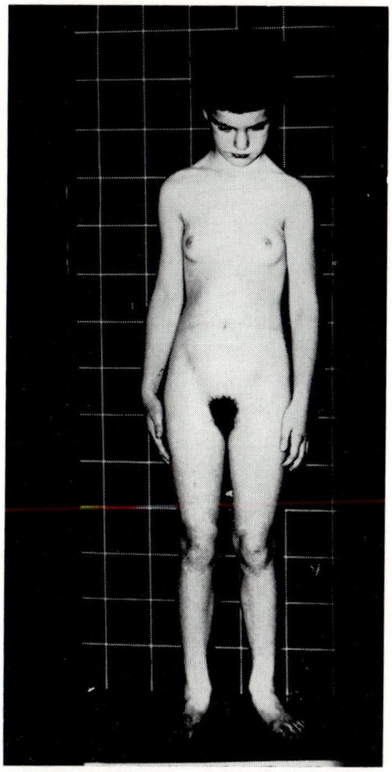

Fig. 4. Patient IBD at the age of 5.6 years

9. SIMMONS, K. and W. W. GREULICH, Menarcheal age and the height, weight and skeletal age of girls 7 to 17 years, *J. Pediat.* 22: 518, 1943.
10. SURTI, N. R., Treatment of constitutional precocious puberty with medroxyprogesterone acetate, *Proc. roy. Soc. Med.* 58: 123, 1965.
11. TANNER, J. M. and R. H. WHITEHOUSE, *Standards for skeletal maturity*, Paris, International Children's Centre, 1959.
12. TANNER, J. M., R. H. WHITEHOUSE and M. J. R. HEALY, *A new system for estimating skeletal maturity from the hand and wrist, with standards derived from a study of 2.600 healthy British children, Part II. The scoring system*, Paris, International Children's Centre, 1962.
13. WHITELAW, M. J., T. N. FOSTER and W. H. GRAHAM, Estradiol valerate: its effects on anabolism and skeletal age in the prepubertal girl, *J. clin. Endocr.* 23: 1125, 1963.
14. WIJN, J. F. DE and J. H. DE HAAS, Biologische ontwikkeling van de adolescent, *Nederlands Leerboek der Interne Geneeskunde*, Amsterdam, p. 710, 1960.

DISCUSSION

Visser: Dr. LARON knows that I disagree completely with him, and I think this has to be said here. As I have said before (p. 253), all the evidence indicates that patients with congenital adrenal hyperplasia can be treated from birth with properly adjusted doses of anti-inflammatory drugs. I have shown one example of a salt-losing patient, who was treated with hydrocortisone, and perhaps prednisone and Doca, who had normal growth and development at the age of 5 years. Recently I have seen a boy 14 months old, with the salt-losing syndrome, who is on $2\frac{1}{2}$ mg hydrocortisone twice a day and has perfectly normal growth and development with Doca treatment. I think that your treatment with a high dose of hydrocorticoid, adding anabolic steroids, should not be performed in those patients. We have seen the loss of potential height by an increase in the bone age. I would say that it is not necessary to keep the ketosteroids as low as shown in your diagram (p. 332). You just lower the glucocorticoids and then the keto's go up a little, it is not necessary that they are 1 mg or less.

Laron: I agree with Dr. VISSER that this should not be the usual treatment, and that there are patients, also salt-losers, who can be treated without any other treatment, but the above case gave me trouble.

Prader: What can one do about the osteoporosis induced by corticoids?

Querido: We have no studies on it, but I have recently had occasion to screen the litterature. I think that from the only two carefully conducted studies available, no evidence can be derived for the view that in the human the demineralizing effect of corticosteroids can be counteracted by anabolic agents.

Stoelinga: In children with long-term corticosteroid treatment, growth is retarded and skeletal development too. I should like to ask if the onset of puberty is also delayed in children. And if so, is it possible to interfere with this onset by anabolic steroids?

Visser: I can give no definite answer. I can only say that I have one girl with bilateral adrenal hyperplasia who was operated, first by total adrenalectomy on one side and subtotal on the other side, and later for removal of the remaining bit. She had a retarded bone age although she showed signs of breast development and pubic hair. This is some evidence that the appearance of signs of puberty can occur when bone age is retarded, under increased amounts of corticosteroids.

Kerrebijn: We have a fairly great number of patients who receive corticosteroids for their asthma. I think that in general puberty is not delayed in such patients, but we now have three patients coming into puberty, as measured by testicular volume and pubic hair, in whom bone age is about 10 or 11 years and who also show a considerable growth retardation. These are observations which we are studying.

Prader: You are only talking about boys now. At what bone age did puberty appear in these boys? Normally the bone age is 13 years.

Kerrebijn: I do not have the figures with me. The boy Dr. VISSER mentioned, is now about 14 years and 6 months, his bone age is about 11 years and his testicular volume is about 15 ml; he also has a fair fair amount of pubic hair.

Van Gemund: We must not confuse bone age with real physiological age. The former only means calcification seen on a radiograph and when we interfere with calcification then we have no correct bone age. When you give thyroxine or cortisone, what we call the bone age may be accelerated or decelerated, depending on the type of interference with calcification.

Prader: I think that when these hormones are given, you still read the real bone age, but your comment may be very important when it comes to rickets.

Steendijk: I have once suggested that it might be possible that in rickets bone age could not be read. Of course you can always see something, and from what I know from my rickets patients bone age is usually in line with chronological age. There is no sign of defective calcification which would cause bone age to appear to be advanced or retarded. I think you would have to give tremendous amounts of cortisone to influence calcification in such a way that the skeletal maturity would appear to be retarded because of peripheral effects on calcification visible on the X-ray. You might see differences in the shape or a difference in calcium content. You might see some abnormal trabeculation of the bones in the wrist, or in the phalanges, but I don't think we can interfere with nature to a large extent in this way.

Sobel: I have seen retarded skeletal maturation in resistant rickets and in a patient with renal tubular acidosis.

Fig. 3 on p. 261 shows the response in bone age as well as in height in a patient with renal tubular acidosis. His bone age apparently advanced very dramatically when alkali therapy was given. I would be inclined to interpret this as evidence that he had some osteomalacia or rickets as a consequence of his renal disease, and that cartilage, which may have matured in accordance with his chronological age, had not ossified and therefore was not visible radiologically. When alkali was given, this already matured cartilage was able to ossify and the bone age appeared to advance abruptly and dramatically. This is purely speculation, I have no evidence that my interpretation is correct. This phenomenon was also observed in a patient described by PRADER et al. (PRADER, A., J. M. TANNER and G. A. VON HARNACK, *J. Pediat.* 62: 646, 1963).

Schwarz: I wonder whether under such circumstances puberty begins at an abnormally early bone age, and whether puberty is associated with a normal growth spurt in such cases.

Steendijk: Well, I have a patient with idiopathic pulmonary haemosiderosis, who has been treated from the age of 8 till the age of 17 years with 15 mg of prednisone per day, which is absolutely necessary to keep the disease in check. I have followed her all through puberty, and she has shown hardly any growth to speak of from the age of 9 years. I think she has increased 2 or 3 cm and she has gone through all the stages of puberty, very slowly the beginning of breast development to the first menstrual period and, under prednisone, menstruations are present. I don't know if she ovulates or not, but the menstrual periods are highly irregular.

Prader: I think that in Cushing's disease there is complete catch-up growth if the disease is fully corrected at an early age. How did your patient develop? It may be that catch-up growth is age dependent.

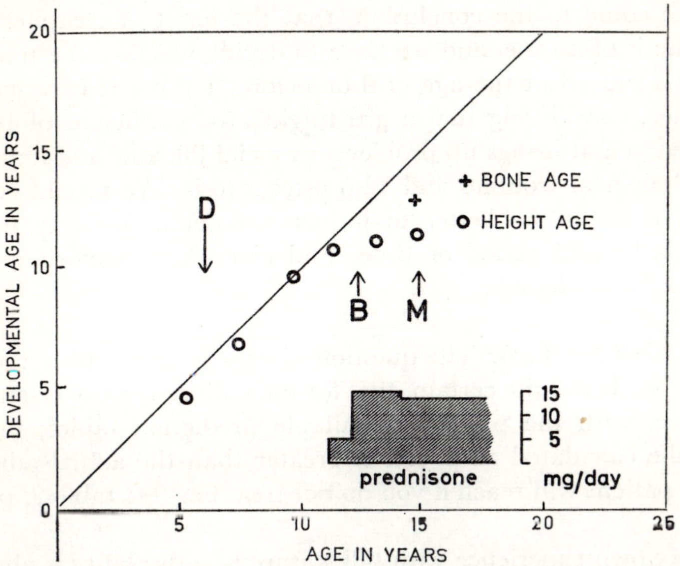

Fig. 1. Curves for height age and bone age of a girl with idiopathic pulmonary haemosiderosis. D = onset of disease; B = breast development; M = menarche

Steendijk: Fig. 1 shows the growth curve of the girl and the D signifies the beginning of the disease. This is a very rare disease which used to be fatal within three years. We have only a few measurements of height before therapy, but by the time of the beginning of prednisone treatment, when she had had a very severe crisis, there was no interference with growth at all. Now during prednisone, nearly always 15 mg per day, from the age of 11 there has occurred only a slight increase in height. Breast development and the first menstrual period were separated by about 3 years. I suppose what will happen now, is that skeletal maturation will go on while there will be very little increase in height.

Prader: There is one important thing lacking in the figure, and that is the bone age when you started to give prednisone. That would be important to answer the question whether her adult height is going to be less than could be predicted.

Laron: I have some experience with the treatment of tall girls.

I have come to the conclusion, that the onset of treatment after menarche is of no use, and we have to decide whether the treatment should be started at the age of 8 or before. I think it is a matter of conscience, considering that a girl might attain a height of 180 cm. Increased height brings up problems in social life and is accompanied by psychological troubles and also osteoporosis. We should consider whether it might be better to induce precocious puberty in these girls for a limited period of time, and give them a more adequate condition for a lifetime.

Van der Werff ten Bosch: The question always is: how tall is the child going to be? It is quite certain, that for tall children one over-estimates adult size, with the presently available prediction tables; in other words, the calculated adult size is greater than the actual adult size that the patient will reach if you do not treat her (see table 2, p. 245).

Sobel: My own experience with tall stature as a disability is obviously very limited. I have, however, women colleagues who do feel that their tall stature was a disability in early adolescence and also in adult life. In my experience, girls with tall stature usually come for evaluation when it is much too late to make any effort to treat them because they are already very close to the end of their growth. If I could be sure that use of estrogens would lead to significant reduction of adult stature, I would be willing to induce early breast development and early onset of adolescence in girls of 9 years. I cannot imagine consideration of cortisone therapy for such patients because of many serious problems associated with prolonged treatment with large doses of the cortical steroids. I have had great confidence in the natural and normal variation among healthy people. Sometimes an individual is so unhappy about the natural course of his own growth and development that we should perhaps try to help as long as we can be sure that we do no harm.

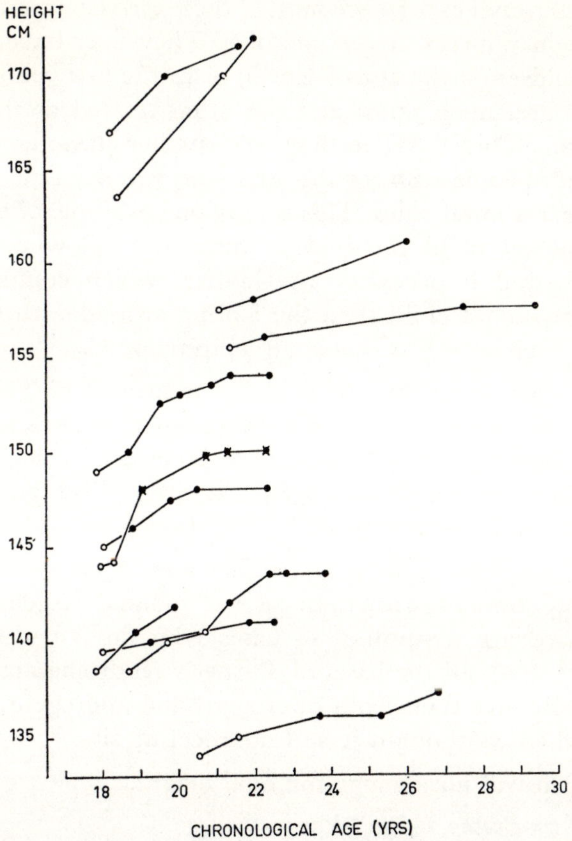

Fig. 2. Curves for growth in height of 11 sex chromatin-negative cases of gonadal dysgenesis after the age of 18 years. ○ = before steroid therapy, • = after oestrogen treatment (since previous measurement), × = after treatment with oestrogen and androgen (from: ENTHOVEN, R. and J. J. VAN DER WERFF TEN BOSCH, *Maandschr. Kindergeneesk.* 32: 466, 1964)

Schwarz: We have seen four girls who were very tall, between 10 and 12 years of age, who had a retarded bone age and whom we have treated with oestrogens. We did not see a growth spurt and I have the impression that we will obtain some reduction in adult height.

Steendijk: In view of what Dr. SOBEL said about the disadvantages that tall women experience, I think what we should do is to stress the fact that rapidly growing children are as important to be seen and followed as slow growing children, because of the psychological set-back. In my personal experience most of these girls enter puberty early; they may begin puberty at the age of 9. They may have difficulties with other children at the age of 4 or 5, or in the first years at school, because they are much taller and are often treated as though they were in fact much older. When they beat smaller class-mates, they get in trouble with people who see this and who will say that a big child should not beat a small child. This is only one example of the psychological trouble the child gets into. I think that follow-up should be psychological, and if necessary psychiatric, which could do much more good for such a child then the fooling around with oestrogens, cortisone or, even worse, orthopaedic epiphysiodesis.

Visser: I am very much interested in the treatment of Turner's syndrome with oestrogens. Could Dr. VAN DER WERFF TEN BOSCH give some comment of this? What does bone age do in such girls, and isn't it interesting that androgens have no effect on growth in those children while oestrogens do?

Van der Werff ten Bosch: I must contradict you. Androgens as well as oestrogens may stimulate growth in cases of gonadal dysgenesis (fig. 2). However, there are a number of cases who do not seem to grow at all. I don't think all the cases of Turner's syndrome are the same. We now usually give them both oestrogens and androgens. But there was a time when we thought it had no effect at all.

Prader: But you will not change the final height.

Van der Werff ten Bosch: I don't know.

Thomson: Excessive stature seems to be a handicap which affects females rather than males, and its symptoms seem to be psychological and sociological. Dr. LARON's suggestion that tall persons may be prone to osteoporosis is the only suggestion I have heard about, of a physical defect accompanying tallness. Presumably the main disadvantage suffered by an exceptionally tall girl is that she has a relatively small supply of potential male partners, and this may produce considerable unhappiness.

INDEX OF AUTHORS

INDEX OF SUBJECTS

8

Biom
Ul

Bio